Second Edition

BROKEN BONES

Anthropological Analysis of Blunt Force Trauma

Edited by

VICKI L. WEDEL, PH.D.

and

ALISON GALLOWAY, PH.D, D.-A.B.F.A.

(With 14 Other Contributors)

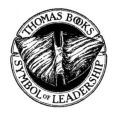

CHARLES C THOMAS • PUBLISHER, LTD.
Springfield • Illinois • U.S.A.

ABOUT THE EDITORS

VICKI L. WEDEL, PhD, is a forensic anthropologist and an Assistant Professor of Anatomy in the College of Osteopathic Medicine of the Pacific and the College of Dental Medicine at Western University of Health Sciences in Pomona, California. She holds a master's in criminal justice from Oklahoma City University and earned a master's of anthropology at the University of Oklahoma. Dr. Wedel completed her doctorate at the University of California, Santa Cruz. Dr. Wedel has been doing forensic anthropology consulting for several California counties since 2001 and since 2008 has been a forensic anthropologist for the National Disaster Medical System's Disaster Mortuary Response Team (DMORT) for Region IX. Dr. Wedel is also a Fellow of the American Academy of Forensic Sciences, and her research focuses on developing new methods of identification for forensic anthropologists and odontologists to use in casework.

ALISON GALLOWAY, PhD, D-ABFA, is a forensic anthropologist and Professor of Anthropology at the University of California, Santa Cruz. She earned her B.A. at the University of California, Berkeley and her M.A. and Ph.D. at the University of Arizona. As Director of the Forensic Osteological Investigations Laboratory, she has consulted on forensic cases throughout California for more than 25 years, working for both prosecution and defense. Her research has focused on trauma and taphonomic questions. Dr. Galloway is a Diplomate of the American Board of Forensic Anthropology. In 2012, the Physical Anthropology Section of the American Academy of Forensic Sciences, of which Dr. Galloway is a Fellow, awarded her its most prestigious award: the T. Dale Stewart Lifetime Achievement Award.

*We dedicate this book to
the people whose remains we have had the humbling
privilege of analyzing. May we never take lightly our
task of giving voice to your lives.*

*To my family and friends for their unwavering support.
VLW*

*To my daughter, who kept me fed and sane
And the EVC staff, who let me keep my day job.
AG*

Published and Distributed Throughout the World by

CHARLES C THOMAS • PUBLISHER, LTD.
2600 South First Street
Springfield, Illinois 62704

ISBN 978-0-398-08768-5 (Hard)
ISBN 978-0-398-08769-2 (eBook)

Library of Congress Catalog Card Number: 2013023909

With THOMAS BOOKS *careful attention is given to all details of manufacturing
and design. It is the Publisher's desire to present books that are satisfactory as to their
physical qualities and artistic possibilities and appropriate for their particular use.*
THOMAS BOOKS *will be true to those laws of quality that assure a good name
and good will.*

*Printed in the United States of America
UBC-R-3*

Library of Congress Cataloging-in-Publication Data

Broken bones : anthropological analysis of blunt force trauma / edited by Vicki
L. Wedel, PH.D. and Alison Galloway, PH.D., D.-A.B.F.A. – Second Edition.
    pages cm
    Includes bibliographical references and index.
    ISBN 978-0-398-08768-5 (hard) ISBN 978-0-398-0876-2 (eBook)
1. Forensic anthropology. 2. Blunt trauma. 3. Fractures. I. Wedel, Vicki L.

GN69.8.B76 2013
614'.17–dc2
                          2013023909

CONTRIBUTORS

BRADLEY ADAMS, PhD, D-ABFA

Director of Forensic Anthropology
Office of Chief Medical Examiner
New York, New York 10016

ALASTAIR BENTLEY, MD

State Pathologist Department
Belfast, Ireland BT12 6BL

SUE BLACK, PhD, OBE FRSE

Professor and Director
Centre for Anatomy and Human Identification
University of Dundee
Scotland DD1 5EH

CHRISTIAN CROWDER, PhD, D-ABFA

Forensic Anthropologist
Armed Forces Medical Examiner System
Dover AFB, Delaware 19902

ALISON GALLOWAY, PhD, D-ABFA

Professor of Anthropology
Director of the Forensic Osteological Investigations Laboratory
University of California Santa Cruz
Santa Cruz, California 95064

GINA HART, MA

Forensic Anthropologist
Regional Medical Examiner's Office
Newark, New Jersey 07103

GWENDOLYN HAUGEN, MA, F-ABMDI

Casualty Analyst
Department of Defense
Joint POW/MIA Accounting Command (JPAC)
Hickman AFB, Hawaii 96853

MERRILL O. HINES, III, MD, DABP (AP, CP, FP)

Assistant Medical Examiner, Program Director, Forensic Pathology Fellowship
Harris County Institute of Forensic Sciences
Houston, Texas 77054

CRIS HUGHES, PhD

Postdoctoral Researcher
Department of Anthropology
University of Illinois
Urbana-Champaign, Illinois 61801

CHELSEY JUAREZ, PhD

Assistant Professor
North Carolina State University
Department of Anthropology
Raleigh-Durham, North Carolina

JENNIFER LOVE, PhD, D-ABFA

Forensic Anthropology Director
Harris County Institute of Forensic Sciences,
Houston, Texas 77054

CAROLINE EROLIN

Medical Artist
Centre for Anatomy and Human Identification
University of Dundee
Dundee, Scotland

GLORIA NUSSE, MS

Instructor, Human Anatomy
San Francisco State University
San Francisco, California 94132
Clay and Bones, Mill Valley, California

VICKI L. WEDEL, PhD

Assistant Professor of Anatomy
Director of Human Identification Laboratory
Colleges of Osteopathic Medicine of the Pacific and Dental Medicine
Western University of Health Sciences
Pomona, California 91711

STEPHEN K. WILSON, MD, DABP (AP, FP)

Assistant Medical Examiner
Harris County Institute of Forensic Sciences
Houston, Texas 77054

LAUREN ZEPHRO, PhD

Forensic Anthropologist
Santa Cruz County Sheriff's Office
Santa Cruz, California 95060

PREFACE

Forensic anthropologists, in general, cut their teeth examining prehistoric and historical human remains to learn how to determine age, sex, stature, ancestry, and describe traumatic or disease-process changes to bone. These bones, which are not of forensic significance because they are older than 50 years, impart wisdom to us, wisdom on what bone quality, dry or exfoliated cortical bone, and macroscopic and microscopic bone characteristics indicate about postmortem interval and how the passage of time affects bone. The bones also often tell us about peoples' lived experiences. If the remains are part of a population study, the bones allow us to learn how to seriate features, which help us better age individuals and place an individual within his or her population. Further, archaeological and prehistoric studies allow us to speculate about quality of life and make comparisons with neighboring or contemporaneous populations. The concern of osteologists examining prehistoric or historical bone is often to tell the story of a person or population's life.

These kinds of stories, though, which are permissible in archaeological reports and prehistoric monographs, are not the kind forensic anthropologists can include in reports submitted as part of medicolegal investigations. We are limited to describing what evidence we see on bones – descriptions of trauma, for example, whose interpretations must be testable scientific hypotheses. We are looking for similarities to documented cases or published trauma research literature. In examining trauma, we rarely have evidence-based literature or actualistic studies on human bone help us in our interpretations. Further, we choose to remain ignorant of knowledge the coroner or medical examiner might have regarding any alleged crime of which the individual whose remains we are analyzing was a victim so as to avoid biasing our analysis. We must train by apprenticeship to gain the knowledge and experience needed in examining one person's remains and to rely on skeletal features and measurements to best contextualize individuals in relative to known ancestral populations.

The present work provides a discussion on how to train for a career in forensic anthropology and offers guidance on how to complete a thorough trauma analysis. It also provides the labels given to different kinds of fractures and the biomechanical forces required to cause bone to fail and fracture. Chapter 6 provides a theoretical framework both for evaluating published trauma studies and designing new ones. Experimental trauma research is an area ripe for research, and criteria to consider in choosing which non-human species to use in an actualistic study are offered. This discussion touches on the ethical considerations of using human cadaver bone versus animal bone, and if animal bone is chosen, whether a homologous or analogous species would be better. Further, the range of histological variation both within one non-human species and within a single individual is often underestimated. The range of variation present within one bovine histological thin section is included to demonstrate how overly simplistic some descriptions of non-human bone are (e.g., non-human bone is plexiform). In Chapter 7, common circumstances in which blunt force trauma is encountered are described. Information is provided on variety of causes of death due to blunt force trauma. These causes range from accidental deaths to homicides due to blunt force from motor vehicle accidents, falls, strangulation, child and elder abuse, among others. Epidemiological information on whom is most likely affected by these various kinds of blunt force trauma is drawn from both the clinical and forensic literature.

The meat of this book is contained in Chapters 8 through 11: bone by bone, fracture by fracture, we describe what to call each kind of fracture, what is known about how much force is required to break the bone that way, and fracture specific epidemiological information. These chapters provide an invaluable reference source for forensic anthropologists and other osteologists to consult when looking at and trying to classify a bone fracture.

Case studies are included to bring the book full circle back to considering the micro and macro bone changes that are seen when bone fails and fractures. The case studies are illustrative both of the concepts described through the book and of the high quality analyses forensic anthropologists contribute to medicolegal investigations of death every day. The case studies demonstrate the kinds of stories forensic anthropologists tell: those of a person's death.

Vicki L. Wedel

ACKNOWLEDGMENTS

In the creation of any work, there are many people to whom thanks are owed, and this work is no exception. This book is an update to the first edition, which became a work commonly used by forensic scientists faced with bone fractures to understand. We thank Charles C Thomas Publisher for suggesting a second edition and for Mr. Michael Thomas, our editor, for his patience and guidance.

Fifteen collaborators contributed case studies for inclusion in this book. Their endurance in the lengthy production of this work is most appreciated. The cases our contributors submitted demonstrate the high caliber work forensic anthropologists do on a daily basis.

Each editor's scholarly efforts are university supported. Dr. Wedel was gently nudged towards progress by Dr. Jim May, Chair of the Department of Anatomy at Western University of Health Sciences, and he is to be thanked for his guidance. The members of Western's Paleontology, Anthropology, and Anatomy Research Cluster are a cohort of tenure track faculty whose common goal helped move this manuscript along by providing collegiality, camaraderie, and encouragement.

The University of California, Santa Cruz supported this project by providing Dr. Galloway with the flexibility she needed to write. UCSC and Western University's unfailing support for the forensic anthropology laboratories is greatly appreciated. The University of Arizona, particularly Drs. Walter Birkby and Mary Ellen Morbeck, laid the foundations for this volume.

Finally, both editors owe a debt of gratitude to Dr. Lauren Zephro for her extreme patience and constant mentoring though this process. She was with us all the way and we knew it.

CONTENTS

Section II. Fracture Patterns And Skeletal Morphology

Section III. Case Studies

ILLUSTRATIONS

Tables

BROKEN BONES

Section I

TRAUMA ANALYSIS

Chapter 1

TRAUMA ANALYSIS: TRAINING, ROLES, AND RESPONSIBILITIES

Vicki Wedel, Alison Galloway, and Lauren Zephro

"The game's afoot" is a Shakespearean quote the omniscient detective Sherlock Holmes says with gusto when he sets out to solve a murder mystery. Sherlock Holmes is always portrayed as a one man, crime-solving machine. In reality, identifying victims of crime and determining their cause and manner of death is much more of a team sport. While death investigations are not games, for sure, the analogy of forensic science as a game is conceptually not that far off the mark. Within every death investigation, there are several players: the police and detectives who investigate the circumstances of the death, the forensic scientists who collect and analyze the evidence, and the forensic pathologists who determine cause and manner of death. Ideally, these interdisciplinary players work collaboratively. They abide by rules, some of which include investigation policies and procedures, criminal statutes and laws, and rules of evidence. Further, these team members work together in pursuit of a common goal: identification of the victim and his or her cause and manner of death.

Among the players who collect and analyze the evidence are forensic anthropologists: forensic scientists who are invited by forensic pathologists and coroners to collect and examine human remains when the remains have been buried, become mummified, been cremated, or have otherwise become so completely decomposed that soft tissue is not available or adequate for autopsy. Forensic anthropologists are also asked to evaluate skeletal material when autopsy reveals skeletal trauma that requires the expertise of a forensic anthropologist to describe and explain what type of force caused the particular defect.

The contributions forensic anthropologists make to medicolegal investigations of death are numerous, and on-going research in the field is slowly increasing the court-vetted methods available for skeletal analysis. Forensic anthropologists are qualified to exhume or otherwise recover remains from death or disposal scenes, but this aspect of forensic anthropology is described in a variety of different sources (Dupras *et al.* 2006, Connor 2007, Pickering 2008). When presented in the morgue or lab with a set of remains, forensic anthropologists always determine how many individuals are present and then proceed to determine the biological profile (sex, age at death, stature, and ancestry) of each individual included in the assemblage. Most cases involve the bones of only one individual, but this must be confirmed by making sure that joints articulate, there is no duplication of elements, and the size and morphology of bones from the left and right side of the skeleton match unless pathology is presented. Once the biological profile has been established, the remains must be examined grossly and under magnification for evidence of trauma or disease. How this is accomplished will be described further in Chapter 2.

In 2008, the Federal Bureau of Investigation along with the Department of Defense Central Identification Laboratory began the development of a series of documents to provide guidance on best practices within the discipline. These documents are the results of collaboration by a wide spectrum of forensic anthropologists under the umbrella of the Scientific Working Group for Forensic Anthropology (SWGANTH). Their documents are being developed and presented to the forensic anthropology community at large, via the SWGANTH website, SWGANTH.org for public comment. Comments are discussed and integrated into final versions of the documents, which are available to the public. Of note, is the fact that the SWG documents are living documents that are undergoing periodic reviews and updates. SWGANTH fits into forensic science trends as a whole since there are other scientific working groups co-sponsored by the FBI for a virtually all of the forensic science disciplines. Within SWGANTH, different subcommittees were assigned the task of providing the principles and best practices in a number of different areas including that of trauma analysis. The present volume is consistent with that text. It identifies the contributions anthropologist make in medicolegal investigations of death including determining the timing of the injuries as to ante-, peri-, or postmortem in nature and establishing the mechanism of injury (projectile, blunt, sharp, thermal, etc.).

This first chapter begins with a description of the education, training and experience a student must pursue to become a forensic anthropologist, a professional member of the discipline of forensic anthropology, and a Diplomate of the American Board of Forensic Anthropology. The second half describes the roles and responsibilities of forensic anthropologists when asked to examine a set of remains for evidence of trauma.

TRAINING AND QUALIFICATIONS

To become forensic anthropologists, students need to have an extensive background in contemporary human osteology and anatomy, an understanding of the legal system in which they will function, and experience with actual casework to provide the context within which we provide our services. These are not skills that can be acquired through a short course. These skills are also not readily adapted from other fields. Typically, students must complete a bachelor's degree followed by graduate school to earn a master's or doctoral degree. Undergraduate students usually complete the requirements for an anthropology major, which includes the traditional four-field anthropology courses: biological, cultural, linguistic, and archaeological anthropology. Archaeological field schools teach students the concepts that practicing forensic anthropologists use in recovering scattered or buried remains. College-level courses in crime scene investigation, offered through criminal justice or public safety programs, are also helpful because they can orient and educate budding anthropologists about how to recognize, document, and collect non-skeletal evidence. The ability of forensic anthropologists to recognize the myriad types of evidence is critical since the crime scene recovery of human remains usually involves contact or discovery of physical evidence. Knowledge of physical evidence, its significance, and potential use will help the forensic anthropologist to work more effectively as a team member in a forensic investigation and not accidentally destroy, contaminate or otherwise mishandle evidence. The inclusion of formal, traditional crime scene training cannot be overstated in importance for forensic anthropologists. In addition to college classes, law enforcement-based training in crime scene investigation may also be an option. Consultation with local agencies for training opportunities is encouraged.

Additionally, students often complete the array of courses included in pre-medical curriculum: chemistry, physics, and biology. This background becomes an asset in graduate school because studies of decomposition are based on chemistry, bone biomechanics and the physical principles of bone fracture, and bone, both as a tissue and an organ, are all fundamentals of biology. If a foreign language is a requirement for the anthropology major, Latin is one good choice, since most of the anatomy and osteology terms professional anthropologists use are Latin-derived. Many of the major founding texts within the field were developed in Germany, so German is another option. Spanish is always helpful in that many leading forensic organizations are located within Spanish-speaking regions of the world.

Successful graduate training in anthropology involves formal coursework, apprenticing a professional forensic anthropologist on actual forensic cases, and completion of an original research project, written up as a thesis or dissertation. Graduate courses in human skeletal biology teach the student how bone develops, replenishes itself, and heals from injury. Osteology courses provide hands-on training in identifying each of the 206 bones of the human skeleton, both intact and fragmented, and how they appear in infants and children. Successfully mastering human osteology and being able to identify highly fragmented skeletal elements requires memorizing the joint surfaces, muscle attachment sites, foramina through which blood vessels and nerves pass, and contours of each individual bone. This skill also requires one to think in a three-dimensional manner, since the fragments often do not appear normally aligned in the position in which we see them in textbooks.

Additional methods courses and mentored experience in determining the age, sex, ancestry, and stature of skeletons in teaching collections are necessary. Exposure to real human skeletal material of all ages and demographics hailing from forensic, historical and archaeological contexts is essential for understanding human variation. We can only estimate biological profile and differentiate between bone modification due to trauma if we view the bones within a framework of how bones vary between individuals, how bone tissue varies in the body, and how bone strength changes with age and configuration. To be a forensic anthropologist requires the ability to recognize and interpret normal variation, temporal and geographic variation, pathologies, anomolies, and to be accountable for the human body from the fetal period into old age. To do this effectively, a forensic anthropologist must have been mentored and had exposure to a wide variety of known skeletal material.

Specific to this book's topic are the kind of methods training where a student is taught to recognize and describe trauma. Students gain experience in recognizing and describing trauma, be it sharp force, blunt force, gun shot, or a mixture thereof, by first watching and often scribing for their advisor while he or she systematically examines each bone and bone fragment both with the naked eye and under magnification. The graduate student then proceeds to conduct mock examinations of teaching cases and case reviews with his or her advisor. Senior graduate students may then be asked to collaborate with their advisor on actual cases from start to finish: conducting the gross and microscopic examination, taking the kind of detailed notes that comprise a case file, and co-authoring the case report. This kind of supervised, but actualistic, experience is irreplaceable in the advisor being able to certify that his or her graduate student will be ready after graduation to take on cases of their own. In making this assessment, mentors also have the responsibility to ensure that the personal and professional conduct of their students meets the standards expected by the law enforcement community.

Participation in the analysis of remains from forensic contexts is one aspect of preparing a forensic anthropology graduate student for professional work. Equally important is the completion of an original research project in the form of a thesis or dissertation. Theory courses in anthropology help prepare students to undertake their own research project by exposing students to the seminal historical literature of the discipline and helping students learn how to read and critically evaluate the current literature. Formulating a testable research question forces students to employ the scientific method and includes selection of the appropriate materials and methods. Choosing what materials to use involves evaluating what autopsy series, museum collection skeleton, imaging techniques, or animal models are available and applicable; how many specimens to include; and how widely applicable the results of the research will be. Institutional requirements for accessing autopsy or museum specimens also require a student to critically examine how they have developed their design to meet ethical and statistical guidelines.

The process of completing a thesis project also helps students develop the skills that will be necessary throughout their career when case reports must be written. Taking on a project with the scope of a thesis or dissertation is formative in helping students learn to complete projects that in the real world will have time constraints and will require them to be able to describe their work in language their peers will understand. Research also trains one in investigating previous work, determining if it is applicable to the question at hand and synthesizing information from many streams. Defending the results of their research helps prepare students for the kind of peer review they will experience after graduation and to some degree simulates what court testimony will be like: extemporaneously answering questions in defense of their results and the methods used to achieve them.

BECOMING A MEMBER OF THE PROFESSION

Students in accredited anthropology programs can become trainee affiliates of the American Academy of Forensic Sciences (AAFS), the largest and most reputable body of forensic scientists. At the annual meetings of the AAFS, results of the latest research are presented for peer review. Workshops provide continuing education opportunities. Advancement in the Academy is partially based on forensic anthropology case review and/or publications. By advancing in membership status from trainee affiliate to associate member to member to fellow demonstrates for the forensic science community that a forensic anthropologist is a lifelong learner who is making measurable contributions to the field.

Forensic anthropologists should also seek specific certification in the discipline. The most common certification is available through the American Board of Forensic Anthropology (ABFA). Other agencies may offer a certification, but interested parties should be careful to check the reputation of the agency supporting the program. Exact requirements for the application to the ABFA should be checked as these are subject to change, depending upon the incorporation of new standards or inclusion of a broader range of applicants. Qualified individuals for the ABFA can apply to sit for the board examinations. All applications are reviewed for the quality of their case reports, the clarity with which their findings can be interpreted, and their knowledge of the field. The board examination consists of written and practical components. Passing the boards bestows upon the candidate the title "Diplomate of the American Board of Forensic Anthropology." Once certified, all active members must continue to engage in forensic work; report on their casework, reports, and court testimony; and maintain an acceptable level of continuing education.

RESEARCH IN TRAUMA ANALYSIS

Forensic anthropologists may be asked to evaluate a set of skeletal remains to document and describe the defects and then render an opinion about the origin of those defects. This is just the first of many ways forensic anthropologists contribute to trauma analysis. Because the ways a skeleton may be impacted by a blunt instrument are too numerous to list (or even conceive of), our role in publishing case reports (e.g., Wedel *et al.* 2013), once cases have been adjudicated, is of the utmost importance in educating our peers. Further, the role of the forensic anthropologist in designing research projects that further our understanding of how the skeleton reacts then fails when struck is paramount. We cannot solely rely on the research that has been done to date; we must experiment in ways to simulate or model blunt force trauma, determine the validity of the experimental media or models we are using, be mindful of technological changes that alter how trauma is imparted to the body, and publish our findings in order to advance our current knowledge base. Thus the forensic anthropologist has the responsibilities of conducting the skeletal analysis, publishing case reports when possible, and furthering the knowledge generated by conducting trauma research. Each of these roles and responsibilities is discussed in the coming chapters.

Skeletal trauma, especially from blunt force, is highly variable and each case presents a unique set of challenges in the interpretation and reconstruction of the events that produced them. The aim of this volume is to present the framework in which trauma analysis occurs in the forensic setting, provide guidelines that may help facilitate the process of evaluating blunt force trauma, and provide documented support for this growing area of trauma research and its application within forensic anthropology. The care given to the documentation of observed skeletal defects and the depth of work in reconstruction of the events that produced them quickly becomes evident in the quality of the written report and subsequent court testimony. It is upon this foundation that we can advance our influence within this exciting area of forensic analysis.

Chapter 2

PROCESSES AND PROCEDURES FOR TRAUMA ANALYSIS

ALISON GALLOWAY, VICKI WEDEL, AND LAUREN ZEPHRO

Forensic anthropological analysis usually begins with an assessment of the biological profile. This work includes a determination of sex, assessment of age and ancestry, estimation of stature, and identification of those characteristics that could assist in identification of the decedent. In court, the biological profile is rarely contested. Instead the analyses dedicated to trauma and postmortem interval are more critical to the outcome of the trial. The former addresses whether a crime has occurred and the latter when it occurred.

The anthropological assessment of traumatic defects follows three stages that cover the handling of the remains and the context under which the remains exist and their usability in court proceedings. The first stage includes the pre-analytic procedures of recovery, autopsy, initial documentation, and skeletal processing. Second, the anthropologist conducts the analysis of the remains for skeletal defects and, when necessary, develops experimental studies to test interpretive models. Third, the post-analysis phase includes the production of a final written report, preparation for court, and the actual testimony.

Running parallel to these stages is a line of documentation known as the "chain of custody." This set of records allows the material to be tracked through each stage from the point of recovery to that of final disposition. At all stages, the anthropologist is responsible for the integrity of skeletal evidence, and information about the measures taken to secure the remains must be reconstructable. Signatures, dates, and reasons for interaction with the evidence must accompany each transfer of skeletal material into or out of the care of the anthropologist.

Courtroom presentation of forensic analysis rests on a foundation of work done in the field and in the laboratory. If that foundation is shaky, the excellence of a presentation can fall apart. Therefore, the level of attention and quality of documentation must be consistent throughout the work, from the recovery and receipt of the material to the storage of records. The following chapter will examine the processes and procedures for analysis of skeletal material with an emphasis on the analysis of trauma.

PRE-ANALYSIS: RECOVERY, TRANSPORTATION AND PREPARATION OF THE REMAINS

Field Recovery and Autopsy

The forensic anthropologist should become involved in the analysis as early as possible (Maples 1986, Black *et al.* this volume). While inclusion in the scene recovery is preferable, attendance at the autopsy can also be extremely beneficial (Love *et al.* and Love, this volume). In the field, the anthropologist is able to assist in recovery of the remains, assess the completeness of the material, locate and recover small bones and fragments, and assess the environmental conditions that may have affected the taphonomic changes to the remains.

Blunt force trauma may result in unusual patterns of decomposition, which are evident on the body at initial inspection. In most instances, insects invade the body through the normal openings on the face (i.e., eyes, nose, mouth, and ears) or in the ano-genital region in preference to areas of trauma (Cross and Simmons 2010). Massive trauma may, however, provide an additional avenue of entrance. When blunt force results in extensive soft tissue damage, insect activity can be intense. Since there is frequent involvement of the head in blunt force injuries, decomposition of the face or cranial vault may be accelerated.

In the rush to recover material and clear a scene, law enforcement may resort to heavy equipment. This approach should be used with extreme caution as massive postmortem damage may occur and make identification and reconstruction more complicated. When co-mingled remains are present, rapid excavation can result in the jumbling of individuals. Slower and more methodical excavation will allow separation of different individuals and location of other evidentiary items in context. The sequence and position in which body or bodies were placed within the grave can be established, possibly corroborating other lines of evidence.

Fragmentation of the remains resulting from blunt force trauma often leads to dispersion of the various pieces of bone. The pattern and process of dispersion can be compounded by the action of scavengers, roots, rodents, and rainwater. Since the recovery of small fragments may be essential to interpretation, recovery techniques that focus on maximization of recovery of the overall remains are critical. Various guides to such techniques are available (Dupras 2006, Connor 2007, Pickering 2009) and basic techniques will not be discussed here. However, when blunt trauma is involved, a second examination of the crime scene to search for fragments may be necessary and is encouraged if there are any missing fragments discovered during reconstruction.

Locating the original site of deposition and decomposition is often the key to recovering the smaller bones and bone fragments. This site may not be evident if the body has been moved subsequent to decomposition by scavengers or other agents. Cadaver dogs are helpful in locating this site if the remains have been moved. These initial decomposition areas are marked by the presence of decomposition fluids and hair masses. Often teeth, small items of jewelry, clothing fragments, bullets, and pocket contents may be located in the area.

Accurate measurements of the locations of bones and field identification of the remains allow subsequent reconstruction of the movement of the body or body parts following the original disposal. Recording of the microenvironment is also important. Temperature and humidity comparisons between the recovery site or sites and recorded weather station data may be essential in assessing the postmortem interval. Soil, botanical, and entomological samples should be collected as appropriate.

If possible, the forensic anthropologist should also be present during autopsy. At this time, total body trauma can be appraised while specific insults (e.g., hemorrhage surrounding fracture sites) can be scrutinized with the forensic pathologist. The sequence in which soft tissue is removed can be documented. The anthropologist can also gain important information from examination of soft tissue, although descriptions on any soft tissue defects should be kept in general terms. For example, discoloration should be noted but not attributed to bruising or hemorrhage. Additionally, with regard to complex or subtle trauma, like child abuse, even when remains are not skeletonized, the involvement of a forensic anthropologist may be critical in discovering and documenting skeletal trauma (see Love, this volume).

During autopsy, any marks on the bone left by the pathologist or technicians can be noted and documented. The association of soft tissue damage with underlying skeletal defects may be useful in linking the reports of the forensic pathologist and the anthropologist. The perspective gained from such observation is also extremely important for the continuing education of the forensic anthropologist and other investigators. Bodies should also be radiographed for documentation of injury, metal, or other radio-opaque materials. This process is critical in recording the presence or absence of bullets or other projectiles, which may be passed to the anthropologist's custody along with skeletal material. Radiographs also, given appropriate comparative antemortem records, may be key in establishing positive identity.

Receipt of Materials for Analysis

Forensic cases arrive at the laboratory in many different conditions. Bodies are found at different levels of decomposition, may have been autopsied, frozen, segmented for testing, and then transported. Whatever the situation, the chain of custody must be maintained. Delivery is accomplished by a number of methods including sheriff/coroner, funeral services, or a tracked delivery service. Occasionally, the anthropologist will collect the material from the agency requesting services. Practicing forensic anthropologists must establish internal policies and procedures for the receipt and handling of skeletal material in their care.

When the anthropologist receives the remains, he/she should obtain the names and identification of the delivering party, begin a case file identified with the case number, and obtain a signed transfer of evidence form. For the forensic anthropologist, it is useful to have such a form on hand as it is not uncommon for remains to arrive without paperwork, especially when no foul play is suspected. The transfer form should include the names of delivering and receiving parties, affiliation, case number(s), and time and date of transfer (Figure 2-1). Copies should be included in the case file and one copy returned to the delivering party. If the anthropologist is providing the transportation, then the information is obtained and the file started at the time the material is collected from the originating agency. Communication with agencies before they require services is critical. It is important to set expectations, provide forms, fee schedules, etc. prior to an agency requiring anthropological services. As a general rule, anthropologists provide analytical services after the body has been examined for physical evidence by a forensic pathologist, fingerprint technicians and similar personnel. Anthropologists should not be accepting personal items or other recognized physical evidence when they take custody of a body. If physical evidence is discovered during the analysis of human remains, it should be documented in context with the remains, collected and packaged for return to the agency.

If remains are sent through a commercial mail delivery service, the case folder should include the label(s) from the package and any enclosed paperwork. The tracking systems available through major suppliers form part of the chain of custody.

The time of delivery is also the occasion to clarify the purpose of the examination. Ideally, the case should be accompanied by a laboratory request indicating what analytical work is being requested, whether DNA has been collected, if remains are identified, etc., and a primary contact(s) with the requesting agency. If this is not provided, the forensic anthropologist should contact the authorizing agency for specific instructions and record this information with the case file, including date and name of the individual providing the instructions.

FORENSIC ANTHROPOLOGY CASE SUBMISSION FORM		
Submit only one case per form. **Print clearly or type all entries**	New	Resubmittal

AGENCY AND CASE INFORMATION**

Requesting Agency _____ Case No._____ Date of Offense _____ Offense (s) _____

Investigating Officer _____ Phone No. (   ) _____ E-mail _____

Is priority analysis requested? _____ Reason? _____

ADDITIONAL INFORMATION AND/OR SPECIAL INSTRUCTIONS
1. HAS A DNA SAMPLE BEEN COLLECTED? Y / N , IF YES, SAMPLE _____
2. HAVE THE REMAINS BEEN POSITIVELY IDENTIFIED? Y / N , IF YES, METHOD_____

Attach additional sheets as necessary.

EVIDENCE SUBMITTED (Please list item numbers as well as evidence description)

Item #	Description	Work Requested

PLEASE NOTE: Evidence items, such as personal items (jewelry, watches, etc.), clothing and bullets, should be retained by the submitting agency. Examples of work requested include full skeletal analysis, trauma analysis, identification and postmortem interval. Requests for postmortem interval estimation should be accompanied by crime scene photographs and associated documentation. Requests for identification should be accompanied by the relevant known antemortem records of the individual(s) to be compared to the skeletal case.

CHAIN OF CUSTODY (Please fill this section out completely and legibly)

Item #	Received From	Method of Transit	Received By	Date

CASE RESULTS

	Skeletal remains are not human
	Skeletal remains are non-forensic
	Please see laboratory report for results

DISPOSITION _____

Anthropologist:_____ Signature:_____ Date:_____

Laboratory use only:
Case Notations:

version 1.0 rev. 08/2012

Figure 2-1. Case submission form. Designed by Lauren Zephro.

However the delivery occurs, the receiving party should be prepared with adequate facilities to store the remains securely. Working surfaces that can be covered with disposable plastic or sterilized after use are critical. Such surfaces should be prepared so that the delivery can be concluded expeditiously. Laboratory facilities must include secure areas for macerating, curating, refrigerating, and freezing human tissues.

Photography is a critical part of the intake process. It provides a record of the integrity of the remains, the type and security of the packaging, the presence of labels, and other markers on the packaging. Photographs should cover the overall remains with additional photos of labels, zipper ties, locks, and other features. An easily visible scale bar and label with the case number should be included in at least one version of the overall shots.

Remains that are fleshed should be photographed from many angles systematically. These images will be critical to the documentation of postmortem interval through total body scores (Megyesi *et al.* 2005). Remains also often arrive in many separate evidence bags with separate identification numbers. In these cases, each bag should be treated separately in terms of photography with the remains photographed in proximity to the label on the respective bag. Separate bags are often tied to separate locations of recovery, so maintaining a record of which bone is linked to which identification number is important.

In particular, the condition of any obvious skeletal defects should be noted such as inclusion of decomposition materials or decayed body fluids within the defects. This may be critical in the determination of perimortem versus postmortem injury. Such evidence may be lost or obscured by further cleaning. Missing portions should be documented. Later recovery of these portions may allow determination of initial areas of injury or decomposition, which can be essential to the reconstruction of the series of events leading to the recovery of the victim's remains. Incomplete recovery may jeopardize trauma interpretation, and it may be necessary to revisit the crime scene to look for missing pieces.

With the advent of digital photography, the expense of photography has decreased so that it is feasible to take more photos than absolutely required. Also, images can be quickly checked to ensure accurate focus and lighting prior to moving to the next step of analysis. Macroscopic lenses allow for attention to detail that may not be easily seen without magnification. It is critical that scales be used for examination quality photos. Most importantly with systematic photography, a combination of overall, mid-range, and close-up photographs (with and without a scale) should be used to document trauma. Each close-up photo must have a context so that its position, size, and anatomical location can be reconstructed.

Forensic digital photography carries risks and responsibilities since images can be digitally altered, images blurred through multiple compactions, storage corrupted or deleted, and storage mechanisms become obsolete. Original copies of all images are part of the evidentiary package and should be retained (see also Record Retention below). Contact sheets can be produced to include in the case folder. It is recommended that archive procedures for any forensic laboratory be documented, and that multiple copies of case photographs be maintained and stored in different locations.

Initial Observations

Initial observations of the remains should be done with photographs and written notes. Notations should be made of the wrappings and/or in which the remains were received, whether there was associated paperwork or clothing, and any special instructions from the agency requesting services. Also at this time, obvious defects should be recorded. These notes are important in showing that the defects predated the cleaning process.

Cleaning and Preparation of Remains

Forensic cases frequently require cleaning to allow full exposure of traumatic osseous defects. The general principle is that the amount of cleaning done should be the minimum required for visualization. In most cases, the remains will be returned to the family and not retained in the laboratory. Therefore, it is not necessary to clean the bones to the level that we would use as anatomical specimens, a process that often includes bleaching of the bone to remove grease and produce a whitened coloration.

Personal protection equipment is essential in any laboratory. Scrubs, gloves, disposable overalls, plastic aprons, face masks, eye protection, hairnets, and shoe covers are among the basics to have on hand. The level of protection varies with the condition of the remains, but even bones should not be handled without gloves. Lab coats are often recommended but may not be practical with material that is decomposing. Similarly, disposable overalls will require either longer gloves or taping of the sleeves at the wrist to prevent or limit contact with decomposing material.

While decomposed human tissue is generally more odious than dangerous, the handling and cleaning of human remains entails some inherent dangers to those who work the bodies. Complete and up-to-date vaccinations for hepatitis and tetanus are required in addition to safe handling practices. The remains received by forensic anthropologists usually come from unknown backgrounds and may bring with them a number of pathogens. Most infectious agents are relatively unstable and dissolve during autolysis and putrefaction (Galloway and Snodgrass 1998). Some, including some forms of hepatitis, are more resistant to destruction. Double latex gloves both inhibit the transfer of odor as well as provide added protection. All injuries to team members while handling the body should be thoroughly cleaned, tended, and logged. As workers' compensation or other forms of liability are often involved, medical attention and documentation of the injury is valuable.

Human remains should be clearly labeled during processing as to case number. Material such as decomposing flesh, which will not be used in analysis, should be bagged in labeled biohazard bags and stored securely.

Fleshed Remains

The amount of flesh or decomposing tissue on the bones will vary significantly from case to case. While maceration in water or the use of natural decomposition techniques, such as dermestid beetle colonies, may be preferable for removing soft tissue, the length of time required may be incompatible with the needs of the agency requesting the anthropologist's services.

For most cases, cleaning is done in baths of water and detergent (Fenton *et al.* 2003), which requires that the body be segmented and the bulk of the tissue removed prior to placing in the bath. This work is accomplished with scalpels, taking care to keep away from both the bones of the deceased and the hands of the anthropologist. Rat-tooth or other gripping forceps are essential in this work.

Recovery of bone fragments in cases of blunt force trauma is essential. In many instances, this entails sifting through masses of soft tissue, which are in various stages of decomposition. Small splinters of bone are easily lost within maggot masses and can be rapidly transported away from the initial location. It is necessary that as many fragments as possible be recovered.

Once the body is segmented, the segments or bones are immersed in a hot water bath with added detergent. The pots should be left to simmer but never boil (Fenton *et al.* 2003). Incubators have been used with great success in the cleaning process (Love 2011). Periodically, the remains are rinsed with hot water and the soft tissue that has become loosened is removed. Although some texts recommend that this be done with wooden instruments, nylon bristle brushes, or spatulas (Maples 1986), such tools may make little progress and careful use of scalpel and forceps is more effective. Soft tissue should be placed in biohazard bags and stored frozen for return with the rest of the remains. If bones are damaged during processing, it must be documented in the case file.

Bleaching to obtain a whiter appearance is not encouraged because bleach can degrade the bone's cortex. A heated mild ammonia bath can diminish the surface grease, making the bones easier to handle. Bone also is susceptible to damage with sudden temperature changes, so immersion of a cold bone into hot water or rinsing hot bones under cold water will produce significant damage.

Once the remains are cleaned, they should be allowed to slowly dry. Rapid drying will produce longitudinal cracks and fractures in the bones, complicating the interpretation process and the report preparation. However, if drying takes too long, mold frequently grows on the bones and they must be recleaned.

Bodies that have been burned are extremely fragile and require special care in handling to prevent production of post-burning fractures. Documentation of the body's appearance upon arrival is even more critical, and fragmentation of burned sections of bone is almost inevitable during cleaning. Recognition of pre- and post-fire fractures can be accomplished by patterns of burning, position of the bone ends at the time of recovery and understanding the varieties of thermal damage seen in previously undamaged bone (Pope *et al.* 2010).

Regardless of the condition the remains are in, if positive identification is to be determined by DNA, selection of an appropriate sample should be done in consultation with the originating agency and DNA laboratory prior to cleaning the remains. This bone can have flesh removed and be bagged and stored separately.

Mummified Remains

Remains that have undergone significant dehydration are often the most difficult to process. The soft tissue can be extremely tough, making dismemberment difficult. Attempting to pull apart segments or cut through the dehydrated tissue can produce defects on the bones in the form of fractures or cutmarks. While these can be easily distinguished from perimortem defects, they open up challenges as to the care given to the overall analysis.

For mummified cases, use of a dermestid beetle colony may be appropriate. If the colony is well maintained, this process can be relatively rapid. Unfortunately, in some cases, particularly in cases where drugs or other chemicals are present in the remains, beetles will take considerable time to make progress. It is often necessary to add some moisture to the remains to make them palatable for the colony. Colonies also need adequate ventilation of the area and a heat source if the ambient lab temperature is low.

Skeletonized Remains

Skeletonized remains may be examined without cleaning or may require a minimum of preparation. Frequently light brushing or a rinse under running water is sufficient. Soaking already cleaned bones is not recommended due to the cracks that can occur during the drying process.

In most cases, trauma to skeletonized remains is relatively easy to see. Fractures, cuts and other defects are often associated with early decomposition and the remaining soft tissue pulls back from these areas during the dehydration process. However, decomposition fluids can become embedded in some defects and these features become obscured if left uncleaned.

Reconstruction of Fragmentary Material

When the remains are fragmented, whether due to perimortem violence or postmortem damage, reconstruction is often required to correctly interpret the evidence. Prior to reconstruction, all fragments should be photographed. Fracture edges should be examined as to gross appearance and under oblique light to reveal the topography of the fracture. In some cases, these edges should be replicated with Microsil or other fine-grained casting material. These edges may yield information on the force of the impact, the nature of the bone when fractured, and the direction of impact. Once reconstructed, these surfaces will no longer be easily accessible for further analysis, including that done by experts consulting for opposing attorneys.

Bone fragments are laid out in the rough order for reconstruction. Pieces can be dry fit prior to applying adhesive to check articulation. Morphological fit is the most important. Fracture surfaces should show close attachment of the fracture surfaces, particularly with perimortem fractures. Similarity in the size and thickness of the bone should also be considered. Coloration of the surfaces may differ significantly if the fragments have undergone different taphonomic processes. For example, bones on the surface of the soil may be light colored and show some bleaching while adjacent pieces may be darkly stained from the soil.

Reconstruction order often is determined by the ability to articulate larger pieces, although it is often best to start with attaching smaller pieces to larger pieces rather than working to articulate the largest pieces. All too often, one is close to completion only to realize that the smaller pieces can no longer be inserted into the correct location and the reconstruction must be dismantled. Unfortunately, cranial vault reconstruction can be complicated by warpage of the bone so that a completely articulated reconstruction is not possible. In such cases, the intervening gaps can be stabilized with rods but bone should not be modified to achieve a fit. Hot Shot® glue or a similar type of cyanoacrylate catalyst-activated adhesive is extremely useful to quickly reconstruct fractures. The rate of setting can be greatly accelerated with a finishing spray. The use of a sand tray or tape can be very useful to articulate multiple pieces without adhesive, especially useful for "testing" refits before gluing. When time is less of an issue, water-based glues are sufficient for reconstructing dry, non-greasy, skeletal material. Glue is applied to the fracture surface and the bones articulated. Tape should also not be used for bone that has a friable surface.

Three-dimensional scanning and imaging of bone fragments provides another option for skull reconstruction. Individual pieces can be scanned and these digital fragments then "reconstructed." Alternatively, scanned pieces can be printed and the resulting prints assembled into the completed bone. This approach has the advantage of allowing copies of the fragments to be sent to other experts for consultation.

ANALYSIS: EXAMINATION, DOCUMENTATION AND CASE REPORT

The analysis of skeletal trauma is an area where the forensic anthropologist can greatly contribute to the reconstruction of the circumstances of death. It is also an area that is emotionally charged. As one begins to comprehend the magnitude of the violence or the deliberation with which it has been imparted or the vulnerability of the victim, it may be hard to resist the tendency to align oneself with one adversarial party against the other. The "golden rule" of the expert witness is that they are not personally involved in the case. The interpretation of the results is based solely on the material analyzed and must not be adjusted according to the desires of the party requesting the anthropological analysis. The expert is being compensated for the time they devote to the analysis; their opinion is not being bought.

Analysis

The analysis of trauma should begin, as noted, prior to cleaning with documentation of visible defects. Following cleaning, each element is reassessed both by visual examination and low-level magnification. Trauma is documented as having occurred during one of three periods: antemortem, perimortem, and postmortem (See Chapter 4 for full discussion). Antemortem trauma includes bone damage prior to death and is characterized by clearly recognizable signs of healing. These signs include the initiation of callus formation through woven bone adjacent to the fracture, erosion of bone at the line where the periosteum was damaged and became necrotic, and rounding of the fracture margins (Barbian and Sledzik 2008). Perimortem skeletal trauma displays fracture characteristics consistent with fresh bone with no indications of healing. In most cases where crushing has not occurred, the margins can be rearticulated easily. Skeletal perimortem trauma may include bone trauma that occurs up to about two weeks before death and after death until postmortem fracture characteristics or events can be discerned. Postmortem trauma is defined as bone damage that occurs after the bone has lost the characteristics of fresh bone. Coloration differences are common. Decomposition fluids usually stain the external cortex, whereas the newly fractured surface is not.

The documented trauma should also be described in terms of (1) defects, including fractures and (2) insults or impacts (Galloway and Zephro 2005). A defect is an imperfection on the bone, a failure or absence of bones or bony features. A fracture is a specialized type of defect in which there is traumatic rupture of the integrity of the bone. Defects should be individually identified and examined. Beveling, the presence of tags or spurs of bone, amd fracture intersections should be observed and documented.

The anthropologist should then identify the minimum number of events that occurred to produce the observable damage to the skeleton. As noted in the SWGANTH section on trauma, determination of the maximum number of impact events is not appropriate as not all impacts may leave skeletal markers.

An insult or impact is the causal event of one or more defects. In order to reconstruct these events, the relationship between defects must be analyzed. Defects that originate at one point should be combined into a probable single impact. For example, a single blunt force blow to the side of the head may well result in multiple fractures, both radiating and concentric. These fractures/defects should then be grouped together. Likewise, if the side of the head opposite to the impact was on an opposing surface (i.e., the floor or roadway) in relation to the impact, fractures may be present opposite the impact site. Both suites of fractures, therefore, represent the same traumatic event as the fractures from the direct blow to one side. The anthropologist should also be aware in this analysis of the possible range of movement of the body. It is important to note that damage in one area may have been simultaneous with a blow to another area of the body. For example, a massive fracture in the upper arm may also be associated with underlying rib fractures. It is critical that observable trauma be related to anatomy, body position, trauma type, trajectory, and context.

Direction of the impact can be interpreted in some aspects but rarely pinpointed in blunt force trauma. Again, anatomical movement must be taken into consideration. Analysis of direction of impact must first be confined to the information available from the skeleton. It is possible that requesting agencies will ask specifically if impact could have come from a specific direction, but that assessment must be made independent of the initial evaluation.

The Written Report

The report by the anthropologist is a legal document and therefore must clearly outline the analysis, conclusions, and limitations of the analysis. This document is usually provided to the agency who engaged the services of the anthropologist, in most cases the coroner or medical examiner, and from there, to the investigating agency and the prosecutor's office. In the event that the case goes to court, this report will be provided to defense counsel. Care must be taken in discussion of trauma to distinguish between observations and interpretation.

Observations of skeletal defects should note each instance of a traumatic defect on the bone. This catalog should not make reference to the relationship between defects or to the reconstruction of the events that produced them. Reports should detail the number of defects, characteristics, and location. Supporting documentation includes diagrams and photographs linked to the description. This serves to lay the foundation upon which the further interpretations are based. This listing should be specific enough to allow easy recognition of the defects by others examining the document or the remains.

Interpretations include the professional opinion on the type of force used, the direction and force of delivery, and the number and sequence of incidents that gave rise to the overall trauma. Links between individual injuries should be discussed so that the minimum number of blows, shots, or cuts can be calculated. It is within this context that the experience of the forensic anthropologist, the results of experimentation and discussion of limitations must be laid out. These interpretations must not address either cause or manner of death, which is the purview of the medical examiner/coroner. Instead, they must be limited to the skeletal material. Relationships between the overlying or underlying soft tissue should be kept to general terms, as noted above. Pathological descriptions or interpretations of soft tissue should be avoided.

Supporting Documentation

The forensic anthropological report should specify what documentation such as photographs and/or radiographs have been prepared and where they are retained. Some of these may be later used in court testimony or in preparation of the attorneys for examination. Photographs of adjudicated or unadjudicated cases, including unidentified cases, should not be used for teaching or public presentations unless explicit written permission is requested by the anthropologist and is granted by the originating agency.

Figures that show the skeleton and views of the skull (Figures 2-2 and 2-3) are extremely useful to accompany photographs. The particular features needed to correctly interpret the trauma may be obscured or difficult to identify on a photograph. Providing accompanying charts allows the requesting agency, opposing counsel's experts, and a jury to familiarize themselves with the basis for the anthropological interpretation. In cases of extensive skull trauma, providing photographs that parallel the six views of the chart, allows quick and direct comparisons.

In some jurisdictions, the medical examiner/coroner will support retention of those skeletal elements that exhibit traumatic defects. This may be particularly useful in subsequent re-evaluation and may reduce possible conflicts over admissibility of anthropological testimony. It may also prevent the problem of future exhumation.

Unfortunately, there is a tendency to assume that bodies should be automatically reburied. In part, this is due to the lack of adequate storage in many jurisdictions where centralized morgue facilities are lacking. All efforts should be made to prevent the cremation of unidentified remains or remains, which show evidence of homicidal trauma. While buried remains can be exhumed for later study, cremation destroys all possibility of retrieving additional and possibly critical information.

The availability of three-dimensional scanning and printing techniques promises better ways of presenting evidence of blunt force trauma to the court. These systems allow for the duplication, with varying levels of detail, of

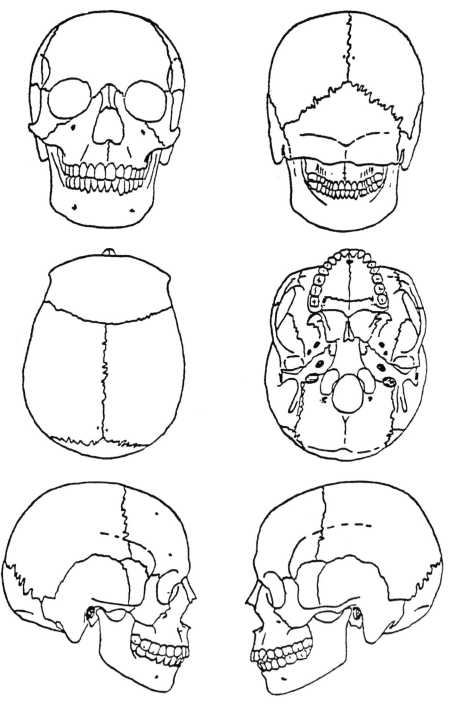

Figure 2-2. Skull chart on which defects and fractures may be drawn. Figure by Walter Birkby.

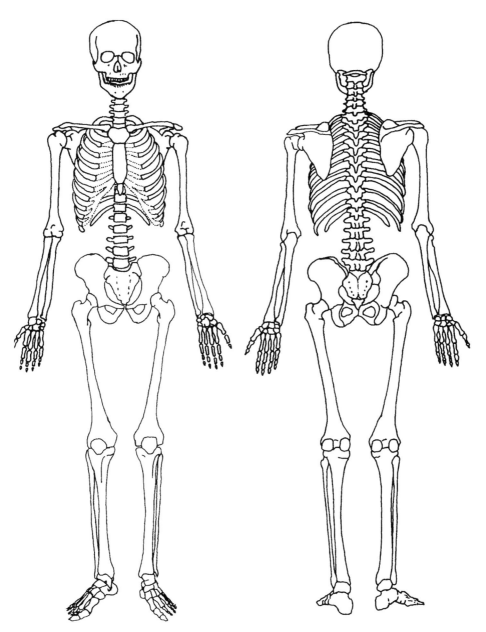

Figure 2-3. Skeleton chart on which defects and fractures may be drawn. This chart can also be used as a skeletal inventory where elements present are shaded. Figure by Walter Birkby,

the skeletal element in question. This methodology will not fully replace the necessity of retaining skeletal material for future re-analysis by consulting anthropologists but will allow retention of information when preservation is not possible.

Peer Review

Peer review and verification of results is a requirement in other forensic disciplines. Within some forensic anthropology laboratories, this activity occurs with each anthropologist independently assessing the material and then collaborating on a report, which is then co-signed. However, the majority of anthropologists work alone or with students. Therefore, the requirement of verification is not met. Both parties should be journey-level practitioners, not students. Alliances between professional anthropologists are another option in which reports are sent between individuals who are separately established. The Society of Forensic Anthropology (SOFA.org) is a group of professional forensic anthropologists, the majority of which are employed as forensic anthropologists with in a coroner/ME office or other law enforcement setting. SOFA offers a peer review network of anthropologists that have been vetted to peer review cases. The need for the peer review service was specifically geared towards forensic anthropologists working in a laboratory setting with only one anthropologist.

The coroner or medical examiner must approve any outside peer review, both for the electronic sharing of documents and the comparing of opinions of any observed defects. One complication, however, is that such consultation effectively eliminates the reviewing expert from serving as a witness for the opposing counsel. However, this does not eliminate the need for a second review of a case by another journey-level forensic anthropologist. Indeed, this step, as a quality control measure, may prevent future disagreements when a case goes to trial.

Experimentation

Occasionally a question will arise during an investigation for which there is insufficient published information. At other times, the information that has been published appears to be inadequately grounded in data and/or does not appear consistent with the interpretation suggested by other factors. The anthropologist may need to conduct experiments upon which to base a decision.

The decision to conduct this work should not be taken lightly. A well-designed experiment may well upset commonly accepted knowledge and may result in questioning the existing interpretation of the case. A poorly-designed experiment that artificially supports or refutues the interpretation degrades the integrity of the discipline.

In many, if not most, cases, there is a span of years between the analysis of a forensic case and appearance in court. Typically this is of the order of two years, sufficient time to conduct a study and have the results close to, if not fully, presented at meetings and published. Chapter 3 presents the theoretical framework for experimental work.

POST-ANALYSIS: COURT TESTIMONY, DEPOSITIONS AND DEFENSE CONSULTATION

How and when injuries to the decedent occurred is often the critical issue should a case come to trial. Information on the injuries are central to whether or not a homicide occurred and the timing and sequence of injuries may influence decisions to either file charges against accomplices or add the gravity of the preliminary charges.

While usually raised in cases involving criminal charges, analysis of trauma is increasingly addressed in civil suits over wrongful death. In both criminal and civil cases, sequencing of events and determining the timing of antemortem, perimortem, and postmortem injuries are important. Reconstruction of the events in relation to other victims or with contact with possibly defective materials is often addressed in civil suits.

The key to good expert witness testimony often lies in the care devoted to pretrial preparation. This is particularly true for how analyses of trauma, which may lie at the heart of the dispute regarding guilt or innocence, are presented. Pretrial conferences should review every aspect of direct testimony, the possible areas of approach for cross-examination by the opposing attorney, and how to counter any misconceptions generated during re-direct questioning.

Given that many attorneys have not worked with an anthropologist before, be prepared with a list of qualifying questions that establish your expertise and inform the court about forensic anthropology in general. In discussing the qualifications of the anthropologist to establish expert witness status, specific work on skeletal trauma, such as the number of previous cases in which trauma was analyzed, research on traumatic injuries or experimental projects, should be highlighted. Pretrial discussions are the ideal time to review these with the attorney.

The anthropologist must make the attorney aware of links between the testimony regarding the skeletal material and that on the cause and manner of death. Since the anthropologist's work inevitably raises questions about how the victim died that the anthropologist will not be able to answer, the attorney must be ready to address these points in his or her examination of the medical examiner/coroner. It is the responsibility of the anthropologist to prepare the attorney for this situation.

Preparation of photographs, diagrams, or models prior to trial are important, as these may be the clearest way to show the jury how the events are best explained by the anthropologist's interpretations. In most cases, references to soft tissue should be avoided. These visual presentations may be ruled inadmissible due to their possible inflammatory nature. Preparation should, therefore, include alternate means of conveying the necessary information.

The issue of consultation fees should be raised with the attorney if these have not already been established. In addition to actual testimony time, consultation, including telephone calls, should be logged and charged. Expenses such as travel, hotel, and communication charges should be included in the cost of hiring an expert witness, in addition to the hourly or daily rate. Often expert witnesses charge the hiring agency for all the time required from when they leave their place of business to attend a trial until they return. Attorneys need to understand this and arrange their budget and schedule accordingly.

Once in the courtroom, the anthropologist will be sworn in as a witness. The witness is seated in the witness box, facing the counsel and usually next to or parallel to the judge. It is helpful to have a glass of water available as questioning may be lengthy.

Testimony typically begins with a discussion of the qualifications. These questions include education, publications, types of cases worked, any certifications associated with the professional organizations, and prior testimony. Opposing counsel may wish to stipulate to these items, but a brief review is almost certainly to be expected. Then the attorney for whom the anthropologist is working will usually ask how the expert became involved with the case, when evidence was examined and the report written.

After this point, the testimony begins to reach the core of the issue. Typically, the basic biological profile is reviewed, in most cases to show the jury to quality of the assessment and the knowledge and expertise of the expert. Then the attorney will proceed to the issues of trauma and postmortem interval. Attorneys also have very different ways in which they approach court testimony from expert witnesses. Some prefer to allow the expert to speak at length by responding to very broad questions, while others prefer to "walk through" the material with short answers to very specific questions. In the latter case, it is essential that the important areas be covered well during pretrial conference as the attorneys may not grasp the critical importance of some key point. It is best to coordinate when and how the illustrations and other supporting items will be introduced.

Questioning frequently centers on the actual events of the death with particular attention to the weapon or weapons believed used in the homicide. In essence, the anthropologist must guide the jury through the evidence and provide an impartial assessment of what can and cannot be determined from the defects on the remains. This must be done in such a way as to not prejudice the jury but without detracting from the information being provided.

In actuality, this balance can be difficult to attain. The prosecution or defense attorney is interested in providing a case in support of their perspective in this highly adversarial situation. They may wish to focus on things that the anthropologist considers irrelevant but will portray the victim or the accused in a particular light. A frequent ploy is to ask hypothetical questions that test the limits of interpretation. For example, if a fracture pattern suggests a relatively broad impact area, an attorney may begin asking if the weapon could have been a baseball bat but then ask about the probability of a succession of weapons of decreasing size.

The anthropologist should be well prepared for the testimony, reviewing not only the specifics of the case in terms of injuries but also when and how they were contacted, what was discussed prior to testimony, and when new lines of evidence were introduced, such as a confession or the report from another expert. While notes are allowed in the courtroom, they may be held as evidence and it is often difficult and time-consuming to fumble through files trying to find notes on a specific conversation. If you need to refer to your notes during testimony, you must request permission from the judge. For complex cases, organizing and making labeled tags for your case file is helpful to quickly find the specific information you require.

Illustrations, when used in conjunction with the testimony, should be clear and large enough to be easily seen in the courtroom. Often it is good to show an overall image of the skeleton with the bone indicated alongside the photograph you wish to discuss. The use of color to highlight portions of the charts is often helpful as long as gaudy colors or color combinations are avoided. Photographs should allow members of the jury to quickly determine the orientation. Video depictions of the results, such as matching an alleged weapon to the trauma or diagramming the sequence of shots through animation of the radiating fracture patterns, may be useful.

Courtrooms come equipped with varying levels of media for presentation. In most cases, large easels are used to mount panels that are visible to the judge, jury, and attorneys. Increasingly, digital images are used to reduce the need for large paper collections on each case. Slides, overheads, and overhead cameras may also be available, but this fact should be established prior to testimony. While a specific order of illustrations may be used in the initial testimony, it is often necessary to work back and forth between a number of illustrations later in the testimony.

Retained skeletal material may be brought to the court at the discretion of the judge. Often, if a pressing question or dispute arises, the anthropologist can offer to demonstrate to the jury how interpretations were made using the actual bone. The outcome in such cases is either (1) the opposing counsel will relinquish their objections to the interpretation for fear that the jury will be exposed to the remains or (2) the skeletal material is used and the point can often be made relatively quickly and clearly. Three-dimensional replicas of the bones showing the defects of interest may be used if they are locally admissible.

If the actual bone or a three-dimensional print is not to be presented, it is often helpful to have plastic models of specific areas such as the skull or pelvis, where the complex three-dimensional shape is difficult to illustrate. These models are available from anatomical supply companies, as well as establishments that cater to the needs of attorneys. Portions that are moveable or easily separated may be very helpful in demonstrating the movements that would occur to produce specific defects.

Cross-examination, re-direct, and re-cross can consume as much time as the initial testimony. Cross-examination is designed to either show flaws in the anthropologist's work or find ways in which this work supports an alternative interpretation. Occasionally, the questions from attorney or the defendant (if he or she is acting on their own defense) may seem at odds with standard interpretation or the basic theoretical framework of the discipline. Rarely do these attorneys have as much experience with forensic anthropologists as the person who retained your services, and this may be the first time they have had to question anyone from the discipline. Questions are aimed not only at the work specifically but also at the role of the anthropologist. Often questions attempt to test the limits of what you are saying by asking for you to determine cause of death or degree of disability induced by various injuries. If the anthropologist strays into the area of the forensic pathologist, he or she has left themselves vulnerable to accusations of working beyond their training. Questions are almost always made about the fees charged for analysis and testimony and should be answered openly.

While the bulk of the trial cases handled by forensic anthropologists are derived from the prosecution's perspective, defense attorneys are increasingly utilizing the services of forensic anthropologists as expert witnesses to support the case for the defendant. This poses a difficult situation but one which should be met as a professional challenge. The anthropologist may be testifying in opposition to the prosecution's interpretation of the events as interpreted by their medical experts or another forensic anthropologist. This may be personally difficult since, within the limited community of physical/biological anthropologists engaged in forensic science, people have established strong collegial ties. In addition, there is the problem of accounting for alterations to the bones produced during previous analyses without automatically adopting any opinions established by earlier work. In these cases, it is best to complete one's own thorough examination of the material prior to comparing findings to the earlier work.

A warning for anyone retained for court testimony is to arrive prepared to spend longer than anticipated. Changes of clothing, overnight kits and some reading material are important to pack for any trial that requires more than a short drive. One-day trips often turn into three days spent sitting in a court-house corridor waiting your turn. It is for this reason that "portal-to-portal" fees or "waiting time" fees are charged.

Few attorneys inform the experts they have consulted about the eventual outcome of the case. It is wise to check some time later as to the verdict, to see if your services may be needed for subsequent court proceedings, and whether the case has been adjudicated and you are now free to discuss the case more openly.

SUMMARY

The analysis of skeletal trauma provides an important turning point for anthropological analysis of skeletal material within the forensic context. The dramatic increase in studies and case reports within professional journals documents this shifting focus. Increasingly, the techniques upon which the anthropologist's involvement in a forensic case have traditionally been needed – those for the identification of age, sex, ancestry, stature, and pecu-liarities – are accepted and, in some cases, surpassed by other techniques such as DNA analysis. The anthropological analysis of skeletal trauma is, however, increasingly important as challenges to interpretations become more prevalent.

Skeletal trauma analysis provides a vast area with almost unlimited potential for anthropologists to assist the medical examiner, law enforcement personnel, and the legal community. Strengthening the links between soft tissue defects and those of the better preserved skeletal tissue may be the keystone for a strong case. Likewise, discrepancies between the soft tissue interpretations and those derived from later analysis of the more easily maintained and preserved skeletal material may draw attention to issues that otherwise would have been overlooked.

Skeletal trauma is highly variable and each case presents a unique set of challenges in the interpretation and reconstruction of the events that produced them. The aim of this volume is to present some guidelines that may help facilitate this process and provide documented support for this growing area of research and application within forensic anthropology. The care given to documenting the defects and the depth of work in reconstructing the events that produced them quickly becomes evident in the quality of the written report and subsequent court testimony. It is upon this foundation that we can advance our influence within this exciting area of forensic analysis.

Chapter 3

THE BIOMECHANICS OF FRACTURE PRODUCTION

Lauren Zephro And Alison Galloway

Blunt force trauma consists of damage inflicted through a number of different forces in which the area of impact is relatively large. While there is no specific size at which one can separate sharp from blunt force, the latter is usually thought to include injuries due to fists, sticks, clubs, boards, etc., as well as those induced by motor vehicle accidents, falls, and manual compaction of the body. In general, these impacts are characterized not only by a larger area of contact but also at a much lower velocity than is seen in more penetrating injuries such as gunshots, now designated as high-velocity projectile trauma (SWGANTH 2011).

Skeletally, blunt force trauma is evidenced by a wide range of fracture patterns. These depend, in part, upon the biomechanical properties of bone at the organ and microstructural levels, and the nature of the applied loading forces. The material properties of bone, morphology, structural integrity, mineralization, and density of the skeletal elements add another level of factors that help shape fracture pathways. The shape, mass, and velocity of the instrument with which forces are applied also affect the fracturing. This section of bone fracture, from a mechanical and materials perspective, is divided into discussions of (1) basic terminology; (2) the material properties of bone, including element structure and microanatomy; and (3) the effects of loading onto bone.

BASIC TERMINOLOGY OF FORCE, STRENGTH AND FRACTURE

The study of bone fracture is based on and uses the same terminology as engineering. The following definitions are after Martin and colleagues (1998),

Nordin and Frankel (2001), Currey (2002), and Turner (2006). A *force* is defined
as a mechanical disturbance or load and, therefore, loading is the application
of force. A *force* can move and/or deform an object, and how a force acts on an
object can vary. Forces can be applied internally or externally, perpendicularly,
angled, or tangentially, and may have gravitational, frictional, tensile, compressive, or shear components.

Strength does not have an absolute definition but can be interpreted as the
ultimate load or force a material can bear before breaking. *Stiffness* is the ability
of material to resist deformation when a force is applied, and *toughness* refers
to the work or energy required to cause failure and /or resistance to crack
growth.

Two important factors in relation to bone breakage are *strain* and *stress*, the
former referring to the bone itself while the latter applies to the force. *Strain* is
defined as the deformation of an object in response to an external force, while
stress is measured as the load or force per unit area. Stress (σ) is calculated as
the applied force divided by the cross-sectional area:

$$\sigma = \text{Force}/\text{Area}$$

Stress is usually measured in MN/m^2 (meganewtons per square meter),
MPa (megapascals), or pounds per square inch (psi) (McElhaney *et al.* 1976;
Carter *et al.* 1985; Cowin 1989a). Strain (ε), the actual change or deformation
in the shape, is described as the ratio of the change in the dimension (length,
width, height, area, angulation) to the original form (Currey 1970; McElhaney
et al. 1976; Carter *et al.* 1985; Cowin 1989a; Harkness *et al.* 1991).

$$\varepsilon = \text{Deformation}/\text{Dimension}$$

The change in dimension may be negative or positive, depending upon the
direction of the force.

The *modulus of elasticity* or *Young's modulus* is a *stress/strain* curve for a material,
such as bone, in tension or compression, indicating the load a material can
bear before failure and the deformation experienced prior to fracturing
(Figure 3-1). Three regions of response for bone are noted on the chart. *Elastic*
deformation occurs when an object can return to its original shape after the
release of the stress. *Plastic* deformation occurs when an object cannot return
to its original shape and is marked by the yield point. In material science, this
includes *creep*, when a viscoelastic material is loaded at a constant rate and
held at that stress. The material will continue to deform, showing an increase
in strain, but that deformation occurs at a steadily decreasing rate. When
loading attains the ultimate tensile strength, the object fails or fractures and is
noted as the failure point. The steeper the initial part of the curve, the more
stiff a material is, indicating that the material is better able to resist deformation
prior to failure. It is important to note that the Young's modulus of a given-

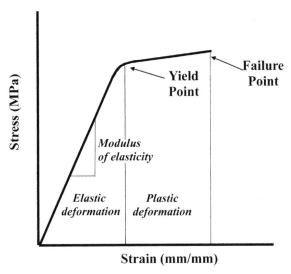

Figure 3-1. Graphic representation of the relationship between stress and strain, also known as Young's modulus or modulus of elasticity.

material is derived from cuboid sections of a material and not, in the case of bone, from whole elements. However, it is evident that bone can absorb considerable energy under elastic deformation and a small further amount under plastic deformation before it fails completely and fractures.

A *fracture* is defined as a disruption in the continuity of a bone and is dependent on the direction, energy, loading rate and duration of the load (Hall 2006). Additional variables that play into bone fracture dynamics include the health and maturity of the bone. Growing bone, for example, with its higher proportion of organic components, is less *stiff* than mature bone, which has a higher mineral content. Similarly, during the postmortem interval, as bone undergoes a variety of taphonomic alterations (loss of organic materials, microbial invasion, diagenesis, etc.), its material properties change.

The forces that produce fractures are tension, compression, and shear (Figure 3-2). In addition, these forces can also produce bone failure in bending, torsion, and multiple other scenarios of loading with combinations of multiple forces. *Tensile* forces are produced when equal and opposite loads are applied to a material, pulling it apart. *Compression* occurs when equal and opposite loads are applied to a material, pushing it together. *Shear* forces are produced when a load is applied parallel to the surface of a material. During fracture propagation, bone tested in tension fails by debonding and microcracking of the osteons along cement lines, while the yielding of bone in compression is seen as cracking of the osteons (Nordin and Frankel 2001).

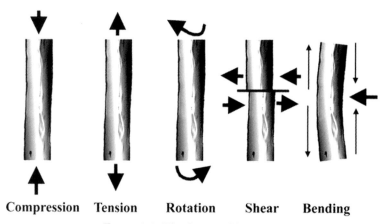

| Compression | Tension | Rotation | Shear | Bending |

Figure 3-2. The forces of fracture.

Bending produces combinations of tensile, compressive, and shear forces. Bending applies tensile forces along one side of the material while the opposing side experiences compression. Shear forces are produced within the middle. In the case of adult human long bones, initial bone failure results first on the side of the bone in tension, with the fractures propagating under shear and finally failing under compression on the opposite side. Clinically, in a human long bone fracture, a triangular fragment of bone will frequently result.

Torsion results when a load is applied to a structure causing it to twist around an axis and causing torque within the material. If a material is weaker in tension than in shear, like bone, the resulting fracture will be inclined at a 45-degree angle to the long axis of the material. Clinically, in humans, a spiral fracture is defined morphologically as a fracture that propagates around the bone shaft at a 45-degree angle in the same direction of the applied torque, which can be used to determine the direction of twist, also known as "handedness," in spiral fractures (Rosenthal et al. 1984, Porta 2005). As the fracture encircles the bone, the shaft becomes progressively more unstable such that a longitudinal fracture develops, which unites the proximal and distal ends of the 45-degree angle fracture (Porta 2005).

THE MATERIAL PROPERTIES OF BONE

The ability of a material to absorb energy is dependent on the overall shape of the material and the stiffness of a material. If a material is able to withstand stress equally in all directions, the material is *isotropic*. If a material is better able to withstand stress preferentially in one direction, the material is *anisotropic*. Bone is better able to withstand compressive stress than tensile or shear. Thus, bone is considered an anisotropic material. In addition, variability exists between elements and in individual organisms due to the inherent variability in bone quality due to growth and development, aging, species-specific bone architecture, and the condition of the bone at the time of fracture (fresh, dry, etc.). The following discussion provides insight into bone fracture mechanics considering bone as a unit (whole bones), microstructure, rate of loading, condition of the bone, and the complexities introduced by individual and species variation for research on fracture morphology.

Bone Composition and Microstructure

Bone is a heterogeneous material. It consists of both organic and inorganic components. Calcium hydroxyapatite $(Ca_{10}(PO_4)_6(OH))$ forms the bulk of the mineral portion while the organic component consists of collagen along with the non-collagenous proteins. Bone also contains water, amorphous polysaccharides, cells, and blood vessels. Tests of bone that has been embalmed or undergone drying will produce significantly different results from tests of wet bone (Reilly and Burstein 1974).

Many tests of bone failure rates are done on small blocks of bone rather than full bones but do allow some isolation of the effects of microstructure. The ability of any material to resist a force is directly proportional to both the cross-sectional area and the stiffness or springiness of that material. If two blocks of material are constant in stiffness but differ in area, they will differ in ability to withstand loading forces. Conversely, two materials with differing stiffness but similar dimensions will also differ in resistance. Bone is not exempt from these principles. The strains in bone rarely exceed about 3% (Currey 1970).

If a material is able to resist stresses equally in any direction, it is said to be anisotropic. If its resistance is aligned along one plane, the material is called transversely isotropic, but if there is no directional dependence, the substance is isotropic. Bone should be treated as a transversely isotropic material (Reilly and Burstein 1974). Bone has also been considered to be orthotropic, meaning that it consists of layers surrounding a central core such as would occur in a tree trunk (Cowin 1989a, b).

Bone is found in many different arrangements. Woven bone, found in rapidly developing or healing bone, has a high organic component and less mineral content. This is commonly found in infants and in callus formation in humans. Plexiform or fibrolamellar bone is rarely found in humans although it is common in animals, which must be highly mobile from birth. It has greater stiffness and strength but lacks some of the ability to arrest microcracks. Most human bone consists of osteonal bone, either primary or secondary. The latter is also commonly called Haversian bone. Primary osteonal bone is probably stronger than secondary osteonal bone as the latter has undergone internal remodeling via the development of Haversian systems within the bone.

As will be explored more fully in Chapter 6, these microstructural differences become critically important when designing experimental studies. The choice of animal models may give distorted effects on the biomechanics of fracture production. For example, fibrolamellar bone found in large herbivores such as sheep and cattle has a higher tensile strength than bone found in humans (Currey 2002). Vashishth, Tanner, and Bonfield (2000), comparing the tensile crack propagation in human and bovine bone, found that bovine bone had significantly higher numbers of microcracks (longitudinal, transverse, and inclined) than human bone samples and that the distribution of the cracking was significantly different. Human bone samples contained 90% longitudinal microcracks, 9.5% inclined, and 0.5% transverse compared with 44% longitudinal, 44% transverse, and 12% inclined in bovids. They found that, based on the microstructure, bovine bone is better able to distribute loads and that the microcracks actually reduce the energy in the bone, requiring more energy to completely break it. The difference in the proportion of microcrack types is explained by the longitudinal orientation of secondary osteons, resulting in damage being more localized. Further, Carter *et al.* (1976), in a comparison of secondary bone remodeling in bovids, found that the presence of Haversian systems reduces fatigue life by decreasing bone density and creating a generally weaker structure.

The differences would also be reflected in differences in microstructure within a single individual based on turnover rate differences in the tissue. Rimnac and collegues (1993) showed that creep resulting in a complete fracture proceeded about 100 times faster in pure Haversian bone than in pure lamellar bone. Not only will the presence of Haversian systems alter fracture toughness, but also the sizes and distribution of the Haversian systems. This difference can be most clearly seen when comparing bone microstructure between species. Yan and colleagues (2006) attempted to examine the fracture toughness of manatee rib and bovine femur. A manitee rib is a pachyostotic, non-weight bearing bone without a marrow cavity from an aquatic animal, whereas a cow femur is a weight-bearing tubular bone from a terrestrial mammal. The results indicated that although the manatee bone had fewer secondary osteons, the Haversian systems and central canals were larger, making the bone more porous. The bovine femoral bone, on the other hand, had a much higher secondary osteon density, but the structures were smaller and thus the bone was less porous in comparison. The result is that denser bone is tougher than comparatively more porous bone given similar overall size. Although this research compares two non-human species, each with distinct and contrasting microstructural characteristics, we can use relevant information from these studies to describe the bone material properties in humans and how these change due to growth and development, aging, and pathology.

Mathematical models for bone strength and fracture criteria have been investigated with varying levels of success. As Doblare and colleagues (2004) note, there is a general lack of agreement between models, at times even on basic principles. In part this may be due to the inability of computational models to fully replicate the effect of trabecular bone, although they can account for porosity. The models are continually being refined, particularly through the integration of data from non-invasive studies such as quantitative computed tomography and dual-energy x-ray absorptiometry. In addition, information from strain gauges anchored to living bone has provided valuable insights as to the actual loading environments for bone.

Bones Under Strain

The geometry of a bone dictates its mechanical properties. Long bones, for example, are essentially long tubes of cortical bone. However, these tubes do not have even dimensions and they incorporate bends and muscle attachment sites, which also change the overall geometry. Thin bones such as those of the cranial vault, vary in thickness and proportion and orientation of intervening trabecular bone. Bones typically experience forces in which the bones are bent and respond accordingly with architecture that best absorbs these forces.

Under tension and compression, the load to failure and stiffness of long bones are proportional to the cross-sectional area of the bone (Nordin and Frankel 2001). Beyond the simple area, there are vast differences in how that bone is distributed around the neutral axis, comprising the cross-sectional geometry. The area moment of inertia, which measures aspects of the cross-sectional distribution of bone material around the neutral axis, dictates a bone's response to bending. Bones with more tissue distributed farther away from the neutral axis have a larger area moment of inertia, which results in a stronger, stiffer bone that is better able to resist bending and torsion (Martin *et al.* 1998, Nordin and Frankel 2001). For example, a human tibia is more likely to fracture at the distal end, where the cross sectional geometry has a lower area moment of inertia than proximally, where the area moment of inertia is higher. Although in the distal tibia there is proportionally more bone tissue than in the proximal shaft, the bone tissue is distributed closer to the neutral axis. When the bone is subjected to torsional loading, the shear stresses experienced by the distal end are nearly double the proximal section (Nordin and Frankel 2001). However, the impact of cross-sectional geometry has proven to be much more complex than initially imagined. Lieberman and colleagues (2004) experimented on animal models to show that along the length of a bone, there are significant differences in cross-sectional geometry and that specific cross-sectional parameters may be better to use in experimental work between individuals or, more importantly, in using animal models to extrapolate to humans.

Finally, a bone's length influences its strength and stiffness. Bird and Becker (1966) found that whole bones were significantly more impact-resistant than blocks of bone material. They observed cracking and fracture between cubed impact specimens at about 200 fps and whole bone impact at 800 fps, suggesting bone geometry is an important determinant of its failure behavior. The longer a bone is, the greater the magnitude of bending moment with the application of force and, as a result, the longer the bone the higher the magnitude of stress (Nordin and Frankel 2001). Human bones, being relatively long and gracile for body size, are susceptible to fracture at lower loading points than similar bones from other mammals.

BIOMECHANICAL LOADING

Loading is the application of a force to an object. Loading forces are applied to bone from a number of different sources. When sedentary, such as standing or sitting, the weight of the body itself forms a load on the bones. This weight will vary by body size and composition, and it changes throughout the lifetime (Skedros 2012). The force is determined by the weight superior to each bone and calculated based on the area of contact for transmission of the load. Thus, when seated, the ischial tuberosities can support a substantial portion of the body's weight, consisting of the torso, head, neck, and upper limbs. In addition, muscle contraction can increase the force applied to bone. When the contraction is constant, or the person is at rest, the force is said to be static, meaning that the loading does not change. In routine movement, however, the forces are dynamic, meaning that the force must be calculated as not only the mass but also the acceleration or deceleration with which it is applied. This dramatically increases the load bearing of bones. For example, a woman walking on high heels can be loading the heel at about 700–2000 psi (pounds per square inch), even though she weighs no more than 125 pounds.

Beyond everyday weight bearing, there are forces brought to bear when the body strikes or is struck by an object or surface. These loads are usually not in alignment with the normal weight bearing of the body and as such generate deformations in the body as the tissues absorb the energy transmitted. If the loads are low and applied repeatedly, the body will gradually compensate for the new function (Meade 1989). When these forces are relatively high, they can overwhelm the ability of the tissues to absorb energy without damage. Among the types of injury found are those that affect the skeleton. The focus of this work is on events that result in acute damage rather than long-term acclimation.

Rate of Loading

The energy-absorbing capacity of bone differs with the relative speed of the applied force. When loaded with a high-speed force, bone material acts as a brittle material, and it fails without going through the plastic deformation stage. *Static* loading refers to loading that is constant, which results in creep behavior (Caler and Carter 1989). *Dynamic* loading occurs when a bone is broken very rapidly with a high kinetic energy (Martin *et al.* 1998). In dynamic loading, fractures are much more comminuted. According to Martin *et al.* (1998), under static loading, a resulting crack causes the adjacent bone material to be unloaded, preventing other cracks in the vicinity. In the case of dynamic loading, a stress wave passes through the bone at the speed of sound (about 3,000 m/s), which results in many cracks forming before the individual cracks can relieve one another by absorbing energy. When cracks grow and intersect one another, many fragments result.

The measure of how much a material can deform prior to fracture differs with the rate at which it is loaded. With regard to bone, this is a phenomenon related to its viscoelastic properties. A study by Frankel and Burnstein (1967) found that bone's ability to absorb energy at a low strain rate was 40–46% of a bone's ability to absorb energy at a high strain rate. Thus, bone is stiffer and stronger when rapidly loaded than when it is slowly strained, but when it does break under rapid loading (as explained above), more fragmentation results (Martin *et al.* 1998). Experimentally, using a bone surrogate material (foam based), Beardsley and colleagues (2002) found that the amount of bone comminution or degree of fragmentation, as reflected in fragment surface area, can be measured on a continuum dependent on the amount of energy absorbed. Their results support the intuitive conclusion and real-world observations that higher energy impacts cause smaller, more numerous fragments.

The difference in patterning of fractures between static and dynamic loading can also be seen in the nature of conjoining fractures. As it is subjected to static loading, bone passes through its elastic phase prior to fracturing. That is, if the load is removed, the bone would return to its original shape. If the static loading persists, bone passes into the plastic phase and becomes permanently deformed. The resulting bone fragments may not fit together cleanly, rather they appear "warped." Bone fractured under high-energy dynamic loading reacts as a more brittle or stiff material and experiences little or no deformation prior to fracture, and the resulting fragments fit together cleanly (Nordin and Frankel 2001). Similar to Currey and Brear (1992), Vashishth and colleagues (2000) found that materials with greater toughness display rougher fracture surfaces, supporting the hypothesis that tissues that show extensive microcracking have a rougher fracture surface. However, Adharapurapu and colleagues (2006) demonstrated that under very high loading rates, the fracture surfaces of bovine bone tend to smooth out in appearance, when compared to fracture surfaces produced by lower energy. This likely involves the changing mechanical properties of bone under high loading rates, with bone reacting as a more brittle material. In the Adharapurapu *et al.* (2006) study, the toughness of bone (the energy required to cause failure) also decreased as the loading rate increased and experienced very low fracture toughness at the highest loading rates.

Loading within the Living Organism

While the above-described relationships are relatively simple principles to apply to a material subject to loading in only one direction, they are less simple to assimilate in living bone. The reasons are threefold. Each will be discussed in turn.

First, bone is subject to forces being applied in many directions. Bone is relatively pliable in the longitudinal direction but brittle in the transverse. The picture is further complicated, however, because bone is subject to the forces generated by weight bearing, muscle contraction, and impact upon other materials all acting simultaneously. In these cases, the bone's ultimate strength is reduced. For instance, the maximum tensile or compressive stress that can be withstood is lowered as shear stresses are superimposed (Cezyirlioglu *et al.* 1985).

Second, meeting the needs of all these loading patterns, as well as other functions invested in the skeleton, can require a bone to "comprimise" with regard to form and function. Particularly vulnerable sites such as the femoral neck would need to be quite different in morphology in order to be best suited to load bearing alone. Bipedal locomotion could be jeopardized in such circumstances. The added weight of the "redesigned" bone would also drastically increase the energy expenditures of locomotion. Instead, the evolution of the human skeleton is one of continual compromises resulting in a set of bony elements capable of meeting locomotor and postural needs as well as maintaining the other functions of these organs including anchoring muscles, housing hemopoietic tissue, and serving as a reservoir for calcium and trace elements.

The cells within the bone tissue must be nourished, waste products removed, and the medullary cavity must be supported. Blood vessels and nerves must pass along or through the bone. Any sudden transition in the shape of bone, however, to accommodate these soft tissue components will alter the distribution of stresses producing stress concentrations. Morphological features such as notches, foramina, abrupt changes in surface contours, sulci, and nutrient foramina going into long bones are all likely sites of such concentrations (Currey 1984). Examination of overall bone morphology shows that these features rarely occur in places or take a course that will place the bone at biomechanical risk.

The third reason is that, if the body were impervious to the changes that occur during elastic deformation, the first indication that loads in excess of tolerable levels were being reached would be the onset of plastic deformation and fracturing. Instead, large levels of elastic deformation permit the bone to measure the levels of forces being applied through proteoglycan deformation, piezoelectric changes or microfractures (Chamay and Tschantz 1972, Eriksson 1976, Martin and Burr 1982, Carter 1983). Living bone responds to normal loading by gradually altering the cross-sectional configuration to accommodate these forces but also retain enough flexibility to monitor changes in the forces.

Loading, Age- and Disease-related Changes in Bone, and Fractures

Bone quantity, quality, and shape vary throughout the human lifetime. Woven bone is the initial form that appears in the fetus as well as in the callus of fracture repair. It can be formed quickly and consists of fine-fibered collagen in a random orientation, although there may be preference for alignment with the long axis of the bone. With time, woven bone is replaced by lamellar bone, which is deposited more slowly than woven bone. In lamellar bone, collagen sheets about 5 m thick surround the bone, although the fibrils in adjacent lamellae are usually not oriented the same direction. As humans get older, the lamellar bone is remodeled into Haversian bone, which consists of secondary osteons or Haversian systems, which replace existing bone. Each osteon has a total diameter of about 0.2–0.4 mm and is formed within a resorption cavity formed in the wake of resorption of existing bone. Osteons are aligned to the long axis of the bone.

In part, bone strength is related to the proportions of primary and secondary osteons (Currey 1970, 1984). Secondary osteons weaken the overall bone structure because the canals of Haversian systems decrease bone density (Carter *et al.* 1976). The skeletons of young people contain more water and are less brittle and more porous with larger Haversian canals than the skeletons of older individuals (Rogers 1992). As humans age, osteon numbers increase while individual osteon size decreases. This change allows for an overall increase in the cement lines along which fractures preferentially form (Evans 1975). The periosteum thickens, becomes more elastic and less firmly bound to the bone and, therefore, tends to remain intact when bones break, hinging fragments together (Rogers 1992).

These changes dramatically affect the relationship between force and displacement (Turner 2006). In young individuals, the bones are ductile and absorb a lot of force with significant displacement prior to failure (Currey and Butler 1975). The bones of children will undergo considerably more plastic deformation prior to failure than adults. As people age, the greater brittleness means that less displacement or absorption of energy is possible prior to bone tissue failure (Turner 2006). Despite this shift, bones in adults are able to re-model to maximize resistance by changing the distribution of bone around the neutral axis of the bone. As endosteal absorption of bone removes bone mineral, periosteal deposition increases rigidity.

Maximum bone mineral density, a measure of the concentration of inor-ganic material within a given volume of bone, peaks between 30 and 35 years of age (Grynpas 2003). This peak is followed by gradual age-related loss. Superimposed upon this loss among women is postmenopausal loss, which lasts 5–15 years after menopause. The loss is more severe although for a shorter period in trabecular bone, while more gradual but prolonged in cortical bone. As this rate of loss tapers off, the age-related loss continues. In sample populations of very old individuals, an apparent "leveling off" may be partly due to survivorship effects, rather than an actual slowdown in rates of bone loss.

Peaks in bone strength due to changes in bone mineral density, micro-structure, bone shape, length, degree of mineralization, and cortical deposition are found in the young adult. Small decreases in the modulus of elasticity are expected with age and average about 1.5% per decade after age 20 (Burstein *et al.* 1976). The maximum strain that can be withstood falls more drastically: 5%–7% per decade. Ultimate tensile strength of bone declines about 4% per decade under low strain rates (Melick and Miller 1966). Burstein and associates (1976) found decreases in strength with age under tension and compression in the femur although not in the tibia. Shear strength declined at about 4% per decade. In general, bone becomes less strong and stiff and more brittle as an individual ages, although this is not evenly distributed throughout the skeleton.

Bone mineral density is significantly correlated with fracture risk (Mazess 1987). Fracture thresholds have been established through clinical analysis of the density of the bones of those who have suffered fractures characteristic of osteoporosis. These thresholds vary by bone and location within the bone but show positive correlation within skeletal locations of the individual in most cases (Mazess 1987, Heaney 1989). Risk of fracture is particularly high in the proximal femur, vertebrae, distal radius, proximal tibia, pelvis, and proximal humerus (Cummings *et al.* 1985, Melton and Cummings 1987, Riggs and Melton 1988, Melton 1993, Melton 1995, Riggs and Melton 1995, Lips 1997, Cummings *et al.* 1997).

In many people, especially postmenopausal women, large amounts of bone tissue are lost, leading to the condition clinically termed *osteoporosis* (Mazess 1987, Melton and Cummings 1987, Grynpas 2003). This metabolic disease is characterized by low bone mineral density accompanied by deteriorated microarchitecture of the bone. Osteoporosis predisposes individuals to fracture from relatively low loading forces. Resorption occurs along the medullary cavity and the adjacent cortical bone becomes more porous. This process is often associated with subperiosteal expansion, although this depends upon whether the person maintains relatively high activity levels. The net result is alteration of the modulus of elasticity.

In trabecular bone, gradual elimination of cross-struts weakens the overall structural integrity despite increasing thickness of the remaining trabecular struts. The decreased bone mass increases susceptibility to fracture, often from minimal or no trauma. As healthy trabecular bone collapses, broken trabeculae fill the pores between the bony struts, which increases stiffness. In osteoporotic individuals, there are fewer struts and the pores are greater in volume. This results in greater deformation before the stiffness due to in-filling of the spaces builds to the point when further collapse is halted. These changes are not confined to a simple loss of density. Although it is likely they will occur with greater frequency in situations leading to forensic examination, osteoporotic fractures will be noted but not directly addressed in this volume.

Pathological changes in bone, such as those induced by diabetes, Paget's disease, Cushing's disease, rickets, osteogenesis imperfecta, scurvy, renal disease, neuromuscular disorders, rheumatoid arthritis, osteomyelitis, benign tumors and metastasizing cancers and the use of exogenous steroids, may increase the risk of fracture. Abuse of alcohol and certain illicit drugs have also been linked to changes in bone quality, either directly or through associated poor nutrition. Strokes or traumatic paraplegia will affect the ability to load the limbs. Muscles will atrophy and this atrophy will be accompanied by bone mineral loss although there are longer-term changes as well (Grynpas 2003). While these may also occur in circumstances leading to forensic analysis, the presence of other bone pathologies (Ortner and Putschar 1981, Aufderheide and Rodriguez-Martin 1998) should alert the anthropologist to the possibility of weakened bone requiring substantially lower than normal forces to produce fracturing.

Chapter 4

DIAGNOSTIC CRITERIA FOR THE DETERMINATION OF TIMING AND FRACTURE MECHANISM

ALISON GALLOWAY, LAUREN ZEPHRO, AND VICKI L. WEDEL

This chapter reviews anthropological studies that investigate how to distinguish when a fracture or break occurred in a bone and how to identify blunt force trauma from other similar patterns of fracture. The first section presents methods for the determination of bone condition, (ante-, peri-, or postmortem) at the time of fracture or breakage. The second section presents on research and criteria for determining the fracture causation and trauma type.

DIFFERENTIATING ANTEMORTEM FROM PERIMORTEM BONE FRACTURE

Antemortem trauma is defined as trauma that occurs prior to death (Sauer 1998). With regard to skeletal analysis, antemortem trauma cannot be recognized unless visible evidence of healing is observable on the bone. The process of healing is highly variable and depends on the age and health of the individual, the location of injury, and the severity of the injury (Galloway 1999, Claes 2012).

In the living body, healing will begin immediately after injury when blood flows into the injured area from disrupted blood vessels (Doblare *et al.* 2004, Hall 2006, Claes 2012). In cortical bone, the blood supply is more limited than in marrow or periosteum. Cortical bone is, therefore, more susceptible to necrosis (Rogers 1992). Granulation tissue formation follows at the fracture site, attracting osteoclasts, the immune system-derived cells that will dissolve bone tissue. Following the invasion and activity of the immune-system cells, the cell population shifts to include fibroblasts, chondrocytes, and osteoblasts.

These cells work to form a callus that begins to mineralize within about a week after callus initiation. The duration of active callus formation is highly variable and may progress over weeks to months. The callus consists of woven bone that follows the invasion of new blood vessels into the area. Over the course of the next few years, the callus will gradually remodel to approximate the original shape of the bone, although the healed area remains visible in adults. In younger individuals, active modeling of bone can occur, eventually obliterating much of the evidence of a previous fracture.

Trabecular bone healing is less commonly associated with noticeable callus formation (Jarry and Uhthoft 1971, Claes 2011). Trabecular fractures are usually compressive in nature and, while the sequence of inflammation, repair, and remodeling parallel those in cortical bone, the stabilization consists of an increase in the number of new trabeculae across the fracture line.

Callus formation will vary by the location and severity of the injury (Rogers 1992, Claes 2012). Because there is greater blood supply metaphyseally, bone formation is often more rapid. Callus formation is exaggerated when there is greater fragmentation of the bone or when the fragments are displaced. Where the blood supply is limited or where infection becomes an issue, healing can be problematic. If bone fragments are missing or where displacement is pronounced, callus formation is slowed. Sequestration of dead bone tissue must be integrated into the healing process. Where there is movement between fragments, the callus may form with a larger proportion of cartilage than mineralized areas. In some such individuals, callus formation fails to reunite the bone segments and healing does not progress well. Instead the portions of the still-viable bones will heal independent of each other to form a *pseudarthrosis* or false joint.

Surgical intervention will affect the healing process (Rogers 1992, Claes 2012). External fixation will immobilize the various fragments of fractured bone and accelerate the callus formation. However, internal fixation may actually hinder or eliminate much of the callus formation where the device itself forms the callus. Moderate forms of inter-fragmentary movement are a positive stimulus for new blood vessel development and callus formation, and elimination of this factor inhibits healing. However, primary cortical bone requires a lower level of inter-fragmentary movement to facilitate healing (Perren 2002).

For the forensic anthropologist examining dried bone, the identification of a bony callus is relatively simple. More problematic is the identification of the very early signs of healing. In a study of cranial trauma in the remains of Civil War soldiers, Barbian and Sledzick (2008) measured the indicators of healing that formed between the time of injury to the death of the individual, at which point the cranial samples were collected. They report significant temporal variation in observable osteoblastic and osteoclastic responses, with healing observable in as quickly as five days with others taking longer. All specimens showed a visible healing response within six weeks following bony injury. The first indicator to appear is usually osteoclastic activity, marked by pitting of the cortical surface and possible exposure of underlying bone structure. Osteoblastic activity follows with the formation of new bone and is part of the periosteal response process. Small areas of new bone that do not show strong integration with the underlying cortex are common. Histologically, there will be spicules of new bone within the soft tissue callus (Ashurst 1992). Both Barbian and Sledzik (2008) and an earlier study by Murphy *et al.* (1990) noted a line of demarcation, often found adjacent to the fracture area. This line may represent the beginning of necrosis of the periosteal membrane and/or the underlying bone. Finally, there may be areas of sequestration where necrotic bone is being resorbed. This process may be marked by a color difference but was not found in all fractures in the study.

In some cases, the forensic anthropologist may be working from radiographic or CT images. Repair is seen on radiographs as a blurring of the bone margins (Rogers 1992), but this may take many days to become apparent. The callus formation will be accompanied by an apparent widening of the gap between the bone fragments. CT scans will show the formation of a hematoma if soft tissue is still present as well as the gradual callus formation (Burke 2012).

If a visible healing response is observed, the bony injury is categorized as antemortem. In most cases, the presence of antemortem fractures are helpful in identification but of less forensic interest with regards to the circumstances of death. In some cases, however, a pattern of abuse is seen with repeated injuries, especially when there are different stages of healing, indicative of different episodes of physical violence. In these cases, healed injuries are critical in the development of criminal charges.

DIFFERENTIATING PERIMORTEM
AND POSTMORTEM BONE FRACTURE

In forensic anthropological analysis, if there is no indication of healing on the bone then the defect is either a perimortem fracture or postmortem breakage. Perimortem trauma is associated with the manner of death (Sauer 1998) although, as noted earlier, this determination lies outside the authority of the forensic anthropologist. More recent discussions of perimortem trauma, however, have expanded the narrow temporal definition to reflect the constraints of interpreting trauma solely from the skeleton. Galloway and Zephro (2004) provide criteria for evaluating perimortem skeletal trauma. They also assert that perimortem fractures encompass the time span prior to the visible signs of healing through the period following death until the bone loses significant moisture, which will change its material properties and, as a result, the appearance of fracture. This time span is therefore variable, dependent on the pace of the healing process, the postmortem depositional environment and bone decomposition, which is affected by bone dehydration and degradation. This distinction is critical because it is imperative that the forensic anthropologist explain to the coroner/medical examiner, legal counsel, and members of the jury that the perimortem period may extend well after the person ceased breathing.

Criteria used by anthropologists to differentiate perimortem bone trauma from postmortem breakage include staining /color of fracture surfaces, anatomical location of injury, fracture pattern morphology, angle of fracture margins, and context dependent damage or clues, such as carnivore modification, excavation damage, weathering, analysis of clothing or skin for bullet holes, *et cetera.* Because determinations of perimortem fracture versus postmortem breakage are inextricably linked to forensic trauma analysis, the discussion of perimortem trauma in a forensic report must detail how and why the designation was made.

Staining of fracture surfaces can be an important clue as to the timing of bone fracture. Bone surfaces that have been buried or come in contact with mineral-rich soil become stained (Sauer 1998). Similarly, through the process of decomposition, exposed bone will become discolored as a result of the release of body fluids (Galloway *et al.* 1999). Other sources of coloration include vegetation, corrosion from metals, dyes from fabric, and other factors. As a result, the fracture surfaces of newly postmortem fractured bone will differ in color compared to the rest of the exposed bone surface. Fracture surfaces stained as the rest of the bone surface are assumed to be contemporaneous with the actual time of death, although this is problematic. Ubelaker and Adams (1995) describe their analysis of a construction site that contained long bones with butterfly fractures, which are typically associated with fresh bone fractures. Taphonomic indicators, however, clearly indicated the fractures were postmortem and, based on direction of force, the bones were disarticulated when fractured. This example highlights the importance of context and the preferential weighting of context over staining in the determination of fracture timing. In reality, using coloration to distinguish fracture timing may be useful to differentiate excavation or post-decomposition damage from older fractures. However, remains with complex taphonomic histories may have had multiple episodes of fracture and deposition, resulting in consistent coloration throughout the bone, which would not indicate injury timing and nature.

Aside from staining, many of the distinctions used to differentiate between perimortem fracture and postmortem breakage entail the features of the fracture patterns themselves. In living or freshly deceased bone, the moisture content is high and the collagen component retains flexibility. Such bone will deform considerably prior to failure (Chapter 3; Lyman 1994). As decomposition progresses, moisture is lost from the bone and the collagen fibers begin to degrade, making the bone less flexible. Bone begins to respond to loading in a manner similar to a purely inorganic block of material and fails at smaller loading forces (Davis 1985). When a force is applied to dry bone, less energy is required to fracture the material, and when it breaks, it does not exhibit deformation as the dry bone does not have an extended region of plastic deformation before failure when measured on a stress–strain curve. As Maples (1986) noted, breaks are less clean and more jagged (Figure 4-1). Fragments are usually smaller and the bone is more likely to shatter. Small pieces of adherent bone, which are common in perimortem fractures, are less frequent in postmortem breakage. Similarly, concentric fractures and radiating fractures are less often found. According to Galloway and colleagues (1999), postmortem bone fracture surfaces may exhibit more crumbling and compressing defects than fresh bone.

Because the changes that distinguish postmortem breakage partly depend on the loss of moisture from the bone, the circumstances of the disposal of remains play a role in the termination of the "perimortem" period. Bodies that are frozen after death will experience a delay in full loss of moisture. Mass graves often accumulate body fluids and moisture for years such that bodies in the lower levels are still fully fleshed while those on the top may be skeletonized. Bodies buried below the water table or those wrapped in plastic will also see delays in moisture loss. However, in waterlogged areas, the bones may become more malleable as the minerals are leached out of the bone tissue.

The majority of anthropological research on the timing of bone fracture stems from zooarchaeology and archaeology, where the goal is to identify bone that was modified by humans versus non-human agents (Johnson 1985, Bonnichsen 1979). Archaeological studies often focus on one type of fracture, percussion fracture, produced when the bone surface is hit directly with a hammerstone or other instrument in order to expose the marrow cavity and extract these nutrients. As Johnson (1985) notes, fresh bone fracture involving this type of dynamic loading typically exhibits a loading point when a hammer stone directly impacts the bone, whereas dry bone does not. While fresh bone is broken to expose the inner contents, dry bone is more likely broken accidentally by trampling. In forensic anthropology, the fracture mechanisms are much more varied (such as bats, bricks, candlesticks, car accidents, stomping, falls, etc.) than the direct hammer stone to bone surface contact scenario seen archaeologically and may involve indirect forces due to bending or twisting of bones. In addition, overlying soft tissue dissipates much of the impact that produces a percussion fracture.

Zooarchaeological studies also suggest that fresh and dry breakage differ with regards to fracture surface and texture. The surface of fractured fresh bone

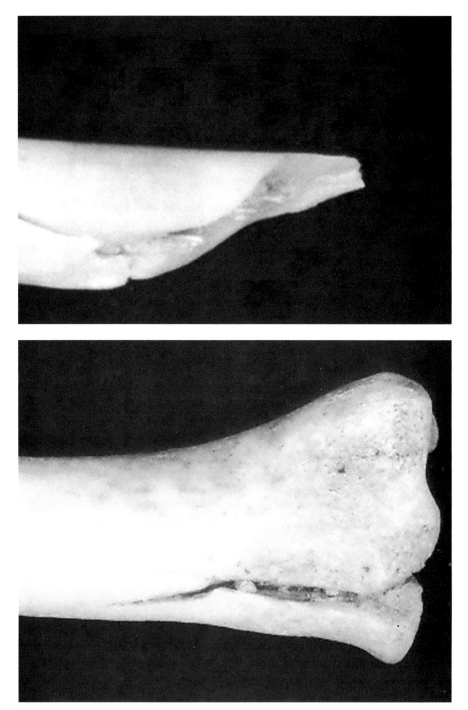

Figure 4-1. Fractures in green and dry Bone. Fractures in green or fresh bone (*top*) are clean while those in dry bone (*bottom*) tend to have jagged torn edges.

is reported as smooth and fracture angles are obtuse or acute. In contrast, dry bone is reported to break at right angles and it has a rough texture (Bonnichsen 1979, Johnson 1985).

Archaeological studies on human bone have also examined the distinction between perimortem fractures and postmortem breakage in order to investigate the possibility of cannibalism. Villa and Mahieu (1991) compared three assemblages of human bone fractured by unique and different agents: (1) breakage from sediment pressure, (2) fractures associated with human cannibalism, and (3) known postmortem excavation damage. Comparing fracture angle, fracture outline, fracture edge (texture of fracture surface), shaft circumference, shaft fragmentation, and shaft length, amongst the bone assemblage sites, Villa and Mahieu (1991) found that the criteria used had statistical significance differentiating bones fractured by sediment pressure from those fractured by hammer stone percussion (fresh) but were not diagnostic at the individual specimen level. Individual pieces broken by hammer stone percussion were only identifiable on an individual level if the bone had visible evidence of impact notches. Fracture edge was characterized as referring to fracture surface texture, which the authors categorized as smooth or jagged. Villa and Mahieu (1991) did not distinguish between longitudinal, transverse, and oblique fracture surfaces, which given the anisotropic structure of bone, may be a complicating factor for assessments of surface texture.

Other studies of alleged human cannibalism have focused on other types of indicators. White (1992) examines evidence of skinning, dismemberment of body segments into manageable components, roasting damage, polish from cooking and stirring bones in a pot, and marrow extraction. Similarly Turner and Turner (1999) use these criteria in evaluating the composite evidence of cannibalism in the American Southwest. In general, these studies show that human remains are treated in much the same way as other large animals when butchered by those who are used to hunting large game. While there may be occasions when these criteria become important in a forensic case, they would be exceptionally rare.

Turning to studies specifically designed for forensic applications, Wieberg and Wescott (2008) examined the changing moisture content of pig long bones over a 140-day period. They correlated changes in moisture content with characteristics of experimental bone fractures produced by a weighted drop tower. They noted that bone moisture rapidly declines for the first two months postmortem and then continues to decline at a slower rate. Although ash weight, fracture surface appearance, and fracture angle all demonstrated a significant positive correlation, the authors note that the correlations were low and there was much overlap in fracture characteristics throughout the study time period. Similarly, Wheatly (2008) conducted a study using deer femora to investigate fracture patterns of fresh (days) versus dry bone (up to 1 year postmortem). Like Wieberg and Wescott (2008), he found that perimortem bone fracture characteristics extend well into the postmortem interval and that determinations about the timing of fracture must be made in combination with other indicators. Wheatly (2008) and Wieberg and Wescott (2008) conclude that fracture surfaces were smoother on fresh fractures and had a "rougher" texture on the fracture surface of bone broken when dry. Like Villa and Mahieu (1991), neither study distinguished texture according to the orientation of the fracture.

Zephro (2012) examined fracture characteristics separately using fresh, frozen, and dry bovine bone samples that had either been fractured by blunt force or projectile impact. Instead of assessing texture directly from the fracture surface, high resolution casts were made, isolating the texture assessment from other indicators of bone condition. Angle measurements were standardized relative to impact sites. Zephro (2012) did not find a statistically significant relationship between fracture angle, cortical bone thickness, type of trauma, or bone condition. The only statistically significant relationship observed was between fracture angle from the impact side of blunt force trauma specimens and bone condition. Fracture surface characteristics did diverge among bone conditions but not for trauma type. However, Zephro (2012) concluded that, for a single specimen, fracture angle and fracture surface characteristics have very limited value in the assessment of bone condition or trauma type. Other observations, such as impact sites and projectile entries and exits, in combination with taphonomic indicators like color, staining, and context should be relied upon to describe and determine trauma type and bone condition.

Postmortem breakage is often the result of carnivore scavenging, and rodent gnawing produces characteristic patterns of damage. Carnivore damage is typically seen as crushing of bone with puncture marks left by the canine teeth (Haglund 1997a). Rodent incisors produce parallel striae on the bones (Haglund 1997b), often on protrusions or margins of bones. These striations may not be present on some bones, especially when the cortex is thin and the bone crumbles under the pressure from the gnawing.

Postmortem fracturing can also be produced by thermal changes, particularly fire (Rhine 1998, Schmidt and Symes 2008, Pope and O'Brian 2004). Fire will often produce fractures of the long bones when the muscles contract because of the heat and the bone tissue is exposed and burns. The outer surface of the skull will exfoliate and fractures may appear in the vault, often caused by falling debris within the fire scene. Because fire consumes the organic components of bone, the remains are more brittle and are easily broken during the post-fire period, especially during the fire containment and discovery periods. Distinguishing pre- and post-fire fractures requires assessment of the location of the damage relative to burning, amount and pattern of charring, and the orientation of the fractured ends to one another. As Pope

(2012) notes, fractures that occur in unburned bone are not associated with fire damage. Post-fire fractures expose the layers of thermal changes within the bone while the surfaces of pre-existing fracture show more even charring. Because of muscle contracture during the fire, pre-existing fractures will allow limbs to "scissor" or significantly displace around the fracture, while limb orientations are more normal when the breaks have occurred after the fire.

In many cases, the mode of discovery also plays a role in production of postmortem breakage. Backhoes used to "explore" or actually excavate buried remains can cause massive fragmentation as well as co-mingling of skeletal material. Similarly, farming activity, such as plowing, can produce extensive damage. In these cases, the distinction between perimortem trauma and postmortem breakage will require extensive and detailed examination of the remains (Ubelaker and Adams 1995).

In practice, the criteria used for determining perimortem fracture from postmortem breakage in forensic anthropology are somewhat ambiguous, and the correct assessment of timing is challenging. Wieberg and Wescott (2008) asked 22 forensic anthropologists to assess 10 fractured specimens their study assessed, to distinguish whether the bones were fractured peri- or postmortem. Correct assessment of the timing of bone fracture ranged from three to 10 specimens, with an average score of 6.8. The study noted that those participants that used fracture surface morphology (smooth, intermediate, jagged) had the highest number of correctly assigned bones. However, as other studies suggest that there is not a reliable set of criteria for judging surface morphology. Anthropologists must rely on the whole suite of available indicators to make this determination.

DIFFERENTIATING BLUNT FORCE FROM HIGH-VELOCITY PROJECTILE TRAUMA

Fracture patterns that differentiate blunt force from high-velocity projectile trauma, commonly referred to as gunshot trauma, are referenced in forensic skeletal analyses. The use of these observations arises when fragmented bones, especially the cranium, are brought for analysis. Reconstruction of the cranial vault or other bones is often required prior to analysis. Fracture surfaces must, of course, be assessed prior to application of adhesives.

High-velocity projectile trauma occurs when a small, hard projectile that travels at a very high rate of speed penetrates the bone. This object punches a hole in the bone surface it strikes, producing a spall from the cone of percussion at the impact point. Often the projectile is deformed by this impact, creating a wider profile for any further impacts. These high-velocity projectiles produce a massive release of energy within the body, with that energy moving from the inside outward. The temporary cavity within the structure expands within the substance of the body, pushing skeletal elements outward with beveling on the outward side of the bone (Figure 4-2).

High-velocity projectile fragmentation of the skull is often readily determinable upon reconstruction due to the presence of "bullet holes" along the path of the projectile. Entrance defects are characterized by internally beveling, while exit defects are externally beveled. Radiating and concentric heaving fractures are often noted.

In contrast, blunt force trauma may be inflicted under a variety of circumstances and by a wide variety of objects, including the human body (kicks, punches). In further contrast to projectile trauma, blunt force trauma produces forces that travel from the outside inwards. Depressed fractures are more likely to be associated with blunt force trauma, however, bullets can also create depressed fractures, particularly when they have lost a significant amount of energy before striking bone or if they strike the bone's surface tangentially.

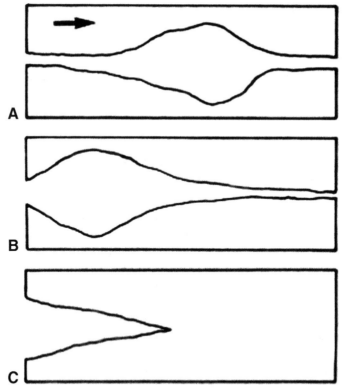

Figure 4-2. Schematic appearance of temporary cavities (cavitation) in gelatin blocks due to (A) full, metal-jacketed rifle bullet, (B) hunting rifle bullet, and (C) shotgun. Arrow indicates direction of bullet travel. After DiMiao (1989).

Using a modern forensic sample of crania for which the type of trauma was known, Hart (2005) tested the hypothesis that blunt force and projectile trauma could be differentiated on the basis of the direction of beveling in concentric fractures. Blunt force trauma is associated with internal beveling on the concentric fractures while high-velocity projectile trauma is associated with external beveling. This pattern makes logical sense as the vault is pushed inward by the impact in blunt force trauma but expanded outward by the cavitation formed following high-velocity projectile impact. While her results supported the hypothesis, her study was limited to the cranial vault and may not be directly applicable to other regions. Other criteria used to identify blunt force trauma include the knapping of fracture surfaces, which is the chipping of fracture margins caused by conjoining fractures rubbing against each other as a result of subsequent blows (Klepinger 2006).

As the material properties of fresh bone vary with the rate of applied force, so, too, does the general morphology of the resulting fractures, a phenomenon that is illustrated by the appearance of conjoining fractures (Harkess *et al.* 1991). As described above, as the speed of the applied force increases, such as in the case of high-velocity projectile impacts, bone's ability to absorb energy increases. When the bone fails, however, it reacts as a brittle material and the resulting fracture damage is catastrophic. In this scenario, the conjoining fractures fit together cleanly, and there is little to no plastic deformation of the bone fragments. Alternatively, with a slowly applied force, bone reacts as a viscoelastic material and, prior to failure, will deform in shape to accommodate the stress. Under this scenario, bone can be compared to a rubber band: when you slowly stretch a rubber band, there is a point at which the stress is removed, the rubber band will no longer return to its original shape. The range under which the bone can be strained but still return to its original shape is the region of "elastic strain." When the applied stress exceeds the region of elastic strain, permanent deformation of the rubber band results, known as "plastic strain" (Harkess *et al.* 1991).

With regard to bone fracture interpretation, bone fractures that exhibit plastic deformation are typically associated with blunt force trauma, while more catastrophic fracturing combined with cleanly fitting conjoining fractures is attributed to high velocity projectile trauma (Berryman and Symes 1998). Characteristics used for differentiation are summarized in Table 4-1.

Similar to the assessment of fracture timing, actual determination of blunt trauma versus ballistic trauma can be complicated, as objects differ in size and amount of applied force, calibers range in size and velocity, and intermediate targets can change the properties of a bullet (direction of travel and fragmentation). The most problematic issue is the incomplete recovery of involved skeletal material. In forensic anthropological casework, some cases involve whole skeletons but many involve only fragments. When the bones are

| | TABLE 4-1 |
| PUBLISHED CRITERIA AND THEIR USE IN DISTINGUISHING BLUNT FORCE AND BALLISTIC TRAUMA |

Type of Trauma	*Blunt Force*	*Ballistic*
Depressed FX	Yes	No
Plastic Deformation	Yes	No
Knapping	Yes	No
External/ internal beveling	No	Yes
Presence of metals	No	Yes
Fragmentation	Low	High

Criteria selected from Berryman and Symes (1998), Galloway (1999), Klepinger (2006).

fragmented by perimortem fracturing, taphonomic processes often disperse these fragments. Recovery is often more difficult and critical portions of the remains may be forever lost.

Chapter 5

CLASSIFICATION OF FRACTURES

Alison Galloway, Lauren Zephro, and Vicki L. Wedel

Fractures are initially classified based on the degree and pattern of breakage. Medical literature also takes into account the soft tissue damage, particularly as it relates to blood supply, and the best management of the damage to promote the optimal healing. The terminology used by the anthropologist is associated with the degree and pattern of fracture. These terms should be used in the forensic descriptions of fractures, whenever possible, because they provide a universally understood description. Specific fracture classifications differ by bone and are discussed in detail in Chapters 8 through 11. This chapter lays out the basics terms in describing a fracture depending on the completeness of the break and whether the fracture is due to direct or indirect forces.

INCOMPLETE FRACTURES

Incomplete fractures are characterized by retention of some continuity between the portions of the fractured bone (Figure 5-1). These are more common in children than adults (Rogers 1992) due to the higher organic nature of younger bones. They also occur when the impact force is low or the area of impact is sufficiently wide that the force is dissipated. Incomplete fractures are also indicative of high moisture content and decrease in frequency in the postmortem period.

Bone Bruises, Bone Contusions or Occult Intraosseous Fractures

Although generally of little forensic importance, the possibility of bone bruises should be noted, especially in examination of radiographic and

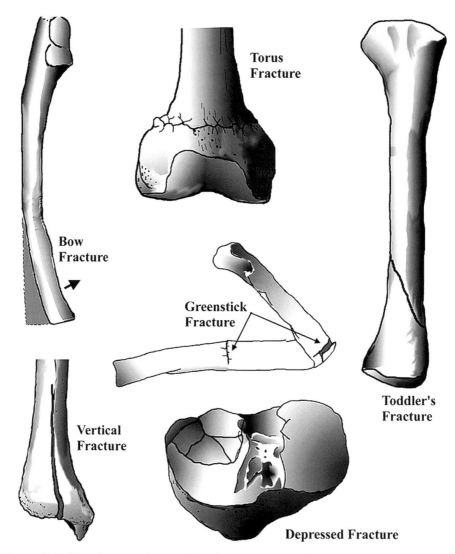

Figure 5-1. Classification of incomplete fractures. Incomplete fractures affect a variety of different bones. This group includes a number of fractures, which occur primarily in younger individuals such as the bow and toddler's fractures. Torus and greenstick fractures are also more common in youth. Vertical and depressed fractures may occur more in older individuals.

magnetic resonance images (MRI) of the bones (Rogers 1992, Mandalia and Henson 2008). A bone bruise is an area of extensive trabecular bone micro-fracturing that results from compression or impaction, accompanied by bleeding and edema. These defects have been classified based on the cortical involvement (Lynch 1989) or on the shape characteristics (Vellet *et al.* 1991).

Bow Fractures or Plastic Deformation

An incomplete fracture commonly found in juvenile material is the bow fracture (Rogers 1992). Here, the bone appears to have an exaggerated curvature, which often encompasses the entire length of the bone. Biomechanically these fractures can be explained as occurring between the yield point at the termination of elastic deformation and prior to the failure point. Bow fractures can occur during longitudinal compression (Chamay and Tschantz 1972) and bending (Mabrey and Fitch 1989). Histologically, they are seen as a series of oblique microfractures induced under both compression and tension (Jones 1994). While such fractures can occur in any of the long, tubular bones, they are most common in the forearm.

Toddler's Fractures

Rarely seen in forensic settings, this fracture occurs in infants and toddlers who suddenly demonstrate a severe limp, possibly without any clear history of specific injury or only relatively mild trauma (Rogers 1992, Tenenbein *et al.* 1990, John *et al.* 1997). Such fractures are usually non-displaced, hairline, oblique or spiral fractures that may not even be visible radiographically until healing is well established. The distal tibia is most often affected, but the term has been applied to other lower limb injuries.

These fractures of the lower limb seem to occur during the normal activity of young children but, in the medicolegal situation, must be distinguished from those seen with child abuse. These fractures only rarely result in epiphyseal separation and are usually solitary, unlike the multiple fractures more commonly associated with abuse.

Torus or Buckling Fractures

A torus fracture is a buckling of the bone cortex produced by compressive forces. It appears as a rounded expansion of the bone where the cortical bone has been outwardly displaced around the circumference of the bony element (Rogers 1992). In almost all cases, these appear in the ends of long bones, usually at the junction of the metaphysis and diaphysis (Jones 1994). These fractures are usually confined to children since their bones have a significantly higher collagen to mineral ratio (Hart *et al.* 2006). There is some difference in classification in that some authors propose that this term be used only when there is bending producing a unilateral buckle (Solan *et al.* 2002) while others contend that it can occur bilaterally (Harvey *et al.* 2006). In some cases, they may be combined with incomplete transverse fracture of one cortex while the opposite cortex has undergone compressive buckling. In these cases, this type of fracture is often referred to as a "lead pipe" fracture (Rogers 1992).

Greenstick Fractures

The classic greenstick fracture results from bending or angulation forces placing one side of the bone in tension while the other is in compression (Rogers 1992). The result is an incomplete, transverse fracture, beginning on the tensile side, which usually extends to about the midline of the bone. At that point, the fracture deviates at right angles, creating a vertical or longitudinal split in either or both the proximal or distal portions of the bone. The remaining unfractured portion of the bone remains bent or bowed. This type of fracture is more frequently seen on ribs or in the bones of children.

Vertical Fractures

Vertical fractures, while relatively rare, may occur in long bones and run along the long axis. These are generated by compressive forces or, in smaller bones, by direct blows (Rogers 1992). As the cortical bone approaches areas consisting of more trabecular bone, then the linear nature may deteriorate into a number of branches.

Depressed Fractures

Depressed fractures occur primarily in the skull and result from direct blows that cause "caving-in" of the bone's cortex. They may also occur on the metaphyseal areas of long bones where trabecular collapse results in the depression. In the skull, the scale of the injury depends, in part, upon the size of the impacted area and the velocity of the force (Gurdjian 1975). On the cranial vault, where such fractures are more common, this injury will may involve only the outer table with the inner table remaining intact. In other cases, the outer table is broken and crushed with incomplete fractures occurring in the inner table.

As the size of the impact area decreases and the velocity increases, the resulting fracture approaches that of a penetrating injury, and inner damage may exceed that of the bone surface being impacted (McElhaney *et al.* 1976). When the impact is highly localized and is accompanied by considerable power, penetration can be complete. Fracturing is due, in part, to the rapid accumulation of compressive forces and subsequent collapse of any underlying trabecular or porous bone.

The term "depressed fracture" is also used in describing fractures of the tibial plateau. In these fractures, the trabecular bone in the inner portion of the proximal tibia is unable to withstand loading forces. It and the outer cortical bone are pushed inward.

COMPLETE FRACTURES

A complete fracture is one that results in discontinuity between two or more fragments. Radiographically, this type of fracture can be distinguished by determining whether one or both cortices are involved in the fracture line (Rogers 1992). Clinically these fractures are divided according to the extent of soft tissue involvement.

Closed or simple fractures are characterized by no disruption of the overlying skin at the fracture site (Harkess et al. 1991, Rogers 1992). Clinically, there is less likelihood of infection. In some cases, however, there will be additional injuries in the area not produced by the actual fracturing process. Open or compound fracture involves injuries to the skeletal element in which the overlying skin is also disrupted. This provides external organisms and contaminants with access to the injury site (Rogers 1992). The bones most often involved with open fractures are the tibia (46%), followed by the femur (12.5%) and then the radius and ulna (11%) (Gustilo et al. 1969).

In addition, complete fractures can be divided based upon the shape and location of the fracture line. Skeletonized material is usually described by this system (Figure 5-2). The direction of the fracture is typically determined by the longest axis of the bone (Rogers 1992). The length bone is then divided into thirds and the fracture location designated as belonging to the proximal, middle or distal portions.

Transverse Fractures

Transverse fractures run at approximately right angles to the long axis of the long bone (Rogers 1992). They may be propagated in three-point loading such as may occur when blunt force trauma bends a bone. The object imparts a concentrated force producing severe angulation. Bones in these cases are often not under compression from the normal weight-bearing functions since loading along the axis tends to distort the fracture from the transverse pathway.

In these cases, the bone undergoes extreme tension along the convex side while the concave side is under compression (Gonza 1982, Hipp *et al.* 1992, Rogers 1992). Since bone is more resistant to compression than tension, the convex side is the first to yield producing a crack. As the outer layers of bone yield, the adjacent layers bear the brunt of the maximum stress and quickly fail. This process occurs at right angles to the long axis of the bone. This failure decreases the cross-sectional area, magnifying the forces acting on the remaining segments of bone. As the fracture crosses the bone it crosses the "neutral axis," the point where there should be a transition from the tensile to compressive loading. However, since the side of the bone bearing the tensile forces has

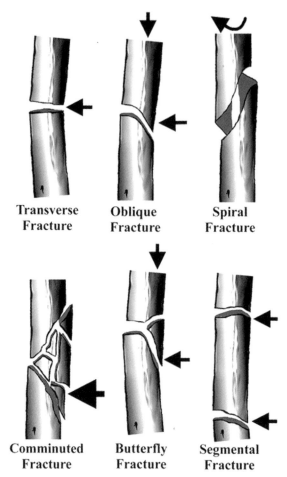

Figure 5-2. Classification of complete fractures. Complete fractures are classified based on the morphology of the fracture. Arrows indicate the direction of the applied force. Compression is a common feature in oblique and butterfly fractures, while torsion is involved in spiral fractures.

failed, the neutral axis has correspondingly moved toward the compressive side. The initial break then quickly spreads across the bone.

Oblique Fractures

Oblique fractures run diagonally across the diaphysis, usually at about a 45-degree angle (Rogers 1992). They usually result from the combination of angulation and compressive forces of moderate force. When this happens, there are several ways in which the fracture can be propagated (Gonza 1982): (1) If the compressive forces are large relative to the bending forces, the bone fails in compression producing a purely oblique fracture; (2) if the bending forces are relatively large then the failure may resemble a transverse fracture; or (3) the more common situation is an oblique transverse fracture that is initiated as a transverse fracture, but, following the initial break, the tensile and compressive forces are magnified on the remaining bone. This process results in shearing as compression forces the remaining bone downward. The result is a bone in which the initial fracture is perpendicular to the long axis while the latter portion is oblique. The magnitude of the tension and compression determine the proportion of transverse to oblique components in the fracture. The impact of the bending load can be determined by the position of the oblique fracture to which it should be adjacent. Oblique fractures can also be produced by a combination of angulation and rotation in the forearm and leg. In these areas, the paired bones act in a manner similar to spiral fractures resulting in oblique fractures in each bone, although at different levels.

Spiral Fractures

Spiral fractures begin as small defects, then the cracks follow the peak of the tensile loading around the bone. In rotational forces, the tensile stresses are oriented at a 40–45-degree angle to the long axis of the shaft and are greatest at the surface and at zero along the axis (Gonza 1982, Rogers 1992). Compressive stresses are greatest at 180 degrees to the tensile stresses and are similarly greatest on the bone surface and zero along the axis. The fracture begins at the point of maximal tension and follows the angle of rotation, approximately 45 degrees until the two ends are approximately above one another. At that time, a longitudinal crack appears and unites the ends. Spiral fractures circle the shaft and include a vertical step. Caused by rotational forces on the bone, these fractures tend to be the result of low-velocity forces. The direction of the spiral indicates the direction of the torsional forces (Gonza 1982) and can be used to reconstruct the events that produced the fracture. Interestingly, a study by Porta and colleagues (1999) suggests a different morphology for spiral fractures depending on the portion of the shaft that is fractured. Under experimentally-produced pure torsion, spiral fractures in the epiphysis has alterations in the helical and longitudinal fracture components. The resulting pattern approximates an oblique fracture, whereas all shaft fractures are true spirals.

Comminuted Fractures

A comminuted fracture is one in which more than two fragments are generated. These can be roughly classed as "slightly," "moderately," or "markedly" comminuted depending upon the severity of the fragmentation (Rogers 1992).

Those in which both the number of fragments and the size are large are more severely fractured. These fractures usually result from relatively high levels of force (Gonza 1982).

In long bones, many comminuted fractures may be classified as consisting of the two segments of bone and a small "butterfly fragment," which is an elongated triangular fragment formed on the concave side of an angulation fracture (Gonza 1982, Carter 1985, Hipp *et al.* 1992, Rogers 1992). This fragmentation results from the combination of oblique transverse fractures produced when angulation occurs in the presence of compression. The protuberance left by the oblique fracture is leveraged against the remaining shaft of bone and a second oblique fracture results. The resulting triangular portion is sheared off the bone. The apex of the triangle indicates the portion of the bone failing in tension and the direction of force (Porta 2005). Previously, the presence of oblique fractures on long bones was attributed to some degree of bending and torsion. According to a study conducted by Porta and associates (1999), oblique fractures were seen as a result of pure bending forces being applied to long bones. Wedge fractures (as described above) and transverse fractures were also observed. Such fractures are most common in the lower extremity, which is often weight bearing at the time of impact by an extraneous object. They are commonly seen in the legs of pedestrians hit by motor vehicles. Butterfly fragments are not common in pediatric victims who, being shorter, are usually pulled under the car and whose bones are more resilient. When they do occur, they are usually limited to the more heavily mineralized areas such as the midshaft of the femur, tibia, or ulna (Jones 1994).

When multiple fractures leave diaphyseal portions separated from the proximal or the distal ends, the intervening segment is called a segmental fracture. This defect may result from multiple simultaneous fractures such as would occur when a bone is hit at two points or by a large surface.

Epiphyseal Fractures

Two categories of epiphyses exist in the long bones: (1) pressure epiphyses, which form the articular ends of bones and (2) traction epiphyses, the origin and insertion sites for major muscles or muscle groups (Salter and Harris 1963). Both are identified by the presence of a cartilagenous growth plate interspersed between the diaphysis and the epiphysis. Both are subject to injury.

The growth plates themselves are substantially weaker than either the surrounding bone or the ligaments and often rupture prior to loss of integrity in these adjacent structures (Wilber and Thompson 1994). Epiphyseal injuries may be limited to the cartilagenous growth plate but may also involve avulsion of adjacent bony structures or crushing of the epiphysis. The growth plate consists of four interdigitating regions. The first two, attached to the epiphysis, are strong, consisting of the resting and proliferating cells. The next region, that of the hypertrophying cells, is much weaker. The final region includes substantial regions of calcification, which provide strength. Fractures, therefore, occur preferentially through the third region (Salter and Harris 1963) or the third and fourth zones of the physes. These are the regions where chondrocytes are undergoing massive hypertrophy and then are gradually becoming necrotic and being replaced by the osseous incursions (Canale 1992).

In children, fractures through the bone are more common than through the epiphysis, even though the latter is structurally weaker (Salter and Harris 1963). The plate is susceptible to only a limited range of forces, specifically avulsive and shearing forces, while the bone is vulnerable to the greater range of loading. Damage to the plate is most often seen at the distal radius, followed by the distal ulna and humerus, radial head, distal tibia and femur, proximal humerus, femur and phalanges. For a variety of reasons, the more distal portions of the bone are more prone to such injuries than the proximal ends (Canale 1992).

Injuries are more common during the periods of rapid growth, particularly in the first year of life and during the adolescent growth spurt. Clinically, these injuries are particularly disturbing as they are frequently associated with disruption of the growth plate (Canale 1992). Blood supply to the areas of the stem cells is essential for maintenance of the growth plate, so destruction of the circulation is important in the genesis of these problems to these areas. Epiphyseal fractures that interrupt the growth plate can terminate growth at this location completely or result in partial loss of growth. The latter condition will, over time, result in angulation of the limb.

The cleavage normally passes through the plate and into the metaphyseal bone, leaving a triangular fragment of the metaphysis attached to the epiphysis. Although these fractures are not easily recognizable in the forensic skeletal record, diaphyseal ends and the epiphyses should be closely examined for signs of avulsion. Since vascular compromise often accompanies these injuries, distortions of the epiphyses due to necrosis may be indicators of prior episodes of violence. These are usually classified by the Salter-Harris system in which four of the five categories involve some osseous damage (Salter and Harris 1963) (Figure 5-3). Type I involves complete separation of the plate without associated fracture of bone and results from shearing or avulsive forces. This type afflicts very young children and is probably not recognizable in the skeletal record. Type II, the most common form, involves a separation that extends through part of the epiphyseal plate and into the bony metaphysis. This form is usually found in children over 10 years of age and results from shearing or avulsive forces. Type III consists of an intra-articular fracture from the joint surface to the weak zone of the plate and is produced by shearing forces. Type IV is also an intra-articular fracture from the joint surface

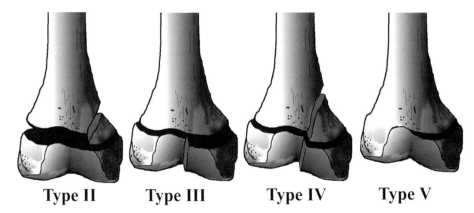

Type II   Type III   Type IV   Type V

Figure 5-3. Salter-Harris classification of epiphyseal fractures. Of the five types of epi-physeal fractures, four will show some form of skeletal damage. Type I involves separation along the cartilageneous growth plate. Type II includes metaphyseal portions, while Types III and IV fracture the articular surface. In Type V, fracture terminates the growth of a portion of the plate.

through the plate but extends beyond the growth plate into the metaphysis. The final type, Type V, involves crushing of the plate due to compression on the epiphysis.

INTERPRETATION OF DIRECT VERSUS INDIRECT TRAUMA

In addition to the simple classification system that describes the morphology of the fracture, a trauma typology compiles fracture morphology by associated biomechanical processes. This classification begins with a division into those fractures derived from direct and indirect trauma.

Direct Trauma

Direct trauma is induced when an object strikes the non-moving or slowly moving body or when the moving body strikes a stationary or slower moving object. This trauma is localized to the point of impact. Skeletally, direct trauma includes only those fractures caused by impact and not by deformation of the bone secondary to impact. Direct trauma produces a range of injuries from tapping injuries to extensive crush fractures.

Tapping Fractures

Tapping fractures result from a small force of slowing momentum on a rela-tively small area of the body. These are transverse fractures, although some may be more obliquely transmitted. When they occur in the forearm or lower leg, only one, and only the weakest or most exposed bone, is fractured. When they occur in the ulna, they are sometimes known as parrying fractures. These fractures are usually accompanied by relatively little soft tissue damage.

Crush Fractures

Crush fractures occur when a large force is applied over a large area of the body. The degree of damage varies from transverse to severely comminuted fractures. In the forearm or lower leg, both bones are usually broken. These fractures are usually accompanied by extensive soft tissue damage and there is often penetration of the skin, which leads to the possibility of infection. On dry or exposed bone, direct trauma produces an impact or loading point (Lyman 1994). This defect appears as an area of incipient ring cracks or crushed bone, often with a crescent-shaped notch. There may also be a rebound point opposite the impact site from the force bouncing back from the anvil upon which the bone is positioned. In the forensic context, this is less of a concern because in most cases, the bone is still enclosed within soft tissue during the trauma.

Indirect Trauma

Indirect trauma results in fracture beyond the site of immediate impact. These can be induced by tension, rotation, and angulation, and often occur while the bone is under some form of compressive loading. Hyperflexion or hyperextension is also a common forms of indirect injury brought on by deceleration or acceleration of the body.

Linear Fractures

Linear fractures often occur in the skull and result from out-bending of large, thin portions of bone as the result of a direct blow of high velocity. They are the result of indirect trauma but frequently extend to the fractures at the impact site. These are characterized by long fractures that usually seek the weakest region of the bone through which to propagate. The production of these fractures is extremely rapid, often outpacing even the velocity of projectiles fired into bone.

Avulsion Fractures

Avulsion fractures produce small fragments of bone that are detached from the bony prominences by the tension produced by the attached ligaments or tendons (Rogers 1992). Extremely tight bonds occur between the Sharpey's fibers (small, anchoring spicules of muscle at attachment sites) and the muscles or ligaments or tendons with which they attach to bone. These bonds preclude rupture at the insertion point, and the nearest weak link is often the surrounding bone itself. These fractures are characterized by detached pieces of bone adjacent to ligament attachment sites and are more frequent in areas where the cortical bone is relatively thin. These fractures tend to be irregular in cleavage.

Traction/Tension Fractures

Traction/tension fractures are an expansion of avulsion fractures and occur perpendicular to the direction of pull. Traction/tension fractures are most common in the patella, olecranon process of the ulna, and medial malleolus of the tibia. Such pure tension fractures are relatively uncommon.

Angulation Fractures

With angulation fractures, the bone is bent so that one side is under compression while the other is under tensile forces (see Figure 2-2) (Burke 2012). As discussed previously, the tensile side is most susceptible to fracture and this results in a transverse fracture. As this fracture approaches the compression side, the bone fails in a shearing fracture to produce a triangular spur of bone, which may become separated from the bone.

Rotational Fractures

In rotational fractures, the bone is twisted so that there are both horizontal and vertical shear forces produced. These are initially seen as a series of small vertical cracks that widen and then are propagated as a spiral fracture (see Figure 2-4). Since the bone is often under compression simultaneously, the length of the spiral is often shortened.

Compression Fractures

Compression fractures vary depending upon the direction of the force and the morphology of the bone. Compression fractures in long bones are identified as longitudinal or "teacup" fractures. Longitudinal fractures can expand down the entire length of the diaphysis but end in a Y- or T-shaped fracture pattern at the metaphysis. This results from the shaft of the bone being driven into the cancellous and less resistant ends of the bone. Similarly, compression fractures of the vertebrae designate collapse the anterior portions of the vertebral body (Bucholz 1994), while burst fractures involve extensive fragmentation of the centrum as the intervertebral disk is driven downward (Rogers 1992).

SYSTEMS OF CLASSIFICATION

The classification of fracture patterns derives largely from the medical literature where determination of stability of the injury, probable extent of associated soft tissue damage, and the prognosis for recovery are the primary concerns. Medical personnel must determine the fractures by external appearance, palpation, and imaging techniques rather than by direct observation of the completely unfleshed skeletal elements. Emphasis is placed not only on the degree of actual breakage but also upon dislocation, or complete loss of contact between articulating surfaces, and subluxation where there is partial or abnormal contact. In some cases, the degree of articulation is evident for the anthropologist in skeletal material, but this is often greatly distorted by taphonomic processes. In addition, the primary biomedical perspective focuses on the damage of joints rather than skeletal elements. The discussion in the following chapters aims to establish a common set of definitions that allows translation between the medical and anthropological sciences with a focus on the individual bones. Dislocations will be discussed when they are a frequent coincident injury to breakage. The focus will primarily be on fractures in adults or within the ossified regions of the bones in subadults since epiphyseal fractures may not be distinguishable in skeletal material.

The validity of the classification systems must be addressed. Numerous, often contradicting, systems have been devised, in addition to the large number of fractures or fracture complexes that have been named for the person who first described them or is identified with their treatment. In an effort to bring some order to this chaos, uniform systems of classifying fractures have also been formulated. These include the Swiss Association for the Study of the Problems of Internal Fixation (AO/ASIF) for long bone fractures (Müller *et al.* 1991) and the Orthopaedic Trauma Association (OTA) (Gustilo 1990). These systems are designed for application to the major long bones, and the correct assignment should be easily identified and interpretable. For example, the AO/ASIF system provides a code for each long bone, which is then subdivided into segments. The "squares method" of defining the distal and proximal ends is adopted in which a portion equivalent to the maximum width of the bone is designated to the end segments. The first two numbers, therefore, localize each fracture within a segment. Additional numbers are given for severity, fracture type, and severity within type. Diaphyseal fractures are classified as (a) simple fractures, (b) wedge ("butterfly") fractures, and (c) complex fractures.

While these systems potentially allow comparison of results between various centers and could permit studies of the mechanism of injury, serious concerns over their utility have been raised. In a study of interobserver variation using the AO/ASIF system, only 32% of the responses were in complete agreement with the final consensus (Johnstone *et al.* 1993). Although all were able to agree on the bone, 7% were in error on the segment and 28% on the fracture type. Similar results were found within the humerus with a comparison of the AO/ASIF system and an older classificatory system for proximal fractures (Siebenrock and Gerber 1993). In this study, even intraobserver reliability was poor. Even with extensive patient history, examination findings, photographs and radiographs, agreement on open injuries to the tibia only averaged 60% (Brumback and Jones 1994).

For this reason, adoption of a straight medical classificatory system is not encouraged for the forensic anthropologist. Instead, all fractures should be charted, using multiple angles if this provides additional information. Photographs of the fracture should include at least one of the complete bone as well as detailed shots of the fracture. All photos should include a scale. Close-up photos should be oriented as to the correct view. Three-dimensional scans are also a good method of recording the complexity of the fracture. The soft tissue trauma associated with skeletal fracture varies by location and severity of the injury, and any interpretation of the extent of such damage from the skeletal injuries should be left to the expertise of the forensic pathologist.

Different bones respond differently to the various forces imposed upon them, resulting not only in different resistance to fracture but also to very different patterns of fracturing. The bones most resistant to tensile strengths are the radius, fibula, tibia, humerus, and femur (Ko 1953). Compressive forces have the least effect on the femur, tibia, fibula, humerus, radius, and then ulna (Yokoo 1952). Unique features of overall morphology, proportions of trabecular and cortical bone, articulation with other skeletal elements, and attachment of ligaments and tendons also result in different fracture patterns in each bone. For this reason and the fact that forensic cases often consist of isolated elements or incomplete remains, in this volume, each bone will be discussed separately.

SUMMARY

The distinct morphology of fractures can provide significant information upon which to base an interpretation of the forces involved, the direction of the loading, and the effect of bone strength. This requires a basic understanding of how the fracture level is reached in bone and where the primary strengths of bone as a tissue reside. Bones vary in strength with regard to the various forces in different areas. Each bone differs from other bones in the body of each individual. Each individual varies throughout his or her lifetime and differs from other members of the population. Despite these differences, patterns emerge in the ways in which bones fracture that enables the anthropologist to begin to understand the suite of injuries that produced the defects seen skeletally.

Chapter 6

THEORETICAL CONSIDERATIONS IN DESIGNING EXPERIMENTAL TRAUMA STUDIES AND IMPLEMENTING THEIR RESULTS

LAUREN ZEPHRO, ALISON GALLOWAY, AND VICKI L. WEDEL

Determinations of the timing and mechanism of injury in forensic anthropology are largely context-dependent and are based on the location and appearance of trauma, hematomas, presence of exit/entrance defects, fracture patterns, presence of metals, examination of clothing, impression of weapon characteristics on bone, and postmortem animal damage. Some have applied experimental studies to gain data derived under controlled conditions, to better understand the sources of variability in intrinsic traits of traumatized bones. An explicit call for more actualistic research has been made (Sauer 1998, Dirkmaat *et al.* 2008). In the 1970s, a similar call within the fields of paleoanthropology and zooarchaeology was made. Prior to that time, paleo-anthropological and zooarchaeological analyses of perimortem and post-mortem vertebrate remains also relied mainly upon context of the finds, rather than traits intrinsic to bone. Actualistic research, experimental studies of modern analogues for prehistoric materials and their modifications, developed out of the need to clarify the causal agents and processes responsible, thereby advancing knowledge and enhancing contextual analysis. We can learn from these studies as we move to develop experimental data applicable to forensic analysis. Among the issues that warrant discussion with regards to designing trauma research is the following: what type of bone to use, namely whether to use human bone or a non-human analog.

The applicability of non-human bone as a proxy for human bone has not been fully explored, yet non-human bone is commonly used as a proxy for human bone in anthropological fracture studies. Within forensic anthropology, this justification is traced back to Sauer (1998) and Johnson (1985). Interestingly, Sauer's (1998) discussion of non-human bone as an analogue for human bone is limited to a concluding paragraph that calls for continued experiments, which use mammalian bone in trauma and time since death studies. Sauer does not mention a particular species, however, pig bone has been cited as an appropriate analogue for human bone in fracture studies (e.g., Wieberg and Wescott 2008) deriving from Sauer (1998). As an example of a study wherein mammalian bone is used as a non-human analogue, we can look to Johnson (1985) who in her extensive chapter on bone fracture refers to mammalian bone as a category and does not further explore the possibility of species variation. Oversymplifying one's justification for using non-human analogues in trauma studies might invalidate the transferability of the results derived from the animal to humans.

This chapter outlines the basic structure of mammalian bone, human and non-human, and provides a discussion of the benefits and limitations of using non-human bone as a proxy for human bone. Although the current chapter does not offer an experiment to answer the applicability of results derived from non-human bone, it does provide a foundation for questioning and understanding the results generated from studies based on non-human bone. Also provided is the histological morphology of one section of bovine cortical bone, from the periosteal to the endosteal surface. This series of images demonstrates the variability in histological structure in one bovine bone, thus serving as a reminder that even within a species there are microstructural differences at the level of the individual.

VARIATIONS IN MAMMALIAN BONE STRUCTURE

Microscopically, mammalian bone structure can be categorized into four types: woven, lamellar, Haversian or secondary lamellar bone, and plexiform or fibrolamellar (Currey 2002). Woven bone is composed of randomly-, loosely organized, and mineralized collagen fibrils. It contains approximately four times the number of osteocytes as lamellar bone and has a lower mineral content (Buckwalter *et al.* 1996a). In contrast to woven bone, the organization of lamellar bone is very consistent. The collagen fibrils vary less in diameter and organization, laying in tightly organized, parallel sheets with almost uniform degree of mineralization (Buckwalter *et al.* 1996b). Haversian or secondary lamellar bone is composed of secondary osteons formed through the process of bone remodeling (Figure 6-1).

Plexiform bone (Figures 6-2 and 6-3) is characteristic of fast-growing, large mammal bones, including those of bovids, pig, and artiodactyls. Differences in maturation rates explain the differences in bone microstructure between

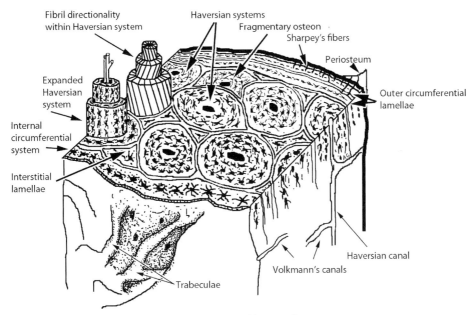

Figure 6-1. Schematic diagram of human bone microstructure.

humans and other animals; for example, bovids attain full body size at approximately two years of age, compared to 16 years in humans (Carter *et al.* 1976). Plexiform bone can be laid down quickly and in an organized manner, which allows for periods of rapid growth (Martiniakova *et al.* 2006). Parallel-fibered (woven) bone is laid down parallel to the long axis of the bone and there are fairly large spaces left between successive layers of new bone. These spaces are then filled with lamellar bone and the combination of the two is referred to as fibrolamellar or plexiform bone (Weiner and Wagner 1998).

Though plexiform bone is primary bone, secondary osteons do occur in cows and they increase in number with age. In humans, however, woven bone only characterizes bone formed during active growth, fracture repair, or as a result of certain pathological conditions, such as Paget's disease.

All normal human cortical bone is lamellar bone (Liebschner 2004). Secondary lamellar bone is characterized by the basic multicellular unit (BMU), which replaces or repairs previously existing bone (Currey 2002). Concentric layers of lamellae (compact bone tissue form osteons around a central canal (Haversian canal) through which the blood vessels and nerves run. In contrast to secondary osteons, a cement sheath does not demarcate primary osteons. Secondary osteons are characterized by a cement line and appear to drill right through the lamellar bone rather than merge with it (Currey 2002). Plexiform bone is present in and largely characteristic of large mammal cortical bone. Species identifications based on bone microstructure can be made with a

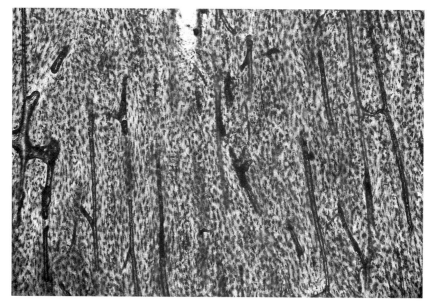

Figure 6-2. Transverse section of bovine long bone cortical histology showing plexiform bone. The thin section (150µm) was harvested from a cow that was approximately 18 months old at the time of slaughter. Micrograph taken at 10× magnification. Micrograph by Lauren Zephro.

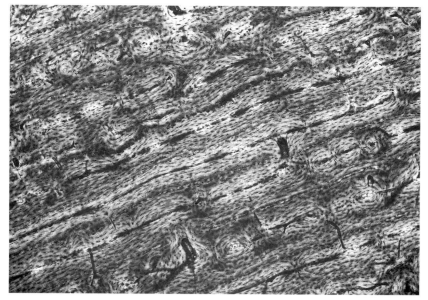

Figure 6-3. Longitudinal section at 10× magnification of bovine long bone cortical histology showing plexiform bone. The thin section (150µm) was harvested from a cow that was approximately 18 months old at the time of slaughter. Micrograph taken at 10× magnification. Micrograph by Lauren Zephro.

relatively high degree of confidence. For example, Martiniakova *et al.* (2006) depict the difference between pig and cow bone, while Benedix (2004) does the same for select Southeast Asian mammals.

SELECTION OF NON-HUMAN MODELS

Far more experimental research exists on how non-human bone fractures than on how appropriate non-human models should be selected for use in musculoskeletal research. This lack of theoretical consideration and actualistic demonstration of how different animal models can be from human bone indicates a fundamental lack of the non-human studies controlling for variables as thoroughly as they ought to have. While the growing body of experimental research on bone fracture that uses non-human bone as a direct proxy for human bone is expanding, the use of inappropriate non-human models will inevitably lead to "useless, irrelevant, or more seriously, misleading information" (Liebschner 2004:1708).

Currently, no standards have been established in bone biomechanical testing for choosing non-human models (Liebschner 2004), and the selection of non-human animals for biomechanical research on bone appears to be based on one of two factors: how convenient it is to acquire the non-human analogue or how familiar the study's author is with how species can vary (Neyt et al. 1998). According to Davidson and associates (1987), there are two types of non-human models, those based on analogy and those based on homology. Davidson and colleagues (1987) suggest that the selection of a non-human model should be subject to the following considerations:

1. appropriateness of an analogue,
2. transferability of information,
3. genetic uniformity of organisms, where applicable,
4. background knowledge of biological properties,
5. cost and availability,
6. generalizability of the results,
7. ease of and adaptability to experimental manipulation,
8. ecological consequences,
9. ethical implications.

Surprisingly, research by Neyt *et al.* (1994) found few studies that compared the ability of non-human models to reproduce human disease in the musculo-skeletal system. They surveyed studies of musculoskeletal and medical research for the use of non-human models published in major journals between January 1991 and November 1995 and for studies, which compared different mammals as non-human models for a single condition, published in major journals between between 1965 and 1995. They found that little consideration was given to the limitations or generalizability of non-human models before the results derived from using the non-human models were extrapolated and put into clinical practice.

According to Wang and associates (1998), to effectively use non-human bone as a proxy for human bone, the non-human bone analogue should reflect similar age- and disease-based biological changes, which would result in similar changes in the material properties of bone. In their study (Wang 1998), they compared the structural and material properties of five species (humans, baboons, canines, bovines, and rabbits), and they found that there were significant differences in the fracture properties among species. The study found that fracture toughness (longitudinal orientation), as measured by a single-layer compact sandwich (SCS) specimen, demonstrated that human and baboon bone shared the most fracture properties. Canine bone was found to have the highest value of fracture toughness, followed by human, baboon, rabbit, and cow. Baboons and rabbits were found to have similar bone density values to humans, with canines and cows having comparatively higher bone densities.

Further, the authors used scanning electron microscopy to compare the bone microstructure and fracture surfaces produced in the SCS specimen tests (Wang 1998). Their results indicated that bone microstructure was most similar between humans and baboons. These species exhibited similar osteon size and distribution. Rabbit SCS specimens consisted of primary bone, and cows exhibited primarily plexiform bone (Wang 1998). SCS specimens from canids exhibited intermediate microstructural characteristics, with secondary osteons present in the center and plexiform bone adjacent to the endosteal and periosteal margins. SEM examination of fracture surfaces, especially at higher magnifications (>1500×), indicated that differences in gross micro-structural appearance demonstrate variation amongst species, especially with regard to the appearance of long collagen-mineral bundles, which were seen on the surfaces of human, baboon and canine bones, but not on cow or rabbit fracture surfaces.

The following ten figures are micrographs of the cortical bone histology of one bovine specimen, which was approximately 18 months of age at the time of slaughter. Figures 6-4 through 6-13 were taken using a Nikon D-80 SLR camera mounted to an Olympus BX-41 transmitted polarized microscope at 10× magnification. The thin section of cortical bone was 150μm in thickness and the transverse distance from the endosteal to the periosteal surface was 9mm. As the figures demonstrate, the bone histology differs markedly from the periosteal surface to the endosteal surface. A higher number of secondary osteons are present closest to the endosteal surface and transition to a majority of plexiform organization towards the periosteal surface. Although a more

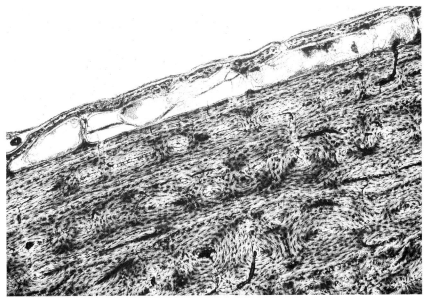

Figure 6-4. Transverse section of bovine cortical long bone, starting from periosteal surface and moving to endosteal surface. Thin section (150µm) harvested from cow that was 18 months at time of slaughter. Micrograph taken at 10× magnification. Micrograph by Lauren Zephro, number 1 of 10.

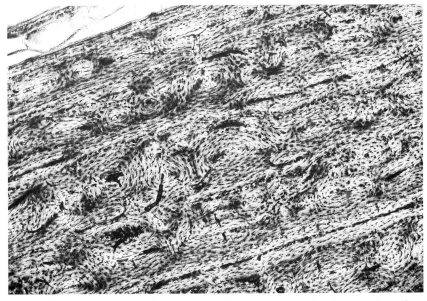

Figure 6-5. Transverse section of bovine cortical long bone, starting from periosteal surface and moving to endosteal surface. Thin section (150µm) harvested from cow that was 18 months at time of slaughter. Micrograph taken at 10× magnification. Micrograph by Lauren Zephro, number 2 of 10.

Broken Bones

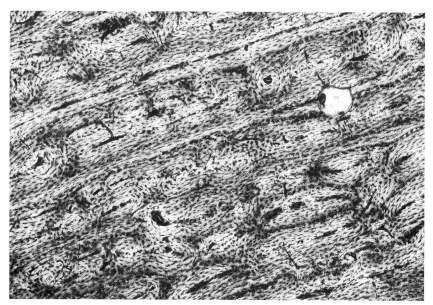

Figure 6-6. Transverse section of bovine cortical long bone, starting from periosteal surface and moving to endosteal surface. Thin section harvested (150μm) from cow that was 18 months at time of slaughter. Micrograph taken at 10× magnification. Micrograph by Lauren Zephro, number 3 of 10.

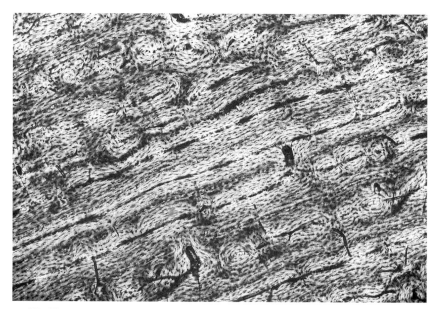

Figure 6-7. Transverse section of bovine cortical long bone, starting from periosteal surface and moving to endosteal surface. Thin section (150μm) harvested from cow that was 18 months at time of slaughter. Micrograph taken at 10× magnification. Micrograph by Lauren Zephro, number 4 of 10.

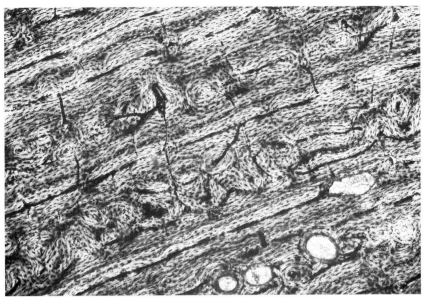

Figure 6-8. Transverse section of bovine cortical long bone, starting from periosteal surface and moving to endosteal surface. Thin section (150μm) harvested from cow that was 18 months at time of slaughter. Micrograph taken at 10× magnification. Micrograph by Lauren Zephro, number 5 of 10.

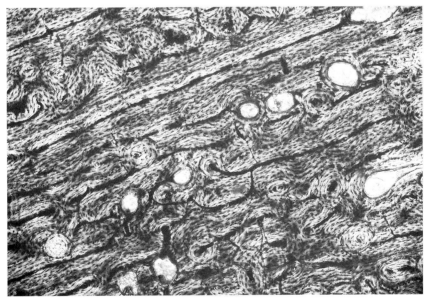

Figure 6-9. Transverse section of bovine cortical long bone, starting from periosteal surface and moving to endosteal surface. Thin section (150μm) harvested from cow that was 18 months at time of slaughter. Micrograph taken at 10× magnification. Micrograph by Lauren Zephro, number 6 of 10.

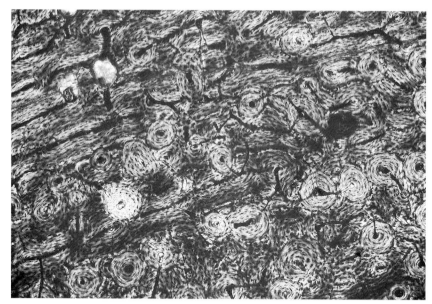

Figure 6-10. Transverse section of bovine cortical long bone, starting from periosteal surface and moving to endosteal surface. Thin section (150µm) harvested from cow that was 18 months at time of slaughter. Micrograph taken at 10× magnification. Micrograph by Lauren Zephro, number 7 of 10.

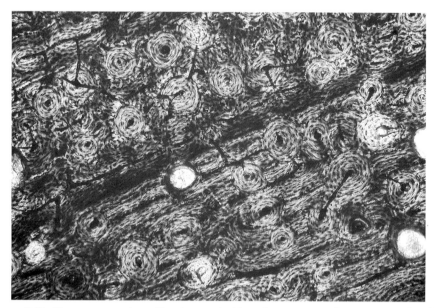

Figure 6-11. Transverse section of bovine cortical long bone, starting from periosteal surface and moving to endosteal surface. Thin section (150µm) harvested from cow that was 18 months at time of slaughter. Micrograph taken at 10× magnification. Micrograph by Lauren Zephro, number 8 of 10.

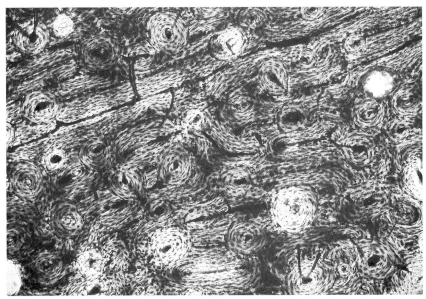

Figure 6-12. Transverse section of bovine cortical long bone, starting from periosteal surface and moving to endosteal surface. Thin section (150µm) harvested from cow that was 18 months at time of slaughter. Micrograph taken at 10× magnification. Micrograph by Lauren Zephro, number 9 of 10.

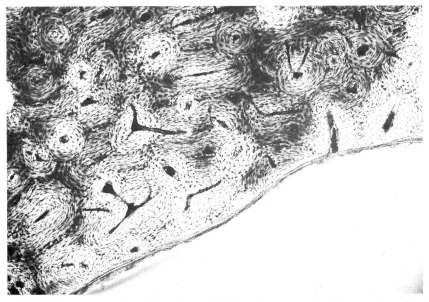

Figure 6-13. Transverse section of bovine cortical long bone, starting from periosteal surface and moving to endosteal surface. Thin section (150µm) harvested from cow that was 18 months at time of slaughter. Micrograph taken at 10× magnification. Micrograph by Lauren Zephro, number 10 of 10.

thorough study including sections from more specimens would be useful, the microstructural differences from the periosteal to the endosteal surfaces of this one cow's cortex demonstrates that the stereotypical description of non-human mammalian bone microstructure as being uniformly plexiform is overly simplistic. This finding is in agreement with other published studies, which report that the compacta of artiodactyls is composed of plexiform bone nearest the periosteal surface that transitions to dense Haversian bone to-wards the middle and endosteal sections of the cortex (Enlow and Brown 1958, Martiniakova *et al.* 2006). One would expect differences in bone histo-morphological sections taken from different species at different ages because bone growth, maintenance, and stress/strain differ by which bone and at which location the a section is taken and at which point during an animals' life cycle the sample is harvested.

Importantly, bone fracture properties are influenced by bone microstructure and ultrastructure, which includes the mineral and collagen bundles that differ amongst species and throughout the life cycle. The bovine micrographs published here and the published studies cited demonstrate that we have insufficient grasp on how widely non-human bone microstructure differs from that of humans. Non-human analogs must be contemplated with care.

ANTHROPOLOGICAL FRACTURE RESEARCH AND MAMMALIAN BONE VARIATION

In anthropology, the availability of non-human specimens countered by the ethical considerations of using human bone has made non-human bone fracture studies the primary examples of fracture research. The following discussion highlights actualistic research and places it with in the context of using non-human models for extrapolating human bone fracture patterns. Highlighted in the following section is the difference between homologue studies and analogue studies. Zooarchaeologists are predominately concerned with non-human bone as homologues, whereas bone-focused anthropologists, including physical and forensic anthropologists, are looking for analogues.

ZOOARCHAEOLOGY

Fracture studies in zooarchaeology are concerned with two primary issues; (1) understanding the mechanism and timing of failure based on fracture patterns, and (2) recognizing patterns in bone fracture so that, if possible, in-ference about human activity can be made. Moreover, logistical concerns are paramount as zooarchaeologists are tasked with describing and categorizing large fragmentary bone assemblages quickly, accurately, and meaningfully (White 1992). Zooarchaeological research is explicitly focused on middle range or actualistic research (see Binford 1981 or Gifford 1981) and is, with rare exception, almost never interested in human bone fracture. The fracture literature reflects a focus on experimentation and, unlike the biomechanical research, is concerned with responses of whole bones. For the purpose of this discussion, a brief review is included of key publications on fracture papers with an emphasis on research addressing differences in fracture patterns among elements and species.

The ultimate goal of zooarchaeology is to interpret past human behavior. Much of the fracture description in zooarchaeology is very goal (usually archaeological site assemblage) specific. To the zooarchaeologist, a bone fragment or fragments pose the causal question: human or animal modification? An actualistic study is designed specifically to answer that question for the assemblage at hand (e.g., Sadek-Kooros 1972; Haynes 1983; Davis 1985; Johnson 1985; Lyman 1994; Marean *et al.* 2000; Outram 2001, 2002; Pickering *et al.* 2005). Most classification schemes make an explicit attempt to describe and classify fractures without implying the cause, so that assemblage patterns can be analyzed objectively. Generally, zooarchaeological studies seek to distinguish whether a bone was fractured for marrow extraction by hammerstone percussion or fractured by carnivore modification (Capaldo and Blumenschine 1994, Pickering *et al.* 2005, Davis 1985). With the exception of Davis (1985), the methods used to induce bone fracture have not been tightly controlled and are not identical between studies, making comparison of individual study results difficult.

In the zooarchaeological literature, the main sources of biomechanical information are primarily those of Morlan (1980, 1984) and Johnson (1985), yet these papers proposed somewhat conflicting criteria for what is the most important factor in bone fracture propagation and morphology. Johnson (1985) argued that microstructure is the most important determinant in governing bone failure. In contrast, Morlan (1980, 1984) asserted that while fractures may follow cement lines and other microstructure, they may also diverge from microstructure in unpredictable ways, based on macrostructure, in the case of long bones, based on their cylindrical shape.

Perhaps more interestingly, neither Johnson (1985) nor Morlan (1980, 1984) investigate the properties of plexiform bone versus secondary Haversian bone, or the differences in micro- and macrostructure based on mechanical usage. Had either done so, it would have lended credibility to their respective arguments. The most problematic aspects of these studies is their small sample size, their use of biomechanical research based on the solely on the properties of bone as a material, and the lack of a controlled fracture methodology. Johnson (1985) did not provide the specifics of her study sample, but does note the use of a 14-year-old male bison for experimental butchering and long bone fracture in her acknowledgements section. Morlan's experimental study sample consisted of one elephant carcass. The liberal use of the biomechanical literature is likely the most problematic by Johnson (1985) and Morlan (1980, 1984), because the subtleties of bone material properties were (and are) still being refined. The results of their analyses are challenging to compare or extrapolate from given the inherent complexity of extrapolating material properties to the level of whole bone.

With regard to species or element differences in fracture patterns, some divergences have been noted by Noe-Nygaard (1977) between tibiae, femora, and metatarsals; Morlan (1980, 1984) about elephant bone variation, Davis (1985) among elements of artiodactyl bones, Gifford-Gonzalez (1989) about young zebra bone, and Outram (2002) regarding bovid metapodials. These studies show, overall, the importance of element shape and configuration of the cortical bone as strong influences on fracture propagation. Davis (1985) also found statistically significant relationships between fracture morphology and type of loading. Dynamic loading produced fewer than expected oblique fractures and more than expected mixed and parallel fractures, while torsional loading (twisting) produced the inverse pattern. Static loading was intermediate, producing fewer mixed fractures and more parallel and oblique.

Villa and Mahieu (1991) discussed non-human bone fracture patterns and their applicability to human bone. Noe-Nygaard (1977) found that when fractured under similar conditions, tibia and metatarsals broke into two main longitudinal pieces with oblique outlines, while femora broke into three main pieces consisting of the two articular ends and the diaphysis. Morlan (1984) considered elephant bone as a special case for fracture characteristics, due to their extremely robust morphology and thick cortical bone. Morlan (1984) argues that fractures to these bones are likely due to human activity because increased force is required to fracture elephant bones and their large size makes most bones inaccessible to gnawing by carnivores. Gifford-Gonzalez noted the high proportion of longitudinal fractures in young zebra bone and suggested that the bones appear to have a "dictated preferentially longitudinal fracture pattern" (1989, pg. 218). She suggested that if the zebra had been older, more spiral fractures would likely be present, thus acknowledging that material properties change as bone matures.

Villa and Mahieu (1991) examined and compared three human bone assemblages and argued that human bone fracture patterns should be derived from and compared with criteria derived from human samples. They argued that although some characteristics, such as cut marks and impact scars, may be independent of species-specific bone morphology, fracture patterns may be related to overall gross bone morphology. This thesis is not explored further experimentally.

Outram (2002) noted a predominance of longitudinal fractures in bovine metapodials, in comparison to other long bones, and he attributed them to the overall morphology of the bones having a "natural division down the center of artiodactyl [metapodials]" (Outram 2002:57). Clearly, these studies suggest that morphological and material differences may somehow contribute to fracture patterns; however, the information is not explored in any more depth.

Davis's (1985) research represents a special case in the zooarchaeological fracture literature because she used a controlled experimental methodology using mechanical means to calibrate the strain to the bones. She was exploring static loading, dynamic impact loading, and torsion on the humeri, tibiae, and femora of variously sized African antelope bones that were fresh or in various stages of weathering. Although Davis did not find a significant relationship between bone size (defined by the live weight of the animal) and fracture pattern, she did find that the amount of force required to produce fracture does vary with element size. Smaller bones required less force to fracture.

Davis (1985) found the types of fractures seen across bovid size categories were remarkably similar, but different fracture types emerged among different bovid elements. A significant relationship emerged between skeletal element and fracture location, orientation, and morphology. Davis found that humeri tended to fracture more anteriorly, tibiae more posteriorly, and femora more medially and laterally. She also found a significant relationship between element and fracture orientation and between element and fracture morphology. Davis explains these relationships as depending on midshaft cross-sectional shape and diameter. She also found statistically significant relationships between fracture morphology and type of loading. Dynamic loading produced fewer than expected oblique fractures and more than expected mixed and parallel fractures, while torsional loading (twisting) produced the inverse pattern. Static loading was intermediate, producing fewer mixed fractures and more parallel and oblique.

It is especially significant to zooarchaeology that oblique fractures were more common as a result of torsional and static loading, because oblique and "spiral" fractures have been used extensively to indicate the condition of the bone at the time of fracture (Johnson 1985) but have not been associated as closely with the type and rate of loading. Overall, Davis's research points to differences in fracture morphology and orientation due to morphological differences among skeletal elements in her experimentally fractured sample.

FORENSIC ANTHROPOLOGY

In contrast to zooarchaeology, forensic anthropology is tasked with interpreting trauma to single elements, to single bodies, and a single species (see

White 1992 for a discussion of general differences in the significance of osteology between physical anthropologists and zooarchaeologists). Fractures may take place under numerous conditions, within the body of a living person or during the postmortem timespan. Trauma also must be interpreted for individuals representing all demographic categories of age, sex, and ancestry. Moreover, the mechanisms of trauma being investigated are numerous and include different rates of loading and loading combinations. Explicit calls for more experimental studies in trauma and taphonomy have emerged (Galloway *et al.* 1999, Iscan 2001), but this is complicated by the fact that all experimental research must meet its final test in a court of law. Under current court admissibility guidelines, such as the 1993 Daubert v. Merill Pharmaceuticals ruling, scientific evidence must meet exceptionally stringent criteria (see also Saks and Faigman 2005):

1. Has the method been tested and is it testable?
2. Has the method been peer reviewed?
3. Hoes it have an error rate?
4. Is the method generally accepted?

For forensic anthropological experimental research to meet Daubert criteria, sample sizes must be sufficiently large, and the methods must be repeatable and quantifiable. Although a growing body of controlled experimental research conducted on human bone does exist, this research is primarily a collaborative effort between forensic anthropologists and bioengineers (e.g., Porta 2005, Kroman 2004, Rabl 1996).

The appropriateness of non-human models as analogues for human bone fracture has been broached but not systematically explored in forensic anthropology. Galloway and colleagues (1999) noted that non-human models have been used, citing Ubelaker's (1992) use of a chicken bone as an analogue for a human metacarpal. The authors briefly discuss problems with non-human models, namely that fracture properties have not been explored across species, and results may thus not be admissible in a court of law. Further, they recommend that the selection of non-human models be based on the similarity in the victim's body size. Possible microstructural variation is noted but not explored.

To understand fracture patterns, forensic anthropology has emphasized bone macrostructure and forensic case studies (Galloway *et al.* 1999). Use of case studies does present problems, possibly introducing unknown variables, but has nonetheless yielded important information. In such cases, demographics are typically known for clinical and autopsy populations. Since bones' visco-elastic properties are known to vary throughout the life cycle, known cases are important to understand bone fracture patterns. For example, the bones of children are less mineralized, more elastic, and less stiff than adult bone. The higher organic component of children's bone means that it can withstand more force before it is permanently deformed, and that it fails in compression first rather than tension, as does adult bone (Pierce *et al.* 2004). In children, unlike adults, fractures are often incomplete, as with greenstick or buckle fractures (Chapter 5 this volume). In the case of children, examination of known cases is essential for forensic anthropologists to explore mechanisms but also to link specific patterns with child abuse (Chapter 7 and Love this volume). Clinical observation can be an invaluable source of information.

For adult bone, fracture atlases testify to the regular influence of gross bone morphology on fracture patterns in humans (Galloway, 1999; Koval and Zuckerman, 2002). Texts are organized by bone and describe the most commonly seen fracture morphologies and fracture locations for given loading conditions. They are primarily intended for or are based on clinical practice and case studies, which are concerned with the diagnosis and treatment of trauma in living people, rather than with postmortem fracture patterns or identification of trauma type.

Given the inherent ethical concerns linked to the experimental use of human specimens and the relative rarity of human bone for research purposes, fertile ground exists for researchers to identify appropriate non-human analogues. When interpolating actualistic fracture experiment results derived from a non-human analogue into an actual forensic case, the forensic anthropologist must at the very least be able to articulate why the particular non-human analogue is appropriate and how the experiment controlled for the variables they are seeing in the remains in question (i.e., sub-adult or adult; fresh, decomposed, or skeletonized bone(s); postmortem environment, etc.). Perhaps the best philsophy to describe incorporating actualistic research into forensic cases is "proceed with caution," since any conclusions drawn in the forensic case based on conclusions interpreted from an actualistic, non-human analogue experiment must be defendable on the witness stand.

Chapter 7

COMMON CIRCUMSTANCES OF BLUNT FORCE TRAUMA

ALISON GALLOWAY AND VICKI WEDEL

Injuries are not random. They result from specific series of events and can be used to interpret from the bone back to the cause of fracture. Blunt force trauma can occur in a number of circumstances. It is a common cause of death in homicidal cases but also produces the primary skeletal damage seen in motor vehicle accidents, aircraft crashes, traumatic compression and falls, blast injuries, and natural disasters like tornados and earthquakes (Lovell 2008, Li 2012). Blunt force trauma is also often seen in the victims of human rights abuses (Ta'ala *et al.* 2006, Kimmerle and Baraybar 2008).

Often blunt force injuries are "bloodless" in that the external skin is not broken or less severely damaged than the internal organs (Adelson 1974, Hiss *et al.* 1996, Vij 2008). Soft tissue may not reflect the underlying damage, and conversely, skeletal elements may remain intact despite extensive soft tissue injury such as contusions, hematomas, and visceral lacerations. Full analysis at autopsy is therefore required and, increasingly, even fresh remains are referred to the anthropologist for examination. Initial determinations of cause of death without anthropological analysis may lead to erroneous conclusions. Cause of death differs by about one-third between the original diagnosis and that at autopsy (Kircher *et al.* 1985, Tavora 2008). For example, cranial and vertebral fractures are often missed in initial trauma analysis or in the emergency room. In about 4% of the cases where initial cause of death is misidentified, the manner of death also differs. Virtual autopsy, utilizing quantitative computed tomography (QCT), promises to show better visualization of skeletal trauma and may allow for more accurate assessment of damage without standard autopsy (Lovell 2008, Stawicki *et al.* 2008). It also provides a lasting three-dimensional record that can be used later for presentation or re-analysis.

The location, nature, and amount of skeletal damage vary with the age of the individual, the nature and severity of the trauma, and the status of the skeletal system (Rogers 1992, Brinker and O'Connor 2004). Because the kinds of activities in which people engage vary by age, so too do the types of injuries seen. In general, younger individuals are more often engaged in high-risk activities than are older people and younger people are more likely to suffer injury during these pursuits. Of course, age alone rarely excludes those who have the desire to experience more dangerous activities. Age-related disabilities may predispose some to accidental injury by decreasing awareness of approaching or impending danger. Similarly, other disabilities, inexperience, drugs or alcohol consumption, or inattention are additional factors that are not evident from the skeleton. One study showed that over half of those arriving at the emergency room with traumatic fractures and dislocations also tested positive for either alcohol or drugs (Blake *et al.* 1997). Therefore, the biological profile can rarely indicate the exact nature of the circumstances of injury but may play a role in suggesting the most likely interpretation of the evidence.

The circumstances through which an individual met his or her death are often difficult to discern once the remains have become decayed, desiccated, burned, or skeletonized. While many times we deal with remains of homicide or suicide victims, this cannot be assumed. Accidental deaths also may involve blunt force, particularly when motor vehicles are involved. This may be the case even if the evidence of such an accident is long since gone. Individuals may have fallen, accidentally or with assistance, and sustained trauma. The scene of the death may be altered, and the investigators may initially attribute the trauma to accidental causes, diverting their suspicions from other causes such as a homicide or suicide.

Anthropological analysis of blunt force trauma may provide valuable information about the circumstances of death. Matched with the pathologist's analysis of the remaining soft tissue, this may shed light on how and why the victim died. For the final determination of the cause and manner of death by the coroner or medical examiner, all potential avenues of investigation should be incorporated. When only the skeletal evidence remains, close examination by a qualified forensic anthropologist is crucial. This chapter reviews the combinations of injuries and fracture patterns associated with homicide, motor vehicle accidents (including trains and airplanes), and falls.

HOMICIDAL INJURIES

Homicidal blunt force trauma requires close contact between the assailant and victim and considerable effort to inflict the injuries. The victim may have the opportunity to resist and possibly transfer trace evidence. The presence of blunt force trauma does not exclude the presence of other forms of violence and beating someone to death is often difficult, leaves evidence at the scene, and may risk injury to the perpetrator.

Frequently, the anthropologist will see other types of damage on the remains along with blunt force. Often the extent of the injuries in undecomposed remains are hidden by hair or clothing. It is therefore essential that the skeletal tissue be examined to reveal the extent of the damage as well as possibly establish the sequence of blows. Fragments of decomposing remains should be retrieved and the skull reconstructed (Chapter 2). Fracture margins should be carefully checked for the presence of trapped hairs or fibers. From the reconstructed pattern, the anthropologist is able to render an opinion on the location, number, and sequence of blows. In the following section, homicidal assault, suicidal blunt force trauma, abuse of vulnerable individuals, and strangulation and hanging are discussed.

Blunt Force Assault

Fatal blunt force trauma includes blows from a variety of weapons such as clubs, rods, pipes, rocks, hammers, baseball bats, lamps, ornaments, chair or table legs, handguns, and almost any other instrument at hand during a fight (Gonzalez *et al.* 1954, Adelson 1974, Murphy 1991, Rodge *et al.* 2003, Spitz and Fisher 1980, Spitz 2005, Batalis 2012). Death from blunt force can be due to forceful contact of part of or the entire body with an unyielding surface or object. Blunt force can also be delivered by the hands, which usually have less power to produce fractures, or by the feet. The potential for injury depends on the amount of energy transmitted by the blow and the size of the impact area (Chapter 3, this volume). In many cases, both the impacting force and the unyielding surface upon which the victim rested combine to produce a pattern of trauma (McGee 1991).

Blunt force trauma may account for over half of individuals who are victims of homicide and subject to forensic autopsy, particularly in areas of the world where guns are less accessible (Fischer *et al.* 1994). In a U.S. national survey, 17% of the victims of physical violence reported musculoskeletal injuries, excluding gunshot damage (Rand and Strom 1997). Almost 20% of assault victims reporting to emergency room were there because of blunt force assault. Ambade and Godbole (2006), in a review of Indian homicides, found that over 40% were from blunt force trauma, slightly exceeding those from sharp force trauma. Strict gun controls and few guns per capita in India narrow the options for homicide. Of these fatalities, almost 87% were male. In a study of Australian hospitalized victims of assault, the majority (77%) were male (Pleuckhahn and Cordner 1991). Two-thirds of the victims were attacked by a single assailant. Over 80% of all their fractures were facial. Many of these assaults resulted from altercations between two individuals that escalated into violence. Alcohol, consumed by either the victim or the assailant, was frequently involved in homicidal blunt force trauma (Fischer *et al.* 1994).

Even in cases of fatal assault, the attack often does not begin with intent to commit homicide. Rather, weapons are chosen from material at hand and vary widely (Adelson 1974, Murphy 1991). In some instances, blunt force trauma will produce identifiable patterns in the remains (Murphy 1991, McGee 1991, Clark and Sperry 1992, Marks 1999). In these cases, characteristics of the murder weapon should be documented, but it is very rare for any particular instrument to be identified as having been used in a crime. In many cases, the damage is so great that accurate reconstruction of the weapon's signature is extremely difficult (e.g., Black *et al.*, this volume). In some cases, seemingly innocuous items may produce injuries that mimic other instruments. For example, three cases have been reported in which railroad ballast produced depressed fractures similar to those produced by a hammer (Bowen 1966).

Craniocerebral damage characterizes more homicidal injuries than all other portions of the body combined (Adelson 1974, Murphy 1991, Hadjizacharia *et al.* 2009). Partly, this may be due to the head being an obvious target for assault and with modern populations, there appears to be a fixation on hitting the nose (Walker 1997). Walker notes that this preference for blows to the head continues despite the head not being the most incapacitating place to strike, a trend he attributes to the introduction of boxing and its focus on "not hitting below the belt." Chattopadhyay and Tripathi (2010) found that blunt force trauma to the skull, especially trauma forceful enough to cause a comminuted fracture, was more consistently fatal than blows causing fractures anywhere else on the body. In looking at fracture and laceration patterns among individuals at autopsy, Rand (1997) observed that blunt assault resulted in more fractures and fracture/lacerations than falls, while falls were more likely to produce fractures without overlying laceration. Victims may also fall to the floor or against a wall and strike their head. Such injuries result in direct damage but may also produce contrecoup injuries to the brain. In these situations, sudden deceleration of the head causes increases in intracranial pressure (Asha'Ari *et al.* 2011). In fact, these traumas can be more severe than the pressure induced by a non-penetrating direct blow (Fujiwara *et al.* 1989, Drew and Drew 2004). Because the brain is the most vulnerable to trauma, it can sustain lethal damage while similar blows to other portions of the body produce much less damage.

Cranial fractures, as noted previously (see also Chapter 9, this volume), require considerable force to result in a linear fracture of the vault. In some cases, cranial fractures are limited and may only affect the outer table of the bone. This type of injury is often able to reflect the characteristics of the instrument that delivered the impact (Spitz and Fisher 1980, Spitz 2005). The outer table will be pushed inward by the striking object, collapsing the underlying diplöe. Occasionally, the inner table will break while the outer remains intact. As the force increases, the vault is more likely to exhibit linear fractures. In cases of beatings, there are often multiple blows producing a high degree of fragmentation with marked displacement, reflecting damage incurred over the larger area of impact (Spitz and Fisher 1980, Spitz 2005).

Blows to the head occur all around the vault but often are located on the upper regions. This observation gave rise to the "hat brim" rule put forward by Richter (1905) and clarified by Kratter (1921). This line or area has been poorly defined but was recently standardized as an area parallel to the Frankfort Horizontal Plane, the superior margin of this area passing through glabella and the inferior one passing through porion (Kremer *et al.* 2008). As discussed by Fracasso and associates (2011), the rule states that blunt force trauma from falls do not occur above the hat brim line if (1) the person was standing prior to the fall, (2) the fall is the height of the person, (3) the fall was onto a flat floor, and (4) there are no intervening objects. In a five-year-long retrospective study of deaths due to falls down stairs, falls from standing height, and homicidal blows, Kremer *et al.* (2008) found that both homicidal and fall-related fractures occur at the hat brim line, however homicidal blows are more commonly found above the hat brim zone. These fractures are accompanied by a higher number of lacerations than fractures sustained in either kind of fall. The blows from assault are also more frequently found on the left side of the skull, probably reflecting the handedness of the assailant. A subsequent study found that about 75% of fractures above the hat brim line were associated with blows (Kremer and Sauvageau 2009). Expanding on the work of Kremer and associates, Guyomarc'h and colleagues (2010) found that fractures from falls were primarily linear or radial, while fractures from blows were predominantly comminuted or depressed. Facial fractures were almost never caused by falls but were frequent caused by blows. Their decision tree, while initiated by scalp laceration number and size, terminates on the cranial fracture type and facial fracture presence following the above principle.

Blows to the face often result in fracturing of the facial bones accompanied by avulsion of the dentition. Single-rooted teeth are particularly prone to loss due to their location and also the ease with which they are detached from the alveolar bone. It is important to determine if this loss is perimortem or postmortem. The root sockets of avulsed incisors and canines are often exposed with fracturing observable on the alveolar ridge. Once loosened, the teeth may be lost, especially if the interval between death and recovery of the remains is extended. Recovery of the teeth themselves, if separate from the rest of the skeleton, may indicate the place of the assault. Detached teeth may also be swallowed or aspirated by the victim (Adelson 1974) and so may be recovered from within the body.

Following cranial injuries, the next most common regions for fatal blunt force trauma are the thorax and abdomen. Trauma to the chest results in 25% of all traumatic deaths (Hanafi *et al.* 2011). Blunt force trauma to the upper torso can result in multiple unilateral or bilateral rib fractures (Adelson 1974) or rarely subluxation of the costosternal joints (Liao and Hsu 2011). While rib fractures are often viewed as a relatively minor injury, these fractures can prove fatal due to puncturing of vital organs, development of a pneumothorax, or dissection of the descending aorta (Hanafi *et al.* 2011). Loss of integrity of skeletal structure of the thoracic cavity also can inhibit the ability to breathe. The contraction of the diaphragm may simply cause in-caving of the chest wall rather than intake of air.

A small number of blunt force trauma homicides result from injuries to the neck or extremities. Neck injuries may be produced indirectly from head trauma but also may result from direct blows. Fractures of vertebral elements vary in the types of medical complications they cause. Pull ter Gunne and colleagues (2010) surveyed adult cervical fracture victims' records and determined that blunt trauma to the cervical vertebrae was most likely to be lethal if the vertebral structure (lamina or facet of C3, C4, or C5 especially) impacted compromised nervous system control of the diaphragm or if the patient were of advanced age. However, Rhee and colleagues (2006) noted that blunt assault often resulted in cervical spinal fractures but involvement of the cord was more frequent with gunshot or sharp force trauma.

There may be damage to the structures of the throat. The latter may be seen skeletally as fractures in ossified/calcified thyroid or cricoid cartilage, sharp edges of which may penetrate the pharynx or esophagus (Hagan 1983). Death may result from a number of injuries including compression or damage to the spinal column/brain stem, obstruction of respiration or loss of blood due to rupture of major blood vessels. Examination of the neck should, therefore, be detailed.

While death attributable to blunt force trauma to the extremities is not common, it does occur. Usually the trauma affects major blood vessels leading to death by exsanguination (Carli *et al.* 2012). Non-lethal trauma to the extremities is more common in homicide victims and often accompanies lethal injury to the head or torso. The hands and arms are, however, often injured as the victim attempts to mount a defense (Adelson 1974). The classic defense indicator is fracture of the ulna (Judd 2008), usually on the dominant arm. In these cases, the hand is pronated and raised to shield the head and body. In such a position, the ulna lies closest to the source of violence. In addition to fractured long bones, fingers may be traumatically amputated by crushing blows to the hands when they are used to ward off impact (Mohanty *et al.* 2007).

Offensive injuries to the hands, such as fractures of the fourth and fifth metacarpals, may also be found, indicating that the victim may have been a vigorous participant in the fight leading to his/her death. Such information may be important when cross-checking the alleged perpetrator's version of the events with the available evidence.

The use of blunt force trauma has also been reported in cases of human rights abuses. Probably the most notorious was the routine killing associated with the Cambodian killing fields (Ta'ala *et al.* 2006, 2008). In this case, the mode of execution was a single blow to the lower back of the skull producing gaping fractures in the occipital bone. Blunt force is also reported in torture of victims prior to being killed (Vogel and Brogdon 2003, Kimmerle and Baray-bar 2008, Delabarde 2008, Maat 2008). In these cases, documentation of the healing fractures along with those that may have occurred around the time of death and during disposal of the remains is crucial.

Although extremely uncommon, suicide by direct blunt force trauma cannot be excluded (Hunsaker and Thorne 2002, Theirauf *et al.* 2012). In one reported case, the individual eventually died from cerebral edema as a result of repeated blows to the cranial vault (Hunsaker and Thorne 2002). The skeletal evidence alone, however, would have supported an interpretation by the coroner as a homicide. Investigation of the scene added to the individual's psychiatric history led to a revised interpretation.

ABUSE OF CHILDREN, VULNERABLE ADULTS AND THE ELDERLY

In some cases, the biological profile of the victim is important in understanding the circumstances of death. Certain individuals, due to age or infirmity, may be extremely vulnerable to abuse, often from those who are closest to them. Often the abuse is evidenced by healed or healing fractures in addition to the perimortem defects. A complete skeletal analysis is critical in such cases as, even if homicide cannot be proven, prosecution may proceed on the basis of both the individual's status as a vulnerable individual and the history of abuse. In some forms of abuse, it is the relationship between the victim and the perpetrator that identifies the abuse and these patterns are less distinguishable from the skeletal injuries or biological profile. A classic example is that of intimate partner violence (Lovell 2008, Juarez and Hughes, this volume).

Child Abuse

Child abuse was first described in 1946 by Caffey. The syndrome was defined and the cause identified in 1962 by Kempe and associates, leading to increased attention to the problem by the popular press. This syndrome refers to cases in which children are hit, beaten, shaken, thrown, dropped, burned, or suffocated. Such violence may result in the death of the child. Frequently, this syndrome is termed "non-accidental injury" (Clarke *et al.* 2012).

Skeletally, this syndrome is usually seen in children under the age of five years. Eighty percent of the fractures in abused children occur when the child is less than 18 months old according to Worlock *et al.* (1986). Two other studies (Mertean *et al.* 1983, DiMaio and DiMaio 1989) found that about half of the abused children were younger than one year of age. Without abuse, fractures are relatively uncommon in children until about age five years, at which time their increased physical activity exposes them to greater risks, and participation in sports becomes more common.

Analysis of a battered-child death requires assessment of the stage of fracture healing. Victims often exhibit numerous fractures in various stages of healing due to repeated episodes of violence. Multiple fractures in varying stages of healing may be present on the same skeletal element. This feature has become the hallmark of the syndrome in the skeleton (Kerley 1978, Rogers 1992). Fresh fractures often interrupt the callus formation of older healing fractures. Determining the age of fracture healing is very difficult, especially as fracture healing can be rapid in a healthy child. Knight (1991) and Swischuk (1992) suggest that in rib fractures new bone formation takes a minimum of 10–14 days to be seen radiographically. Whether this stage of callus formation will be preserved in the skeletonized material is not certain. Although multiple fractures are the hallmark of this syndrome, about half of the child abuse victims are found with only a single fracture. For as many as 10% of abused children, the second incident brings them to the attention of the medical community and is fatal (Green and Swiontkowski 1994).

While the "battered baby" syndrome can be diagnosed from injuries in various stages of healing, the majority of child abuse deaths are due to sudden, violent acts provoked by an often trivial event, although they may be part of an ongoing pattern of physical abuse (DiMaio and DiMaio 1989). In these cases, the child is often hit severely or thrown about the room.

"Shaken baby syndrome" is a major cause of physical abuse in children (Gilliland and Folberg 1996, Gerber and Coffman 2007, John *et al.* 2012). In these cases, the child is shaken violently causing hyperextension and hyper-flexion of the neck. Death is due to subdural hemorrhage. Ocular hemorrhage is commonly found among the soft tissue injuries. Skeletal trauma is usually confined to bilateral rib fracture. These children tend to be quite young, around six months of age. DiMaio and DiMaio (1989) caution that many, if not all, shaken baby deaths may actually be due to blunt force trauma to the head.

Many cases of physical abuse in children leave no skeletal evidence. Of 24 cases of child abuse leading to death by subdural hematoma, two-thirds had no skull fractures (DiMaio and DiMaio 1989). This study also showed that laceration of the internal organs, often without external evidence of trauma, was the cause of death. However, careful examination of the skeletal elements is warranted when circumstances or history raises the possibility of a pattern of abuse. Love and Sanchez (2009) have outlined the method of examination.

In this volume, the following discussion of child abuse is truncated and readers are referred to the Love chapter in this volume for a detailed description of the skeletal patterns in the ribs, extremities, scapulae, sternum, and vertebral column associated with child abuse. In this section, discussion introduces ribs and extremity fractures but focuses on the skull and clavicles and the types of injuries that may mimic some of the fractures seen with abuse.

Fractures of the extremities and ribs are among the more diagnostic fractures linked to child abuse (Bensahel *et al.* 1986; DeBoeck *et al.* 1986). The fracture pattern will shift with age. Infants suffer more skull and rib fractures as well as more fractures of the lower limbs than abused toddlers (Worlock *et al.* 1986). One study showed that when fractures were present, the extremities were involved in about 77% of cases (Merten *et al.* 1983). Long bone fractures are most often diaphyseal. Fractures of the hands and feet are rare. Rib fractures are found in less than one-fifth of the cases, but when they do occur, multiple ribs are often involved, often occur bilaterally and are considered highly diagnostic of child abuse (Feldman and Brewer 1984, Worlock *et al.* 1986, Swischuk 1992). Rib fractures often occur posteriorly from the child having been grasped around the chest. Other sites, such as the clavicular mid-shaft, spine (Leonidas 1983; Swischuk 1992; Diamond *et al.* 1994) and pubic rami, are infrequently broken.

After the ribs and extremities, the next most common site is the skull, primarily in the form of simple linear fractures (Green and Swiontkowski 1994, Kemp *et al.* 2008). These cranial fractures are found particularly in the first year of life (Leonidas 1983; Merten *et al.* 1983). Head injuries are the most common cause of death (DiMaio and DiMaio 1989; Knight 1991). Ninety-five percent of serious head injuries are attributable to child abuse, while the rest are due to falls, motor vehicle accidents and other traumatic circumstances (DiMaio and DiMaio 1989). Low-level falls such as from chairs and beds are not considered to be adequate explanations for serious skull fractures. Helfer and colleagues (1977) surveyed the medical records of 85 children who fell accidentally: only one sustained a skull fracture, and this child recovered without serious defects.

Parietal fractures are more common in non-abused children than fractures in other bones of the vault, but linear fractures in other locations are likely more suggestive of child abuse (Rogers 1992). Knight (1991) suggests a common location of abuse-produced fractures is the occipitoparietal area, although the location is not sufficient to distinguish these from accidental fractures. He also notes that the fractures are less likely to cross suture lines in the skulls of young children than in adult skulls. While the fracture line may appear to "stagger" when it does cross the suture, it is more likely that the displacement represents two separate fractures resulting from the impact. Knight also cites bilateral horizontal fractures extending posteriorly from the coronal suture, often continuing into the basilar area as a common finding in child abuse. These injuries may be caused by blows to the top of the head or the child being dropped onto his head. Facial fractures due to direct blows are also found, including those of the mandible (Swischuk 1992).

Fractures of the clavicle, while rare, have been found in cases of child abuse (Knight 1991; Swischuk 1992; Green and Swiontkowski 1994). In neonates, these fractures must be distinguished from those due to birth trauma (see below). In accidents, the clavicular fractures tend to be in the midshaft, but when they occur with abuse, the clavicle breaks due to sudden traction as the arm is yanked, and fractures move away from the midline (DiMaio and DiMaio 1989).

Skeletal indicators of environmental stress often accompany the pattern of fractures due to child abuse. These children often exhibit enamel hypoplasias and Harris lines, defects that are most commonly associated with interruptions of growth due to such stresses as infection or malnutrition (Skinner and Anderson 1991).

Birth injuries should be considered in neonates. While fractures are relatively rare, broken clavicles and, to a lesser extent, skull fractures and long bone fractures, along with loss of a phalanx have been reported (Rubin 1964). The skull fractures typically accompany an instrument-assisted birth and are less common in normal delivery (Dupuis *et al.* 2005). The fractures are usually non-displaced and linear or may be depressed ("ping-pong") fractures (Heise *et al.* 1996, Doumouchtsis and Arulkumaran 2008, Reichard 2008). Depressed fractures appear to result either from asymmetrical compression in the birth canal, particularly with an occipito-posterior delivery position, or from the use of forceps to assist delivery (Garza-Mercado 1982). The cause of the non-instrument-derived fractures has been identified as the maternal 5th lumbar vertebra, sacral promontory, pubic symphysis, ischial spines, or a asymmetrical pelvic girdle (Arifin *et al.* 2012). Some resist calling these defects fractures but instead term them "congenital moulding depressions" (Axton and Levy 1965). Circular elevated fractures can also be found due to the use of a vacuum in extraction of the infant during birth (Hickey and McKenna 1996, Simonson *et al.* 2007). Linear fractures are also a common finding in neonatal head trauma. In some cases, linear fractures occur in the sutural lines, do not resolve, and become growing diastatic fractures (Hansen *et al.* 1987, Huisman *et al.* 1999, Miranda *et al.* 2007). Where there is a living child or remaining soft tissue, age of associated hematomas can help distinguish birth trauma from child abuse but variable signs of skeletal healing will be needed in the skeletonized remains (Patonay and Oliver 2010).

Postcranial fractures also occur during birth. Clavicular fractures are a relatively common finding from vaginal deliveries (Monjok 2008) and usually result from shoulder dystocia. Neonatal humeral and femoral fractures are linked to breech births and can occur even with Caesarian section (Al-Habdan 2003, Alexander *et al.* 2006, Matsubara *et al.* 2008, Sherr-Luri *et al.* 2011).

In older children, other conditions may mimic some of the injuries seen with child abuse. Metaphyseal injuries have been reported to occur in non-intentional cases such as "playing airplane" in which the child is swung by the arms around the adult or older child. The strength of the triceps muscle is greater than the cartilaginous attachment of the olecranon process, and the centrifugal forces generated can result in tearing off the olecranon process. Sperry and Pfalzgraf (1990) report on a child who suffered bilateral clavicular fractures due to "pseudo-chiropractic" manipulations meant to repair shoulders, which were believed to be dislocated.

The dangers of reliance entirely on the skeletal indicators for a diagnosis of child abuse should be emphasized. Fractures usually thought to be specific to abuse are found in low incidence (Merten *et al.* 1983). Patterns of multiple injuries and/or repeated injuries are more strongly suggestive of abuse than the presence or absence of specific injuries. Pathological conditions, such as osteogenesis imperfecta, must also be evaluated when making a determination because some will predispose children to fracture.

In cases of evident abuse, it is possible that the responsible party will be charged and brought to trial on the charge of abuse, regardless of the actual cause of death. Testimony by the forensic anthropologist becomes critical to the support or dismissal of the case, especially if the remains are fully skeletonized. Assessment of the pattern of skeletal damage as well as the extent of healing are important factors in determining the strength of the charges and must be well documented.

Elder Abuse and Abuse of Vulnerable Adults

The concept of elder abuse was introduced in 1975 by Burston as "granny-battering." It is believed to be as common as child abuse, but often the victims never disclose the abuse due to their lack of mobility and confinement within the areas where they are subject to abuse (Brogdon and McDowell 2003). Even at death, cause and manner of death often is attributed to natural causes and little or no investigation occurs. The phenomenon is believed to wide-spread with estimates of around one to two million Americans suffering from some form of abuse annually (Shields *et al.* 2004). Abuse can be physical, sexual, financial, or psychological, or it may involve confinement and/or neglect. The victims are also more vulnerable to injury due to poor skin and bone health (Collins 2006).

Studies show that, in most cases, the abuser is a family member or intimate partner (Cheatham 1983, Kingston 1994, Zhu *et al.* 2000, Collins 2006, National

Center on Elder Abuse 2006, Coelho *et al.* 2010, Friedman *et al.* 2011). Often the abuse follows a familial pattern of abuse. Over 80% of deaths occur in the residence of the decedent (Collins and Presnall 2006).

Among elderly victims of homicide, blunt force trauma occurs more than expected although it is exceeded by high-velocity projectile trauma (Falzon and Davis 1998, Collins and Presnall 2006). In other parts of the world, blunt force trauma may be more common (Coelho *et al.* 2010). Murphy and colleagues (2013) reviewed the literature on injuries from elder abuse. They found that the upper extremities were the most often affected, followed by maxillofacial, dental and neck, then skull, lower extremity, and torso. Almost two-thirds of the injuries were in the first two categories. Fractures often occur in the midfacial area. Death, however, may be due to neglect, natural causes or suicide (Akaza *et al.* 2003, Zephro and Galloway. this volume).

The abuse of vulnerable adults should also be part of any inquiry that shows a pattern of multiple injuries, particularly when there are different stages of healing. Since the reason behind the vulnerability may not be suggested from the skeletal evidence, any such pattern should be reported with enough attention to prompt further inquiry on the part of the investigators. However, since no pattern is fully diagnostic, overinterpretation is always a concern.

STRANGULATION

Strangulation is a common cause of death among homicide victims (Fischer *et al.* 1994). While strangulation is less frequent among males, it is found in close to half of female homicide victims and is a frequent cause of death in children under five years of age. Stangulation may be induced by one of three methods: (1) hanging, (2) ligature strangulation, and (3) manual strangulation. In hanging, the body is wholly or partially suspended. In many judicial hangings, the deceased is dropped with the rope angled under the chin and usually behind the ear (DiMaio and DiMaio 1989). However, hangings can also be accomplished by shorter or no drops and these forms are similar in nature to ligature strangulation. Ligatures usually encircle the neck horizontally while hanging involves a gravitational element with one part of the encircling material higher than the rest. With manual strangulation or throttling, hands, a forearm or other part of the body produces neck compression.

Hanging

The production of fractures in the second cervical vertebra has historically been claimed as the hallmark of judicial hangings involving a long drop.

However, this specific fracture is often not produced in judicial hangings although other cervical fractures may be found (Hellier and Connelly 2009). The length of the drop is determined by the weight and robusticity of the individual to be hanged (Lachman 1972). The goal is to produce a snapping of the spinal column, moving the head back forcefully and abruptly. Excessive drops will result in decapitation while those too short must rely upon strangulation to cause the death. In judicial hangings that proceed according to plan, the decedent loses consciousness immediately and will be dead within a short time. The heart often continues to beat for some time, up to 20 minutes, after the drop.

There is some disagreement as to the cause of death in such judicial hangings. Some argue that the fractured odontoid process is driven toward the medulla, which controls both the heartbeat and respiration, resulting in rapid death (Spitz and Fisher 1980, Spitz 2005). This is achieved by placing the knot under the left side of the jaw, producing a sudden hyperextension of the neck as the body reaches the end of the drop. Others (Lachman 1972) note that the spinal cord may be severed at the level of the fracture. A separation of up to 2.5 inches between C2 and C3 has been recorded. It is felt that the shock of the drop itself induces loss of consciousness, while death is brought on by the damage to the central nervous system or interruption of blood flow through the carotid and vertebral arteries (Hellier and Connelly 2009).

Fractures associated with hanging include the classic "hangman's" fracture or acute traumatic spondylolysis of the second cervical vertebra or fractures of the pedicles or laminae of the third or fourth cervical vertebrae. The likelihood of these fractures in the forensic setting is remote, as a substantial drop and correct placement of the knot is required to produce these fractures. Other causes such as hyperextension of the neck during motor vehicle accidents are the more likely source of injury.

Hyoid and thyroid cartilage fractures may be found with hanging (Spitz and Fisher 1980; Luke *et al.* 1985; DiMaio and DiMaio 1989, Betz and Eisenmenger 1996, Nikolic *et al.* 2003; Spitz 2005). Nonfusion of the greater horns of the hyoid, often confused with a fracture, must be determined (Chapter 8, this volume). These fractures are more common in the elderly and in those individuals in which there had been a substantial drop to the point of suspension. The rate of hyoid and thyroid fractures in accidental and suicidal hangings varies, but careful analysis reveals that single or multiple fractures are common (Paparo and Siegel 1984, Simpson and Knight 1985, DiMaio and DiMaio 1989, Green *et al.* 2000). Some of the discrepancies may be due to different methods of dissection, palpation, or radiography in the analysis of such fractures (Khokholov 1997). Several studies suggest that hyoid fractures occur in about a quarter of suicidal hangings while thyroid cartilage fractures vary between 13 and 37% (Luke *et al.* 1985, Green *et al.* 2000). Green and associates (2000) also noted that fracture patterns did not differ significantly by whether suspension was complete or partial. Betz and Eisenmenger (1996) reviewed cases of accidental and suicidal hanging and noted that fractures were common when the highest point of the noose was anywhere but directly in front of the chin. Nikolic and colleagues (2003), however, found no difference in noose position and fractures. Most studies note an increase in fracture with age in those who were not totally suspended. The thyroid cartilage is usually sufficiently calcified by the third decade to be subject to fracture (Knight 1991).

Ligature Strangulation

Many aspects of ligature strangulation overlap with those seen in hangings in which the drop was absent or insufficient to produce vertebral trauma. Ligatures themselves vary considerably from thin wires to thicker substances. In published surveys, 11–13% of ligature strangulations showed hyoid fractures and these were often associated with fractures in the thyroid and cricoid cartilages (Green 1973; Hansch 1977, DiMaio 2000). Harm and Rajs (1981) found such fractures in over 40% of their 12-case review. Since the hyoid is well protected behind the chin, the more superficial thyroid cartilage would be expected to fracture more frequently. Green (1973) reports more frequent fracture of the thyroid cartilage's cornua occurring in over one-third of cases. The hyoid is more likely to be damaged as the age of the victim increases or as the ligature widens, as well as when it is placed relatively high on the neck (Hansch 1977). The elasticity of the ligature is also a factor in the damage inflicted, since this can accommodate some of the force applied to the region. In addition, fractures of adjacent bones have been linked to ligature strangulation. Mandibular fractures and fractures of the laminae of the cervical vertebrae have been attributed to strangulation with a double wire noose tightened by twisting a solid object in a side loop (Angel and Caldwell 1984).

Manual Strangulation

Manual strangulation has been associated with damage to the bones and ossified cartilages of the throat (Plueckhahn and Cordner 1991, DiMaio 2000). The horseshoe-shaped hyoid bone and winged thyroid cartilage may be fractured (Spitz and Fisher 1980, Spitz 2005). Thyroid cartilage compression usually results in vertical fractures of the cornua (DiMaio and DiMaio 1989). The stronger, ring-like cricoid cartilage is located below the thyroid cartilage. Cricoid cartilage is less prone to fracturing during lateral compression but can be broken when pushed posteriorly against the cervical spine. The line of cleavage is usually vertical and may be at the midline or laterally placed.

While hyoid fractures are most often attributed to manual strangulation, they have been found with judicial, suicidal, and accidental hangings and ligature strangulations (Ubelaker 1992). The reported frequency of hyoid fracture in manual strangulation is variable, ranging from 17% to 71% (Gonzales 1933, Green 1973, Hansch 1977, Harm and Rajs 1981, Line *et al.* 1985, Ubelaker 1992). It is frequently associated with fractures of the thyroid cartilage, especially in the older individual in whom these structures have been ossified. Age seems to be one of the most significant factors, as fusion of the epiphyses of the hyoid as well as ossification of the thyroid cartilage increases with advancing years.

Variability is seen in the fracture patterns. Factors include the magnitude of the force applied to the neck, the precise position of the force and the rigidity of the hyoid and associated throat tissues. Reviews of hyoid fractures also suggest that curvature of the hyoid may be involved (Pollanen and Chiasson 1996; Pollanen *et al.* 1999). Those hyoids found to be fractured tended to be longer antero-posteriorly and more steeply sloping than the unfractured ones, producing an overall U-shaped morphology, rather than a V-shaped form to the bone. Most fractures were unilateral with the fracture site in the posterior or middle portions of the greater cornu. Anteriorly positioned fractures are only rarely found. Other factors, however, such as the level of strangulation on the neck, the force applied and the age of the individual are possibly more significant factors (Pollanen and Ubelaker 1997).

Other Circumstances with Similar Patterns

Hyoid fractures have been reported in deaths due to natural causes (Hansch 1977) or falls/accidents (Dickenson 1991, Dalati 2005, Bux *et al.* 2006). Myocardial infarction or other acute heart failure, which triggers intense contraction of the muscles of the throat, are thought to cause some isolated hyoid fractures. No reported links have been made between hyoid fracture and deaths due to autoerotic asphyxia, although this remains a possibility. In these cases, ligatures or the complex devices to induce asphyxia for non-lethal purposes usually are designed to minimize trauma, relying on body weight to compact the soft tissue (Uva 1995).

For the anthropologist, evidence of asphyxia due to compression of the throat tissue or traumatic rupture of the spinal cord may be difficult to determine. Frequently, no skeletal injuries are produced and the difficulty of having bones with highly variable rates of fusion or ossification complicates the issue. Care in recovery and extraction of the neck elements is critical, and separation of fractures from anomalous instances of non-fusion is essential. It is also important to remember that direct blows rather than constriction could produce fractures to the thyroid cartilage and even the cricoid cartilage and hyoid.

TRAUMA DUE TO MOTOR VEHICLES

Motor vehicle accidents are a leading cause of injury and death at all ages in America (Rogers 1992) and a primary cause of blunt force trauma as seen in the forensic setting (Raasch 1985). Motor vehicle accidents are the leading cause of death for Americans between ages five and 34 years. Deaths peak at age 20–24 years for males while at a slightly younger age in females, 15-19 years (O'Neill 1985). Fatal injuries are inflicted most often on the head and chest, and over half are multiple in nature (Raasch 1985). Drivers, passengers, and pedestrians may all suffer fatalities. These deaths may be induced by impact with other vehicles, stationary objects, or by portions of the occupied vehicle. Passengers of the vehicle will show different patterns of injuries based on where they were seated at the time of impact, whether their legs or ankles were crossed, what restraints they used and how they used them, their own body size and shape and the nature of the impact. People may be thrown clear of the impact and survive or may be thrown into the path of the collision. Modifications of the vehicle design and addition of safety restraints have provided significant improvements in the overall survival ratios but do not eliminate the hazards from critical vehicle failure or the much stronger effects of driver error.

Motor vehicle accidents can be classified by the area of impact: (1) front-end impact, (2) side impact, (3) rear impact, and (4) rollovers (DiMaio and DiMaio 1989). During motor vehicle accidents, there are drastic changes in acceleration and deceleration. When the moving vehicle strikes another object, part or all of the energy from the vehicle is absorbed by the object and deformation of the vehicle. The occupants are, however, semi-independent, traveling at the original speed of the vehicle upon impact. The energy from their momentum must be absorbed by their impact on restraint devices, the vehicle, or other objects. In many cases, the lower body is constrained by the dashboard or seats and the head and upper body are projected forward. In late model vehicles, steering wheel air bags can diffuse some of the potential for the head and upper body to strike the steering wheel, car doors and windows, or dashboard. However, the rapid rate at which air bags deploy has been the cause of nasal and rib fractures, especially in the elderly or osteoporotic individuals (Wallis and Greaves 2002).

In side collisions, victims are "left behind" as the vehicle initially accelerates in a new and unanticipated direction. Victims are thrown to the side that received the blow (Adelson 1974), hitting the interior of the car or being thrown across the car's interior. The neck undergoes lateral flexion, for which it is poorly suited. Superimposed on the injuries that result from these changes in momentum are those inflicted by direct blows to the interior and from the striking object. A similar situation exists with rear-end collisions, where the vehicle is rapidly propelled forward, leaving the passengers behind. Hyperextension of the neck is common.

The vast majority of motor vehicle accident victims are recovered shortly after the event. In some instances, however, anthropological assessment is helpful or even critical. Lack of witnesses may mean that an accident goes undiscovered until the decomposition process is advanced. If a vehicle leaves the road during the accident, it may remain undiscovered for some time. Pedestrians may be thrown off the road or the body moved after the accident in an effort to mask a hit-and-run event. There is always the possibility of fire accompanying the accident, and anthropological analysis may be required to properly recover the remains and facilitate identification and determination of the sequence of events. In two separate multi-fatality instances in Arizona, anthropological analysis at the accident scene allowed for correction of the fatality count, charted each victim's location accurately, and assisted in distinguishing accident-induced trauma from those fractures produced by fire.

Since the trauma of motor vehicle accidents may be extensive, autopsies may focus on only those injuries that are most likely responsible for the death. When the forensic anthropologist is confronted with the often partial and skeletonized remains of an accident victim, it may then be difficult to assess the injuries around death within a context of overall patterns of damage due to fire, fire extinguishment, body retrieval and transport, and autopsy.

The discussion below will examine motor vehicle accidents from different motor vehicle involvement with regard to the victim. Drivers and passengers are partly protected from the impact by the car in which they are enclosed. Motorcyclists lack many of the protective measures available to those inside vehicles. Pedestrians and bicyclists hit by motor vehicles are extremely vulnerable to massive trauma. Vehicular homicide and suicide need also to be considered. Motor vehicles usually refer to autos, trucks and motorcyclists, but trains and various aircraft also produce blunt force trauma during crashes. These various circumstances will be discussed below.

Driver/Passenger Injuries

Motor vehicle accidents cause injuries in drivers and passengers due to direct impact on the body as well as the drastic changes in movement due to deceleration or acceleration (Knight 1991). About 60–80% of accidents are frontal collisions involving another vehicle, a fixed structure, or other object. On impact, the vehicle will experience deformation that partly absorbs the energy produced, providing some protection to the occupants. However, this same deformation may intrude on the passenger compartment inflicting further damage. Safety features within the vehicle structure may also provide mitigating cushioning. The age of the victim also plays a role, with elderly suffering more chest wall injuries and lower extremity fractures (Nagata *et al.* 2010).

Injuries to occupants of motor vehicles are highly variable, especially if they are unrestrained. Head injuries, however, are quite common and injury to the brain is present in about 75% of all traffic deaths (Seelig and Marshall 1985). At speeds typical of motor vehicle accidents, skull fractures typically are (1) penetration/depressed fractures, (2) comminuted depressed, or (3) remote linear (McElhaney *et al.* 1976). These injuries are most dangerous in that underlying structures may be lacerated, particularly the meningeal arteries or the venous sinuses (Seelig and Marshall 1985). Head injuries are particularly frequent among ejectees, usually as the result of striking an object or surface outside the vehicle. Basilar fractures, which run along the petrous portion and through the sella turcica in the typical "hinge" pattern, are commonly found (DiMaio and DiMaio 1989).

Facial fractures are a common feature of motor vehicle accidents (Cormier and Duma 2009, Hitosugi *et al.* 2011, Natu *et al.* 2012). The most common bones to be broken are the nasals when there is a frontal impact followed by maxillary and mandibular fractures. The nose is rarely broken in side impacts. Instead the frontal bone and mandible are the most commonly fractured in side impacts, which often have a frontal-impact component.

Many vehicle passengers, including the driver, suffer damage to the neck from the drastic deceleration and from impact of the head against the windshield or other portions of the interior of the car. Often these injuries occur without any severe head trauma, and actual head impact is not necessary to involve cervical fractures (Shkrum *et al.* 1989, Robertson *et al.* 2002).

Unrestrained drivers experience direct chest impact but also flexion injuries in the cervical and thoracic spine (Blacksin 1993). In most cases, fractures occur at or below the level of the second cervical vertebra, although fractures of the atlas may be found. More frequently found are teardrop fractures of the lower cervical vertebrae. The articular pillars and laminae are particularly prone to fracturing. Whiplash injuries with hyperextension of the neck may also involve some bony damage, usually to the posterior elements of the lower cervical spine. These are most often due to rear-end collisions and may occur either lower in the neck, at about the C5–C6 level, or at the top of the atlanto-occipital joint (Spitz and Fisher 1980, Spitz 2005). The headrests and airbags prevent these injuries (Morris 1989, Mikhail and Huelke 1997).

Fractures also may occur in the upper cervical/occipital complex when there is extension of the neck during motor vehicle accidents (Hadley *et al.* 1988, DiMaio and DiMaio 1989, Shkrum *et al.* 1989). In fact, one survey showed that 68% of the acute atlas fractures were due to motor vehicle accidents and an additional 7% to motorcycle accidents. In these cases, the lateral masses and pedicles of C1 and C2 are the points of greatest leverage between the head and the neck. Classic "hangman's fractures" of the first and second cervical vertebrae are reported and "Jefferson" fractures of the atlas may also occur. The latter tend to be less fatal as damage may be less severe due to the outward splaying of the C1, avoiding extensive damage to the spinal cord, but in other cases the spinal cord may be injured.

Rib and sternal fractures occur in the driver from impact on the steering wheel (Watanabe 1972, Knight 1991, Spitz and Fisher 1980, Spitz 2005). Thoracic compression also may result from the vehicle rolling over an ejected passenger (Adelson 1974). Typical injuries include transverse fractures of the sternum and bilateral rib fractures (DiMaio and DiMaio 1989). Rib fractures become increasingly common with advancing age as rib resilience declines through childhood and the bone density decreases with old age. Rib fractures are often linked to facial fractures in front-end collisions as the person is thrown forward onto the window, dashboard, or a forward seatback.

Pelvic injuries are also found in motor vehicle accidents, particularly when seat belts have not been used. It was noted early in the development of our automobile-based transportation system that there was a suite of injuries associated with motor vehicle accidents that included pelvic injuries and hip dislocations. One study in 1954 reported that hip dislocations went from being a rare occurrence to one relatively common, due to the number of auto accidents, which produced 72% of the hip injuries examined (Stewart and Milford 1954). While these injuries are relatively less common in total injuries, pelvic fractures are more common among fatalities (Walz 1984). Occupants of cars and other vehicles account for two-thirds of the pelvic fractures with the rest found among pedestrians. Injuries to the lower abdomen and pelvic girdle result from either direct blows or through restraint devices (Dejeammes 1984). Direct blows may result in fractures of the anterior pelvic girdle, usually but not always on the side of the blow as discussed in Chapter 11.

The pelvis is particularly vulnerable as it receives forces transmitted from the femora. "Instrument panel syndrome" is one complex of pelvic injuries recognized early in auto safety evaluation (Kulowski 1961). This complex results from the knees striking the instrument panel, driving the femoral heads into the acetabula. The hip joint fractures and there is luxation of the femoral head (Walz 1984). This often begins with patella fracture and a longitudinal split of the distal femur. There may also be fracture of the proximal femur as the body's momentum carries it past the fracture point of these elements. Subsequent to this, the body jackknifes and the head may be thrown into the windshield, steering wheel or dashboard.

Drivers are particularly vulnerable through the pressure they are frequently placing on the brake pedal prior to the impact. This stiffening of the leg drives the hip upward, often resulting in a postero-superior dislocation (Stewart and Milford 1954). Passengers tend to have a hip that is more flexed at impact and is therefore driven downward and back with less damage sustained by the acetabulum. An exception is with passengers in unrestrained "crew seats" such as are often seen on shuttle buses and other vehicles where the seats line the outer edge leaving central standing or luggage room. Eyers and Roberts (1993) reported on 11 of 12 passengers injured in a minibus accident who had pelvic fractures from lateral compression presumably from sliding down the bench into each other in a "domino effect."

Injuries to the lower legs may also be found. These fractures may be due to direct trauma (Spitz and Fisher 1980, Knight 1991, Spitz 2005) or they may be due to attempts by occupants to anticipate the impact forces. Drivers may press hard on the brake pedal, resulting in compression fractures of the foot and ankle. The floorboards may be driven upward and inward, wrenching the foot and producing fractures at a number of points from the foot through to the hip. Portions of the vehicle, such as the engine block, may be rammed inward trapping the lower limbs of the occupants. The seat may also move forward, breaking the ankle. Backseat passengers may be thrown forward while their feet and lower legs are wedged beneath the front seats. This situation will produce bending fractures in the lower tibia and fibula.

In side impacts, fractures will tend to be unilateral, on the side of impact (DiMaio and DiMaio 1989). Arms as well as legs may be broken. Lateral flexion compression fractures of the neck may occur. However, facial fractures are less frequent than in frontal collisions (Cormier and Duma 2009). Furthermore, these facial fractures were even less frequent when the impact was on the far than the near side if the person was not wearing a seat belt. Fractures other than in the neck are not common in rear-end collisions due to the protection provided by the seats and the trunk of the vehicle (DiMaio and DiMaio 1989).

Rollover accidents may produce an array of injuries. Often only part of the body is protruding from the car. This portion will suffer massive damage as the car rolls over it while the rest of the body is relatively untouched. Backseat passengers are vulnerable to ejection and may suffer numerous and massive head, chest, and limb injuries (Knight 1991). In some cases, the ejection is partial and does not involve a rollover. However, protruding portions of the body will exhibit extensive damage or detachment (Morild and Lilleng 2012).

Due to the implementation of mandatory seat belt laws followed by shoulder-lap combinations, air bags and side-impact bags, the pattern of injuries has undergone secular change. Seat belts have reduced the risk of fatality in motor vehicle accidents by 43–86% (Evans 1986, Rivara *et al.* 2000). Upper extremity injuries average 13.7% for unrestrained drivers but decrease by 2–2.5% with seat belts (Petrucelli 1984). Lower limb trauma is more substantial, found in 22% of all injuries for unrestrained drivers. With seat belts, these are reduced by 7–11%. Much of this decrease is the result of preventing impact with the dashboard. Prior to the implementation of car restraints, dashboard and front compartment impact were responsible for 50% of upper extremity and 60% of lower extremity injuries. An additional 20% of the lower limb injuries were inflicted by the floor (Gershuni 1985).

While seat belts responsible for a dramatic lowering in the mortality from automobile accidents, they also produce some patterns of fracture themselves. Lap-type seat belts generate shearing forces during front impact crashes and can produce compression fractures of the lumbar vertebrae along with horizontal fractures in the transverse processes and posterior elements (Haddad and Zickel 1967; Levine 1992). These *chance* fractures are found between T12 and L4 and concentrate in the L2–L4 region. About half are associated with serious intra-abdominal injuries. Shoulder harnesses can concentrate forces on the bony portions of the shoulder, particularly the clavicle and sternum (Johnson and Branfoot 1992). They have been implicated in production of sternal fractures, although these usually are not associated with serious chest injuries (Peek and Firmin 1995). Experimental studies show that rib fractures occur early in chest compression from the body being thrown against the shoulder belt (Kemper *et al.* 2011). In this study, the first fractures occurred at the lower margin of the rib cage, where the belt moves into the abdominal region. Only then were fractures found in the mid-thoracic region.

The introduction of air bags further reduces overall injuries including those of the spine. Used with seatbelts, fatalities in cars equipped with airbags dropped by 48% (Stacey *et al.* 2008). Facial fractures show a dramatic drop in accidents in which airbag and seat belt were in use at the time of impact (Loo *et al.* 1996, Murphy *et al.* 2000, Stacey *et al.* 2008, Cormier and Duma 2009). Similarly, upper extremity fractures are less frequent (McGwin *et al.* 2003). Much of these decreases are due to the effect of the seatbelt, however.

Air bags can, however, inflict their own damage during accidents. Children incorrectly positioned in their car seats are at risk, and elderly individuals (Jumbelic 1995) have been killed by the rapid inflation of the air bag. These devices inflate at a rate of 144–211 mph within one-twentieth of a second from impact. This rapid inflation can produce massive chest damage including rib and sternal fractures, somewhat reminiscent of the steering wheel impacts the devices were designed to prevent. A case was reported where an elderly woman who drew her seat close to the steering wheel was killed by the impact of the rapidly inflating air bag against her chest following a minor accident (Jumbelic 1995). Blacksin (1993) noted that drivers sitting close to the steering wheel force the airbag upward under the chin, producing hyperextension fractures in the neck.

Motorcyclists

Motorcyclists and their passengers are at far greater risk of injury than those in enclosed vehicles (Waller 1985, Knight 1991, Plueckhahn and Cordner 1991, Hinds *et al.* 2007). Aside from a helmet, there is little protection for the motorcycle rider. Most fatalities are among young men in their late teens and early twenties. Excessive speed, inexperience, and alcohol consumption are significant contributing factors (Whittington 1981, Bjornstig *et al.* 1985, Aare and von Holst 2003). The majority of accidents are caused by collisions with other vehicles or with stationary objects (Zettas *et al.* 1979), The extent of injuries depends on the nature of the collision. The increased use of mopeds results similar fracture patterns as seen in motorcycles but the frequency of injury is about twice as high (Aare and von Holst 2003).

Motorcycle accidents often entail head and neck injuries (DiMaio and DiMaio 1989, Knight 1991, Varley *et al.* 1993). Skull fractures amongst motor-cyclists are also typically more severe than in other motor vehicle accidents (Haug *et al.* 1992) and when drivers are traveling at high speeds (Varley *et al.* 1993). Skull fractures, particularly basilar ones including hinge fractures, are frequent as the rider is thrown to the ground or strikes a stationary object. Atlanto-occipital avulsions and ring fractures of the base of the skull may be produced by flexion and anterior traction of the neck during head-on collisions with automobiles (Maeda *et al.* 1993). Transverse fractures across the greater wing of the sphenoids and passing through the sella turcica have been called "motor-cyclist's fractures" (Knight 1991). Cervical fractures are also found. Severe head and neck injuries are also seen in instances where the cyclist was closely following a truck and, at impact, the machine passed under the truck while the motorcyclist was caught by the tailboard. Decapitation may occur in such situations. In general, helmeted riders sustain fewer head, face, and neck injuries in motorcycle accidents than do those without helmets (Waller 1985, Ankarath *et al.* 2002, Murphy *et al.* 2009) and head injury risk is reported to drop by 72% with helmets (Liu *et al.* 2003).

Motorcyclists often exhibit multiple fractures when they have crashed (Robertson *et al.* 2002). They will show isolated injuries less frequently than occupants of a car. Open pelvic fractures also are common with motorcycle accidents, accounting for almost one-fifth to one-fourth of these injuries (Rothenberger *et al.* 1978; Richardson *et al.* 1982). Ankhrath and colleagues (2002) noted higher frequency of lower thoracic/upper lumbar fractures than others of the spine. Robertson and colleagues (2002) also noted high levels of thoracic injuries among those motorcyclists who experienced spinal damage, especially the seventh thoracic vertebra. Rib and clavicular fractures may be produced as the rider hits the ground or other object (Knight 1991, Varley *et al.* 1993). Radial fractures, involving severe intra-articular comminution, are common in some studies to the point that they called "motorcycle radius" (Zettas et al. 1979, Varley et al. 1993). Other lower limb injuries are also common amongst this group (Zettas *et al.* 1979, Varley *et al.* 1993, Aare and von Holst 2003, Murphy *et al.* 2009). Lateef (2002) notes that not only are lower limb fractures more common, but the bones most often injured are the tibia and fibula, followed by ankle fractures, while Ankhrath and colleagues (2002) found femoral fractures followed the tibial fractures in frequency. Foot injuries, while trailing other major injury patterns, are also relatively common, particularly affecting the metatarsals (Jeffers *et al.* 2003).

Murphy and colleagues (2009) compared the fracture patterns between driver and passengers in accidents involving "biker couples." Drivers are more likely than passengers to exhibit scapular and rib fractures. Scapular fractures are themselves associated with more significant fracture patterns in other areas of the body. Otherwise, there is little difference in the fracture patterns between drivers and passengers.

Similar injuries are found with other vehicles in which the driver and passengers are not enclosed. Accidents with all-terrain vehicles may involve drivers too young to legally operate a vehicle on the road (Bolthrop *et al.* 2007, Hall *et al.* 2009). ATVs are prone to rollover accidents, especially as they are used in off-road situations. Like other vehicles, drivers also lose control and collide with stationary objects. ATV accidents are most common among rural males and alcohol use is common and lack of helmets close to universal in these accidents. Unfortunately, spinal fractures are frequent in ATV users with Boltrop and associates (2007) finding about a quarter those brought to a trauma center to have sustained spinal fracture or dislocation. Of these spinal injuries, the majority occurred in the cervical area in some reviews although others place them in the thoracolumbar levels. Spinal injuries are especially common in children (Sawyer *et al.* 2012). Younger children are more likely to have lumbar fractures, while adolescents experience thoracic fractures more often. Other ATV-related fractures include rib, forearm, and leg fractures. Among fatalities, off-road accidents are more frequently due to rollovers, while on-road accidents tended to be due to collisions.

Automobile Versus Pedestrian (AVP) Injuries

Pedestrian fatalities affect all age groups, although school-age children and the elderly seem at particularly high risk (O'Neill 1985, Waller 1985, Demitriades *et al.* 2004). Such accidents represent a significant percentage of seriously injured patients in hospital emergency rooms (Hannon *et al.* 2009). Alcohol impairment is also a common feature in many pedestrian victims (Haddon *et al.* 1961). People are hit as they walk along a road, as they attempt to cross a road despite traffic, as they attempt to retrieve items left in the road, or even when they sit or lie down in the roadway. Adult pedestrians are often hit from behind, but many turn moments before impact so that the initial circumstances may be masked. Multiple vehicles may strike the same individual. For example, one individual was recovered with grease stains on his abdomen made as a car passed over his prone body. It appeared that somewhat groggily, he then sat up to see what had happened and was fatally injured in the face and head by a subsequent vehicle (A. Jones, personal communication). This example illustrates a common feature in that many victims of being pulled under a car are already highly intoxicated (Karger *et al.* 2001).

When a car hits a pedestrian, the types of injuries produced depend, in part, upon the velocity of the car and position of the pedestrian. Other factors include the weight and mass of the vehicle; the configuration of the impacting surface; whether the speed of the car is being reduced; the age, height, and weight of the pedestrian; and the location of impact on the body of the pedestrian. Ehrlich and colleagues (2009) have shown that the changes in front design of cars, incorporating more even and rounded front ends with more yield on impact, have changed the pattern of injuries. Passenger cars in the 1970–80s produced significantly more head injuries, while cars in the 1990s to mid-2000s were less likely to produce head and lower leg injuries, but chest, abdominal, and pelvic injuries increased dramatically. Light trucks have been linked to higher than expected incidence of severe injury although lower limb injuries were similar to cars and vans (Roudsari *et al.* 2004). SUVs and trucks tend to produce fractures higher on the leg (Ballesteros *et al.* 2004).

Injuries can be classed as (1) primary, resulting from the impact with the vehicle or (2) secondary, due to impact with the road (Adelson 1974; Spitz and Fisher 1980; Knight 1991; Plueckhahn and Cordner 1991, Spitz 2005). Pedestrian accidents may also be grouped by the movement of the body with regard to the vehicle. Victims may be "run under" or "run over." They may also be side-swiped by a passing vehicle.

Most pedestrians are actually "run under" since, in the adult, the center of gravity for the body is usually higher than the impacting portion of the vehicle. When struck, the upper portion of the body falls toward the vehicle as the lower legs are "swept out from under" him or her by the bumper. At this point, the victim strikes the front body of the car and then is hurled against the windshield or corners of the car. In some cases, the victim may actually be launched upward so that they land on the roof. The bumper produces the primary injuries on the knees and lower legs, the front of the vehicle strikes on the hip and thigh, the hood produces injuries on the ribs, while the hood/windshield/roof strikes the head. The faster the vehicle, the farther back the pedestrian usually will be thrown before landing on the car (DiMaio and DiMaio 1989). At very high speeds, the car may pass entirely under the pedestrian as they are thrown upwards. The secondary injuries are incurred as the victim rolls off the back of the car and hits the roadway. In cases where the pedestrian was thrown forward, chest and arm injuries may be concentrated on the side opposite that of impact (Knight 1991).

In contrast, when the victim has a lower center of gravity, when the vehicle has a higher chassis or a more vertical frontend such as with a truck, minivan, or

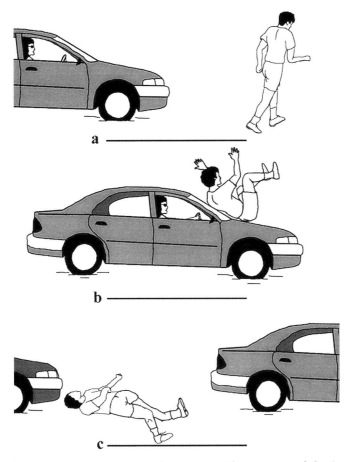

Figure 7-1. Movement of the pedestrian during impact by an automobile. An adult struck by a motor vehicle is typically hit on the legs and thigh, below the center of gravity (a). This causes the person to be thrown upward and onto the front end of the car where they will sustain additional injuries on the head and shoulders as they hit the hood and windshield (b). The victim then usually rolls off the vehicle back onto the pavement, where they may be hit by a second vehicle (c). (Modified from W. V. Spitz and R. S. Fisher, *Medicolegal Investigation of Death.* Springfield: Charles C Thomas, 1980.)

van or when the vehicle is moving more slowly (less than 15 mph), the pedestrian may be thrown forward then pulled under the vehicle in a classic "run over" accident (Spitz and Fisher 1980, Knight 1991, Spitz 2005). This category often includes those hit by cars moving backwards, although at high speeds, the injuries will duplicate those of a car moving forward. Pedestrians who are run over likely exhibit compression, shearing, and crushing injuries. The wheels may amputate limbs, segment the torso, or twist the spine and rib cage to the point of breakage (Gonzalez *et al.* 1954, Spitz and Fisher 1980, Spitz 2005).

The victim may be pinned against the front of the vehicle for some distance before falling to the road. The wheels may pass over the body producing some crushing injuries. If the victim is actually run "over" and the vehicle has a low chassis, rolling injuries may result. The victim may become trapped in the undercarriage and be dragged, on some occasions for considerable distances. The body may become detached from the car well away from the impact site. The bones may then exhibit abrasion marks or even polish from the roadway as the soft tissue is worn off and the bones "filed" down.

Because of differences in body proportions, children often are run over by a vehicle. Small children are more likely to be thrown forward upon being struck, thus sustaining femoral and chest injuries from the initial collision and head injuries from the landing (Wilber and Thompson 1994). They are also subject to being pulled under the car, exhibiting chest and head injuries from contact with the vehicle and lower extremity injuries from the wheels.

Furthermore, young children are prone to accidents with slow-moving vehicles as they may play or walk around cars in driveways and parking lots. These injuries may be almost entirely primary and include considerable compression or bending injuries. Crushing of the thoracic cavity and skull are common among the fatal injuries in these cases. Such injuries may be violent enough to produce extrusion of the brain or internal organs of the thoracic and abdominal cavities. The action of a vehicle passing over a body combines both compression and tearing (Figure 7-2) (Watanabe 1972). The extreme resilience of the bones in children may prevent fracture of the ribs and vertebrae during such compression while allowing for destruction of the internal organs (Spitz and Fisher 1980, Spitz 2005). Shearing forces generated by the tire may amputate body portions.

Distinguishing a victim of a "run-under" accident from one who was, in fact, run over is made more difficult by the subsequent "running over" by other vehicles once the victim of a run-under accident lands back on the road. The main identifiers of victims who have been hit by a vehicle and "run-under" are the glass fragments with the body, car paint on clothing, especially of the lower extremities, and abrasions on the soles of the shoes (Karger *et al.* 2001). Victims who were run over may exhibit tire tracks on the clothing or oil smears. These observations lie within the realm of the scene investigators. The anthropologist should note, however, wedge-shaped or "butterfly" bumper fractures (see below) and traumatic amputations which are associated with impact victims rather than those run over by a vehicle. Both situations result in similar incidence of fracture of head, chest, abdominal, upper limb, and upper leg injuries.

Pedestrians may also be "sideswiped." These victims often lack the more characteristic leg injuries but may sustain head injuries as they are thrown to the side by the vehicle. Because they may be launched off the roadway,

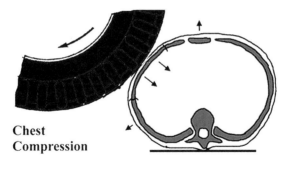

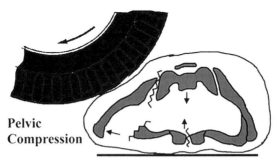

Figure 7-2. Compression of the body during rollover accidents. Passage of a wheel over the body will compress the rib cage or pelvis, producing serious fracture patterns due to the angulation produced. (Modified from T. Watanabe, *Atlas of Legal Medicine.* Philadelphia: J. B. Lippincott, 1972.)

such victims may lie for some time before being discovered if the driver fails to stop.

Head injury is the most common cause of death in car-pedestrian accidents (Chandra *et al.* 1979, Waller 1985). Often these will occur without significant damage to the rest of the body. In most cases, these fractures are found in the cranial vault without damage to the base of the skull. Often, though, injuries are so extensive that discrete patterns cannot be determined. The cervical spine may be hyperextended upon impact producing fractures of the arch (Spitz and Fisher 1980, Spitz 2005). In some cases, these may be the only injuries significant enough to cause the death. In the elderly, the risk of intracranial injury increases dramatically compared to younger adults but the risk of skull fracture appears to remain relatively constant (Richards and Carroll 2012).

While head injuries may be the most common cause of death, multiple points of injury and fracture are seen in automobile versus pedestrian accidents (Gonzalez *et al.* 1954, Watenabe 1972, Spitz and Fisher 1980, DiMaio and DiMaio 1989, Spitz 2005, Hannon *et al.* 2009). Spinal injuries are uncommon in children but increase dramatically with age. Cervical and lumbar fractures are often found with the primary impact (Karger *et al.* 2001, Vives *et al.* 2008), however, these are not exclusive to this category of victim (Teresinski and Madro 2002). As the vehicle hits the body, usually in the lower legs, the cervical and lumbar spine experience overextension/flexion, rotation or shearing forces resulting in damage. When the victim is run over, the crushing fractures are more common in the spine, often the thoracic region. Martos and Jackowski (2012) note that fractures of the transverse processes of the thoracic and lumbar vertebrae are frequent in overrun victims, may occur bilaterally, and usually involve more than one process along the spinal column. Fractures of the spinous process also may occur. The number and complexity is often greater in the thoracic area in overrun victims while infrequent in impact victims. The researchers postulate that these fractures occur when the spine is pressed against the ground by the overrunning car.

Pelvic fractures are common in the pedestrian with car-pedestrian accidents and increase in incidence with age (Demetriades *et al.* 2004). In one large survey, almost 40% of all pelvic fractures were found in occupants of cars, 30% in pedestrians (Rothenberger *et al.* 1978). For the more lethal open pelvic fractures, the rates were only 9% among occupants and almost 60% among pedestrians. About 80% of pelvic fractures in pedestrians are from the initial impact, only 20% from the secondary impact of the ground. These may be of the open type resulting in perforation of major organs or blood vessels (Perry 1980). Since these may be quite severe, death may occur quickly due to loss of blood. Older pedestrians are almost twice as likely to have pelvic fractures, compared to young adults (Demetriades *et al.* 2004, Siram *et al.* 2011). Women are more likely to suffer these types of fracture.

Lower extremity fractures vary by the bumper height and the speed of the vehicle. Faster speeds are associated with tibial and femoral fractures, while lower speeds often affect the knee joint. Femoral fractures are more common in children than adults, presumably because their shorter height places the thigh at bumper level (Demetriades *et al.* 2004, Hannon *et al.* 2009). Tibial fractures are the most common fracture among pedestrians struck by automobiles (Demetriades *et al.* 2004, Hannon *et al.* 2009). "Boot-top" fractures of the tibia and fibula are common due to the bumper of the vehicle striking the legs (Breitenecker 1959, Spitz and Fisher 1980, DiMaio and DiMaio 1989, Teresinski and Madro 2002, Spitz 2005). The more common pattern is for a butterfly fragment to be formed within the tibia with the base of the wedge at the point of impact (Rockhold and Herrmann 1999). Often the fractures are at different heights on the legs, suggesting that the pedestrian was walking or running when hit. Usually, but not always, the higher injury is the one hit while the foot was on the ground. The non-weight-bearing leg is more likely to suffer a transverse fracture than a butterfly or oblique fracture (Knight 1991). A study by Patrick and associates (1968) showed that fractures can be produced at relatively slow speeds. Leg fractures were produced beginning at a speed of 14.5 mph at impact, and, by 25 mph, these were quite severe with multiple breaks.

Matsui's study (2004) on bumper heights also notes the importance of observing femoral and knee fractures. Higher bumpers are more frequently linked to femoral fractures while lower ones are more likely to produce tibial fractures. Unfortunately, bumpers themselves vary in the construction and where on the bumper impact occurs can affect the severity of injury, with impacts on the center of the bumper usually being less problematic that those to the side (Matsui *et al.* 2011). In a review of accidents, the bumpers on newer cars appear to produce fewer and less severe fractures (Otte *et al.* 2007). Some pathologists advocate measurement of the height of the fracture to compare to the suspected vehicle. This, theoretically, can help determine if the car was actively braking at the time of impact if the height of injury was lower than the normal height of the bumper. However, this measurement can be distorted by other factors such as whether or not the pedestrian was wearing boots, in which case fractures often occur at the top of the boot (Eisele *et al.* 1983). There is simply too much variability in fracture height to correlate it to an actual bumper height although gross determinations (high versus low) may be indicated.

An additional injury that does not preserve as well in skeletal material is bone bruising within the bones of the knee (Teresinski and Madro 2002). These defects are often also accompanied by avulsion and compression fractures around the knee and support the contention that the person was upright at the time of impact. Matsui (2005) also notes the importance of knee injuries, particularly through the ligaments. At impact, slower vehicles tend to displace the portion of the leg relative to the next segment (leg or thigh), producing damage at the knee joint while faster ones produce fractures at the impact point. Cadaver studies verify that knee injuries will occur at lower energy levels than femoral fractures (Matsui *et al.* 2004).

Not all motor vehicle accidents involve individuals who have acted predictably. Passengers riding in the back of a pickup may perch on the side, only to be thrown backwards when the truck hits a bump or takes a curve. There are some unusual situations such as fatalities among "car-surfers" who, while strapped to the hood or roof of the car, sometimes obscure the vision of the driver causing them to drive off the road (Kohr 1992). Others lean out of a car to strike or catch something, only to misjudge distance and speed.

Another form of "car-pedestrian" accident involves bicyclists. Bicyclists may also be injured in single-vehicle accidents (Waller 1985). Head injuries are the most common cause of death (Knight 1991, Plueckhahn and Cordner 1991). Males seem to be at greater risk among adults, although, in children, both sexes are vulnerable (Hawley *et al.* 1995). Cyclists hit by vehicles will follow a similar trajectory to the adult pedestrian (Adelson 1974). The exception is that they often have fewer severe leg injuries since the legs are not in a weight-bearing position at the time of impact (Otte *et al.* 2007). Tibial and fibular fractures tend to occur more distally, near the ankle joint, compared to the victim who was standing at impact. However, like pedestrians, bicyclists will exhibit wedge fractures.

Vehicular Homicide And Suicide

True vehicular homicides in which the auto is used as the weapon are very difficult to distinguish from accidental deaths. The scene investigation is often crucial (Copeland 1986) as is the review of the victim's and possible suspect's backgrounds. Documentation of injuries is extremely important as such cases are difficult to pursue for the prosecution while the defense may be able to show high likelihood of lack of intent.

In some cases, attempts are made to disguise a homicide as a motor vehicle accident when, in fact, other weapons were used (Knight 1991). Knowledge of the most common patterns of injury becomes important in identifying inconsistent injuries. For example, injuries to one side of the body may be consistent with a person in the passenger position when it is claimed that they were the driver. Injury impressions may also be useful in either matching or excluding material at the scene as potential impactors. Of course, all of this becomes extremely difficult when working solely with skeletonized material.

Spitz and Fisher (1980) and Spitz (2005) show the importance of linking autopsy evidence to the vehicular damage. In one case, they describe how a man killed his wife by blunt force to the head, placed her in the car, and jammed the gas pedal down. Although the car ran off the road, drifted back across the road, up an embankment, struck a tree, and rolled over, the head injuries were the only damage seen on the body and the car was only minimally dented. The husband was later convicted of the crime.

Vehicular suicide is another possibility that must be considered by the coroner/medical examiner. These may be extremely difficult to distinguish in cases where the interval between death and investigation are lengthy. The clues are more likely to come from the context of the death rather than the types of injuries. Often the circumstances of the death include an isolated location, a lack of skid marks suggesting that there was no attempt to brake, and the vehicle striking squarely on an obvious stationary object. Some "traffic deaths" may be natural deaths that occur while in the car and may have parallels to the above circumstances. Skeletally, injuries are unlikely to allow much distinction of these cases, although most occur with minimal trauma to either the person or the vehicle (Baker and Spitz 1970) and the injuries related to fighting for control of the vehicle or attempting to brake are unlikely to be found.

Several cases of vehicle-assisted suicide have been reported that ended in complete or partial decapitation (Byard and Gilbert 2002, Turk and Tsokos 2005, Morild and Lilleng 2012). In these cases, a rope was tied around the neck and the other end around a stationary object. The individual then drove the car away until the rope cut into the neck causing soft and hard tissue damage.

RAILROAD-RELATED INJURIES

Railway fatalities include (1) those that occur within the train in which the passenger experiences impacts during a crash similar to those of any other unrestrained motor vehicle accident although with greater force, (2) those involving collisions between trains and other vehicles, and (3) those that involve people on or near the tracks. The last of these types of fatalities will produce patterns of injuries that depend upon the position of the victim and the type of accident (impact, running over, etc.) (Watenabe 1972). The mass of the train is such that even glancing blows can produce devastating injuries (Cina *et al.* 1994. In some cases, trains are used to commit suicide (Radbo *et al.* 2005, Silla and Luoma 2012) usually resulting in decapitation (Knight 1991, Cina *et al.* 1994, Lin and Gill 2009). They have also been used to mask a homicide (Murphy 1976) by producing such massive damage to the body that reconstruction is difficult and discerning pre-impact from impact damage from the skeletal remains almost impossible.

In an extensive review of European railroad collisions and derailments (Evans 2011), most fatalities occurred at level crossings and often involved trains hitting vehicles on the tracks. Such events generally had a lower number of fatalities while collisions between trains produced a higher death toll. Fortunately, fatalities involving collisions between trains or train derailments are infrequent and these events attract enough notoriety that investigations are prompt. In such impacts, bodies exhibit a combination of blunt and sharp force trauma due to the fragmentation of the metal structure of the carriage. Thermal damage may also be present (Murphy 1976). In a review of one such incident, non-survivable chest (75%) and head injuries (54%) were found among the victims (Shackleford *et al.* 2011). Spinal fractures were also frequent with 71% of victims showing some vertebral fracture, particularly in the cervical area. In two cases, the victims did not show the massive impact but were trapped under debris and likely died of asphyxia.

A more common occurrence is the vehicle hit by a train, usually at a level crossing (Murphy 1976). Such individuals sustain massive blunt force trauma from the train but also impact from the fragmentation of the vehicle itself. Traumatic amputations are less likely to occur in this group than with pedestrians (Shapiro *et al.* 1994).

The typical pedestrian hit by a train is male and often highly intoxicated (Cina *et al.* 1994, Shapiro 1994, Silla and Luoma 2012). In many instances, victims have been reported to be sitting or lying on the tracks at the time of impact and have been unresponsive to warnings. The injury pattern in general mimics that of car-pedestrian accidents except that the damage is almost always much more extensive and mutilating (Gonzalez *et al.* 1954, Cina *et al.* 1994). The characteristic type of injury is amputation of those portions of the body that extended across the tracks (Watanabe 1972). The skull is often crushed. Traumatic amputation of limbs is common, particularly of the lower limbs (Shapiro 1994). There may be massive segmentation of the remains, which, since moving trains are unable to quickly come to a halt, will be strewn along the track for considerable distances. For example, a relatively obese man overcome by alcohol was hit by a freight train and his body scattered along the track for about half of a mile. At autopsy, investigators were presented with a body bag of limbs, muscle, and fat. It took almost 45 minutes to locate a small portion of the mandible with some dentition, the only bone still adhering to a virtually intact face (Galloway 1996). Rail deaths of pedestrians are often associated with massive damage corresponding to the width of the actual rail (Lin and Gill 2009). The same may be seen with skeletal evidence where an area is unreconstructable due to the pulverization of the bones in this area (Figure 7-3).

A critical decision to be made about train-pedestrian deaths is whether or not they are accidental, suicidal, or homicidal. Skeletal evidence is rarely

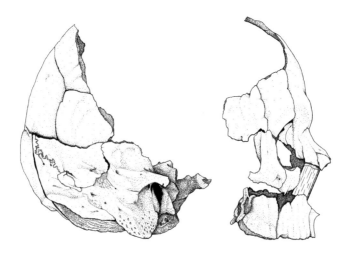

Figure 7-3. Skull reconstruction of an individual on the train tracks. Large gap shows the probable location of the track and remaining cranial fragments were too small to facilitate reconstruction. Illustration by Mathew J. Wedel.

helpful in this determination. A study of the New York City subway system deaths found that suicides were the most common mode of death, most of the deaths due to blunt force trauma from the train rather than electrocution (Lin and Gill 2009). Both decapitation and torso transection were more common with suicides than accidental deaths. Suicidal individuals tend to jump immediately in front of the train, lie down on the tracks, or stand on the track braced for impact. Train surfing, where people ride on the roof of the train, and skylarking, hanging onto the outside of the cars, has also been linked to deaths (Lin and Gill 2009). Usually these are attributable to impacts with structures that are close to the tracks.

AIRCRAFT-RELATED INJURIES

Aircraft crashes can usually be fit into one of six basic patterns: (1) "nose dive," (2) spin impact, (3) spiraling impact, (4) low angle, (5) in-flight disintegration, or (6) wire strike (DiMaio and DiMaio 1989). In a "nose dive," the angle of impact is steep and the plane becomes buried into a relatively small area, sometimes producing a crater. Heavier components are most deeply buried and there is massive compacting of bodies, plane, luggage, and debris. Examples include the Colorado Springs, Colorado crash (Fulginiti *et al.* 1999), the ValuJet Flight 592 crash in southern Florida in 1996, and the 9/11 crash of United Flight 93 in Pennsylvania. If the plane is also spinning during the descent, the airspeed may drop, decreasing the degree of fragmentation. Planes may also be spiraling and usually the wings strike separately, wrenching the craft apart and strewing it over a wide area. When impact is at a low angle, there is usually somewhat less damage to the entire plane. There may be successful landings of the plane as occurred in US Airways Flight 1549, which landed in the Hudson River, or the catastrophic landing of Arrow Air flight 1285 in 1985 killing 256 Canadians. In-flight disintegration may involve explosions such as the Pan Am flight 103 over Lockerbie, Scotland in 1988, or midair collisions such as the El Cerritos disaster in 1986. These events will inflict injuries separate from the impact with the ground. Such events produce widespread distribution of bodies, body parts and debris that may take considerable time to recover. Injuries to those on the ground are also more likely. Low-flying aircraft, such as crop dusters, and planes during takeoff and landing may also experience wire strikes or collisions with other ground-based objects producing a subsequent crash.

Aircraft injuries often are accompanied by massive destruction of the body, bone breakage, and soft tissue fragmentation. Fires from the fuel, cargo, and impact site structures can further destroy human remains. The degree of destruction will depend upon the speed and angle of impact, aircraft size and design, sequence of events such as mid-air collision or explosion, integrity of the vehicle safety features among other factors.

Fatalities in crashes of light aircraft (less than 12,500 lbs) result from blunt force trauma in about two-thirds of the cases (Shkrum *et al.* 1996). About 75% of the blunt force trauma deaths resulted from multiple injuries with the remainder involving major injury to the head and neck. At least half of the deaths were produced by craniofacial, rib, and extremity fractures and internal injuries. Chalmers and colleagues (2000) found similar distributions of fractures. They listed head and chest fractures as the areas most often evident in fatalities. A substantial portion of fatalities had fractures confined to the nose or mandible. Impact is often at the level of the chin or below the eyes (Spitz and Fisher 1980, Spitz 2005). Passengers appeared to suffer a disproportionate number of craniofacial fractures and abdominal injuries (Shkrum *et al.* 1996), whereas cervical spine fractures were found almost entirely in pilots. Thoracic fractures and skull fractures were infrequent. Pilots have also been reported to suffer greater numbers of hand fractures from their attempts to control the craft, presuming they are conscious during the descent. Typical fractures include fragmentation of the carpals and phalanges. Avulsion of the thumb at the proximal joint also fits within the spectrum of skeletal injuries for pilots (Krefft 1970). Feet on the rudder pedals may induce comminuted fractures of the tarsals and metatarsals, and the pedals may penetrate the feet upon impact (Campman and Luzi 2007). Even as early as World War I, it was observed that pilots tended to have more talar fractures while those who died from falls exhibited calcaneal fractures (Anderson 1919). These fractures usually involved compression of the talar head or, less commonly comminuted fractures of the talar body or fractures of the talar neck (Coltart 1952). While some injuries to the hands and feet have been linked to pilots as opposed to passengers, Campman and Luzi (2007) show that the patterns are insufficiently sensitive to differentiate between these two categories. However, Hoyer and colleagues (2012) felt comfortable in making such an assessment based on close examination of the fracture patterns and the damage to the controls in a light plane crash in which both people held a valid pilot's license. While restraint systems provide some protection if the passenger compartment remains intact, they are often ineffectual with the more extensive damage seen in many crashes. Only in about half the cases of light plane crashes are the victims found inside the wreckage.

In larger aircraft, the degree of fragmentation can be immense, produced by the high speeds of impact and the greater mass of the aircraft (Fulginiti *et al.*, 1999, Spitz and Fisher 1980, Spitz 2005). These vessels cruise at altitudes considerably higher than light aircraft and at greater speeds than the approximately 200 mph of the lighter planes. Of reported injuries in commercial aircraft, lower limb fractures are the most common, followed by head injuries

(Baker *et al.* 2009). Other crashes have shown higher numbers of head and chest injuries (Lillehei and Robinson 1994). Head injuries are often found in child fatalities (Li and Baker 1997). In one commercial crash in which about half the occupants survived, decedents had more cervical or thoracic spine injuries as well as head and chest injuries (Barancik *et al.* 1992). Survivors suffered more lumbar fractures. Lower limb fractures were common in both groups.

The speed and force of impact, however, is often so great that all bodies may be torn apart with the largest part found being only one-third to one-fourth of the original body weight (Spitz and Fisher 1980, Spitz 2005). Extremities are particularly prone to detachment. This fragmentation can even occur in slower crashes of large planes such as those occur on landings and takeoff (Dulchasky *et al.* 1993). Usually, however, anthropological examination in these cases is limited to the identification of the victims.

Helicopter pilots may experience segmental, comminuted fractures of the tibia, usually at the junction of the middle and distal thirds of the shaft (Dummit and Reid 1969). These seem confined to craft that land in an upright position and where the pilot is wearing a heavy boot. Since the feet control the tail rotor pedals, pilots often are applying pressure to these in an effort to control the descent. Forces are transmitted through the pedals to the lower leg. These fractures accompany a host of other skeletal injuries including tibial plateau fractures, mid-leg amputation, and rotational ankle fractures.

Combining engineering expertise with the anthropological examination can be critical in assessing the events. In one published report (Snyder *et al.* 1984), such work resulted in a sizable civil settlement against a manufacturer when it was shown that injuries resulted from failure of a recently "improved," seat design. In other cases, examination revealed a mid-air homicide (Gunther *et al.* 1999).

FALLS

Falls are also a common cause of fractures (Rogers 1992) (Figure 7-4). Most are found among young children, although adolescents and young adults are often at risk due to sports activities. Risk levels tend to dip then until old age when both increased osteoporosis and decreased agility and balance take their toll. Rates tend to be higher among younger men than women, but there are dramatic increases in fractures in women after menopause. By very old age (over 85 years), women's risk is almost twice that of comparably aged men and the risks of osteoporotic fractures appear to be increasing (Cummings et al. 1985; Cummings *et al.* 1997; Riggs and Melton 1988, 1995; Melton 1993, 1995; Lips 1997).

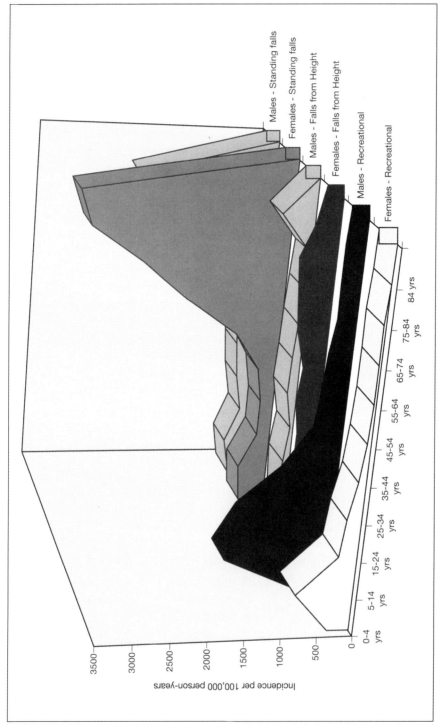

Figure 7-4. Causes of limb fractures. Age and sex-specific incidence of limb fractures as determined by survey of Rochester, Minnesota residents 1969–1971. (Redrawn from Melton and Riggs 1985.

Standing Falls

Falls from standing height include those falls where there is no significant drop between the substrate upon which the person is standing or moving prior to the fall and the level of impact. The nature of the substrate (grass, cement, gravel, etc.) along with the speed at which the person was moving will affect the level of injury. In most cases, the victim will attempt to break the fall by using the hands and arms. Fracture often reflects these defensive movements. Young children are susceptible to neck damage including dislocation of the atlanto-occipital joint with minor skeletal trauma. These tend to occur in toddlers and result from slow forward falls as the child loses its balance (Spencer 1981).

Falls onto the outstretched hand can result in very different fractures depending upon the age of the victim (Rogers 1992). In a young person, under five years of age, a supracondylar fracture of the humerus is likely, while between ages five and 10, a transverse fracture of the metaphysis of the distal radius occurs. In the mid-teens, the most likely fracture is an epiphyseal separation of the distal radius, while in the late teens through early adult years, fracture of the scaphoid or other carpal bones may be more common. After age 40, the effects of age-related bone loss often mean that falls result in a Colles' fracture of the wrist, while in advanced old age, fractures of the proximal humerus are common as well. Clavicular fractures usually result from falls directly onto the shoulder and only occasionally with an outstretched arm (Stanley et al. 1988).

Standing falls tend to result in head injuries that affect the cranial vault circumferentially, usually at about the level where the brim of a hat would lie (Spitz and Fisher 1980, Spitz 2005, Kremer *et al.* 2008, Kremer and Sauvageau 2009, Guyomarc'h *et al.* 2010). However, as noted in the section on homicidal assault, the location of fractures in the region of the "hat brim line" cannot be isolated to either falls or assault. Falls produce contrecoup injuries to the brain that can also yield fractures of the superior orbital plates, particularly in the elderly. These may be seen with falls on the back of the head but are also produced by blows to the top of the cranial vault. Facial fractures are also noted in some cases of falls due to stumbling, with the nose being the area most frequently affected (Zandi *et al.* 2011). Nasal injuries were higher in those that stumbled than those that fell from any height. Stumbles also may produce fracture in the dentoalveolar region. Mandibular fractures from such stumbles also tended to focus on the condylar area.

Only rarely will these injuries be of forensic interest. Fatalities due to the trauma are not frequent and so the individual is less likely to require the attention of an anthropologist. In some cases, however, such falls may explain minor injuries that may otherwise raise suspicions of foul play.

Osteoporotic Fractures from Falls

Falls are the leading cause of fatal and non-fatal injury in those over age 75 years of age (Granek *et al.* 1987). This vulnerability is due to a number of factors including the high degree of bone mass lost due to aging and hormonal changes. Women are more susceptible due to postmenopausal bone loss, which compounds the losses that occur due to aging and reduction in physical activity. Actual risk of falling is increased in those who are using anti-depressants, sedatives, vasodilators, tranquilizers, or non-steroidal anti-inflammatory drugs (Granek *et al.* 1987).

Osteoporotic fractures cluster at particularly susceptible portions of the body. These areas are prone to severe depletion of bone tissue as well as being recipients of heavy loading during falls. Among women, these include both the distal radius and proximal humerus while both sexes are afflicted by higher incidence of hip fracture (pelvic and proximal femur).

Osteoporotic fractures will not be discussed extensively here as they rarely are of forensic concern. It is important, however, to remember that, in the osteoporotic individual, fractures will be more severe with considerably less force. This may explain severe fragmentation in circumstances that would normally be considered only mild trauma.

Falls from Heights

Falls from heights produce patterns of vertical deceleration injury from the impact. Forensically, these injuries are most often seen in urban areas where they have been termed "jumper syndrome," referring to the mechanism of injury rather than motivation (Scalea *et al.* 1986). Cases referred to anthropologists are more likely to come from remote rural areas where remains could go undiscovered for long periods of time after the fall.

The distinction between low and high heights for falls is usually designated as approximately 70–100 feet (35 meters). In a study of 59 falls, distinct differences were seen between falls from low and high heights (Gupta *et al.* 1982). In low height falls, there is a high probability of forearm damage as the person reaches out to break the fall. In these cases, cranial damage may be the cause of death with the rest of the body being subjected only to survivable injuries. A frequent cause of such falls is individuals who lose their balance while working on ladders (Lombardi *et al.* 2011). Usually these accidents involve older individuals who are trying to work on an unsteady ladder.

In contrast, falls from heights over about 35 meters have been shown to result in higher rates of thoracic damage (Gupta *et al.* 1982). Spinal fractures are also somewhat high but head injuries infrequent. This work was corroborated by that of Simonsen (1983) who reported on 10 cases of suicidal falls from bridges. No injuries to the face, mandible or neck were reported. In falls from extreme heights, it is likely that the person will lose consciousness prior to impact so that body positioning and any involuntary response are non-existent. Almost 90% of those who fall from four or more floors suffered multiple fractures, three-quarters of the falls involved spinal fractures, almost entirely in the lower thoracic and lumbar regions (Scalea *et al.* 1986).

Victims of falls from heights in urban areas are more likely to be male (Scalea et al. 1986). About half are accidental falls, while about 40% are suicidal. The remaining fraction is due to homicide. Atanasijevic and associates (2005) found a correlation between the height of fall and suicide, with those falls over 35 meters suicidal as opposed to accidental.

Determining suicide from accidental falls lies in the purview of the medical examiner/coroner. Some studies assert that injury patterns can contribute to that determination. However, other studies show consistency between injury patterns in intentional and accidental falls (Richter *et al.* 1996, Crowder and Adams, this volume).

In children, the larger proportional size of the head often means that this is the first part of the body to hit upon landing (Wilber and Thompson 1994, Eggensperger Wymann *et al.* 2008). Children are also less able to brace themselves or attempt to land on their hands than are adults. Consequently, children suffer a higher proportion of head injuries from falls than would be expected in an adult sample (Mayer *et al.* 1981). Other injuries include fractures of femur, forearm, tibia, fibula, ribs, and humerus (Smith *et al.* 1975, Barlow *et al.* 1983). Fortunately, children tend to be able to survive longer falls than adults.

When a person falls from a height, the damage will depend upon the velocity of the impact, the position of the body at landing, and the surface upon or into which they land. The importance of body position was noted in a retrospective study of 146 individuals for whom landing position was reported by witnesses (Goonetilleke 1980). When the landing is primarily focused on the lower limbs, about two-thirds result in bilateral fractures. Buttock-first landings result in more extensive injuries to the torso including pelvic (82%) and spinal injuries (55%). Side impacts can result in both pelvic and rib damage. In addition, angulation fractures of the spine occur with side impacts. It is important to remember that the victim often strikes a number of objects such as ledges, outcroppings, trees, fire escapes, or awnings before reaching their final resting place. Each additional impact can induce a separate suite of injuries.

Head injuries may occur when the person lands foot or buttocks first, driving the spinal column upwards into the base of the skull. Basal skull fractures, when occurring with impact damage on the lower body, are usually indicative of this type of injury (Goonetilleke 1980). One typical form is the ring fracture with the rim of the foramen magnum being driven inwards as the impact of landing is transmitted from the feet or buttocks, through the spine to the head (Spitz and Fisher 1980, Spitz 2005).

Harvey and Jones (1980) sounded a warning on the interpretation of basal skull fractures. They noted that a common type of basal fracture across both petrous bones usually initiates at the point of impact, as is the case with other fractures. Basal fractures, however, are more likely than other fractures to deviate from this pattern and be due to impacts in other areas of the skull with the basilar component being secondary.

Fractures in the torso are relatively common in falls from heights. Around two-thirds of individuals who have fallen from a height will exhibit thoracic injuries, including rib and sternal fractures (Atanasijevic *et al.* 2009). These fractures increase in frequency with increasing height and almost all individuals who have fallen at least 30 meters will show rib fracturing. Multiple rib fractures are a common finding, with the fragments frequently penetrating the pleural cavity (Lukas *et al.* 1981, Atanasijevic *et al.* 2009). In some cases, sternal fractures accompany the rib damage with increasing occurrence with greater height and with anteroposterior compression of the chest. Less common are fractures of the scapula and clavicle, but these too can be produced by falls from a height. The rib fractures are most often occurring at the point/side of impact.

Falls from moderate heights (up to about 7m) often produce fractures in the upper extremity and pectoral girdle (Lombardi *et al.* 2011). Fallers often suffer from fractures to the hand and forearm (Lowenstein *et al.* 1989).

Falls from heights may produce massive damage to the legs (Spitz and Fisher 1980, Spitz 2005). If an individual lands on their feet, the bones of the leg may be driven down through the soles of the feet. Calcaneal fractures are common in these circumstances. Compression fractures of the ankle, knee and hip joints are also common findings. Femoral and pelvic fractures also occur (Lowenstein *et al.* 1989).

A subcategory of the falls from heights is found among parachutists. In most cases, injuries are nonfatal and are most often to the lower extremity (Barrows *et al.* 2005). Upper extremity and spinal injuries also occur. Serious parachute malfunctions result in freefall and parallel the injuries seen in other falls from heights. Many parachute fatalities occur, however, in landing where there is no parachute malfunction (Sitter 2000, Hart and Griffith 2003). The performance improvements in parachute design can result in landings in which the parachutist can produce a "hook turn," a maneuver where there is a high-speed turn close to the ground (Barrows *et al.* 2005). These turns have produced a significant number of fatalities. In addition, the newer parachutes allow "swooping" whereby the parachutist comes in quickly to the ground but levels out close to the ground, traveling up to a hundred meters just above the ground at high rates of speed (Hart and Griffith 2003).

Section II

FRACTURE PATTERNS
AND SKELETAL MORPHOLOGY

Chapter 8

BONES OF THE SKULL, THE DENTITION, AND OSSEOUS STRUCTURES OF THE THROAT

ALISON GALLOWAY AND VICKI L. WEDEL

The skull is a geometrically complex structure that exhibits a basic symmetry along the midsagittal plane. Functionally, it can be divided into the cranial vault, or neurocranium, that houses and protects the brain and the facial skeleton, or viscerocranium, which is a much more delicate structure. The skull is comprised of eight cranial bones, 14 facial bones, and 29 uniting sutures. The bony structures of the throat and the dentition are included in this chapter. The cranial vault forms a relatively closed structure around the brain, providing resistance to impacts. The facial bones, in contrast, form a complex arrangement that houses not only fragile sensory organs, muscles for the fine movements of facial expression, and the dental arcade but also large sinuses and areas for mucous membranes that provide little resistance to impact. In some areas of the face, forces derived from muscular contraction are minimal while in others, such as around the jaw, considerable strain is generated and the bones are correspondingly stronger.

Head injuries occur in a wide variety of situations. Falls, assaults, motor vehicle collisions, and penetrating missiles are the most common causes of head injuries (Britt and Heiseman 2000). Motor vehicle accidents cause the majority of cranial vault fractures (Haug *et al.* 1992, Saadet *et al.* 2011). Assaults and sports-related injuries are also linked to cranial fractures. The head is particularly vulnerable in all of these situations. Interpersonal violence is of particular forensic interest. In many cases, the head and face are psychologically linked, in the mind of the perpetrator, to the victim's identity, making these areas the focal point of rage (Walker 2001). Furthermore, identification of remains is commonly made initially by visual means, which are followed by positive confirmation from dental radiographs, fingerprints, or DNA comparisons. Identity may be established from radiographic features of the skull (e.g., Marlin *et al.* 1991). Knowledge of this utility of the skull in identification may lead the perpetrator to attempt to disguise the victim by demolishing the face or the entire head. Crushing injuries tend to be massive and devastating and require lengthy reconstruction.

Blunt forces on the skull may be imparted by compression or by direct or indirect impact. These forces can be dynamic or relatively static. The cranial vault can undergo considerable compression in any direction without fracture and may accommodate a decrease in diameter in one direction by an increase in the perpendicular direction. However, because of its spherical shape, compression to the point of failure often results in extensive fragmentation. In static loading, forces are usually dissipated over a larger area, but resistance is calculated to be about half of that withstood under dynamic conditions (Yoganandan *et al.* 2009). The fragile facial bones are more susceptible to damage, and vault deformation may indirectly fracture the facial region.

Because of the placement of the relatively heavy head at the top of the relatively less robust neck, the head is strongly influenced by acceleration and deceleration of the body. In situations such as motor vehicle accidents and falls, the force with which the head strikes an object can, therefore, be greater than that inflicted on the rest of the body. Cervical fractures concomitant with skull fractures are not infrequent. Studies estimate 5–15% of skull and facial fractures are accompanied by neck fractures (Mithani *et al.* 2009, Mulligan and Mahabir 2010).

Skulls vary in bone thickness and robusticity (Law 1993). Female skeletal material is, on the average, more gracile than that of males and, therefore, on average, more prone to fractures. Large intra- and interpopulation variability preclude accurate assessment based solely on sex (Ross *et al.* 1998). Head shape may also play a role but re-examination (Kroman *et al.* 2011) of the studies by Gurdjian (1975) leaves unconfirmed his conclusion that longer heads better withstand compression along the long axis. This finding does not address the question of lateral compression. Head shape is controlled by genetics and environment but internal changes, which affect strength, also occur due to age, including development of pachionian pits or Paget's disease, for example.

In this chapter, the head and throat are discussed in terms of the major segments including some discussion of individual bones. Discussion is divided into the cranial vault, the facial bones, the mandible, dentition, and the bones and cartilage of the throat.

CRANIAL VAULT

The cranial vault consists of the frontal, parietals, temporals, occipital, and sphenoid. Of these bones, the parietal bone fractures the most frequently, followed by the temporal, occipital, and frontal bones (Cooper and Golfinos 2000). Outer and inner tables of dense cortical bone, sandwiching a trabecular diploë, characterize these bones. The bones of the vault are between 2 and 6 mm thick, depending on location (Carpenter 1991, Rockswold 1996). In most cases, the outer table is thicker than the inner. There are also differences in diploë thickness, particularly between males and females (Lynnerup *et al.* 2005). In some areas, this structural arrangement transitions to thinner bone without a diploë, such as is seen in the temporal squama and sphenoid. The cranial vault appears to act isotrophically under loading, meaning that there is little linear organization within the bone tissue itself, which will alter the modulus from one direction to another (McElhaney *et al.* 1976). The compressive strength of compact bone is 24,500 psi while that of the diploë is only 3640 psi. Considerable variation has been noted between specimens (Melvin and Evans 1971, Martin 1991).

The degree of sutural closure also influences fracture pattern (Kroman *et al.* 2011). Infants have open sutures, and trauma to the vault tends to be localized by the inability of fractures to cross the membranes and patent sutures (Blount 1955, 1977; Greenes and Schutzman 1997). The bones of a child are much more elastic than in the adult, which allows for greater tolerance of deformation, at least in terms of bony damage. As the suture lines become joined, energy can be transmitted beyond the area of direct impact. Suture closure and obliteration is a long and highly variable process. Sutures that completely disappear in one skull may still be open in another individual of the same sex and of similar age and population. Due to this variation, the course of fracture patterns will vary. Observation of the suture fusion is essential in understanding the fracture patterns, with the basic principle being that the less unified the bones on each side of the suture are to each other, the greater the chance that a fracture will propagate along the suture rather than across it.

The velocity and mass of the impact are critical in determining the type of injury. Upon direct impact, fractures radiate outward from the point of impact (Kroman *et al.* 2011). In direct impact, the cranial vault accommodates a small amount of in-bending, with out-bending occurring in all areas around this point (Gurdjian *et al.* 1953; Gurdjian 1975; Rogers 1992) but quickly fails at the point of impact (Keaveny and Hayes 1993, Kroman *et al.* 2011) (Figure 8-1). While Gurdjian's work has been considered monumental in the field of forensic experimentation on trauma, more recent studies such as that by Kroman and colleagues (2011) suggest that the original studies were unintentionally biased. Gurdjian (1975) coated dry skulls with a stress coat of lacquer, simulated blunt force trauma, and observed the fracturing in the lacquer. Based on his simulations, Gurdjian (1975) suggested that fracturing initiated away from the site of impact due to bending of adjacent bony areas based upon changes in a stress coat of lacquer applied to the dry skull. However, observational studies on

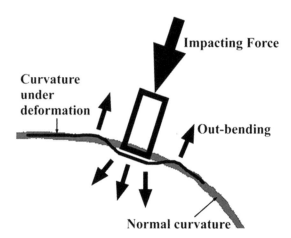

Figure 8-1. Deformation of the cranial vault with impact. The cranial vault is depressed immediately beneath the point of impact. Fracturing begins at the point of impact.

cranial blunt force trauma always identified an impact point with associated fracturing. In replicating the study with fresh intact crania, Kroman and colleagues (2011) found that impact sites were clearly visible and that additional fracturing originated from that point, as seen in high-speed video.

The outer table may be involved more extensively than the inner table because it bears the direct forces of an impact. Fractures seen externally may not have corresponding damage visible internally or such damage may be minimal. In some situations, however, the inner table will fracture without any fracture of the outer table. Such a case has been discussed from the forensic context (Galloway and Zephro 2004). Once a linear fracture has been sustained, relatively little energy applied subsequently will produce additional fractures and complete skull destruction (Black *et al.*, this volume).

Another important factor is the shape of the object making the impact. A pointed impactor will likely produce perforations of the bone resulting in complete penetration. As the area of the impacting surface increases, the likelihood of penetration decreases. As the area of impaction increases still further, larger forces are required to produce fracturing. Depressed fractures occur when the striking object is of moderate size; however, when the impact site extends over much of the cranial vault's surface, comminuted or linear fractures are more common. The principle is as follows: "the higher the velocity and the smaller the mass of the object, the more likely is a depressed fracture" (Rogers 1992: 303).

Another factor involved in determining the amount and form of fracturing is the amount of "padding" on and within the head (Yoganandan *et al.* 2004, Verschueren *et al.* 2007). The retention of the intracranial contents and subsequent drying of bone significantly affect experimental tests on resilience.

The additional material on the skull consists of the scalp's layers and whatever amount of hair the individual retains. A hat or other clothing may augment soft tissue and hair. Additional protection may come from helmets or from other parts of the body used to ward off impact. For example, Johnson and colleagues (1995) found that among 37 motorcyclists involved in accidents where the head was impacted, the only individual to sustain a skull fracture was the one non-helmeted individual.

Since head injuries are often involved in homicidal fatalities, careful preparation of the supporting documents by the forensic anthropologist during the analysis may become critical in presenting the conclusions in court. Features to note are the extent of damage, whether both the inner and outer table are involved, which bone(s) are affected and probable point of impact. If possible, fractures should be sequenced (see Chapter 2, Black *et al.*, this volume). Measurements of fracture lines, detailed charts, photographs, and radiographs complete the documentation.

Classification of Cranial Vault Fractures

Cranial vault fractures are divided into five basic categories based on the morphology of the fracture. The most frequent type is a *linear* form, which accounts for about 70–80% of all skull fractures (Rogers 1992). *Diastatic* fractures, where the fracture follows the suture and causes traumatic separation, account for about 5%. The remaining 15% of skull fractures are *depressed*, *comminuted*, or *stellate* fractures.

Linear or *fissure* fractures pass quickly through the cranial vault and tend to follow the path of least resistance (Figure 8-2). These breaks include any single fracture that passes through the outer and/or inner table. In most cases, both tables and diploë are separated. Linear fractures may be displaced dramatically, forming distinct pieces of bone, or they may be essentially undisplaced. The latter is particularly true in the denser portions of the skull. Because tension inherent in the skull is released by the fracture, warpage of the bone may occur, and it may be very difficult to refit the fragments (Nusse, this volume). Dense bone may re-route the fracture line. Any pre-existing fracture or open suture can terminate a fracture by dissipating the energy that is propagating the fracture. Linear fractures are rarely straight, as the name may seem to imply, rather they may diverge in some areas, especially when there is an incomplete fracture. Often, there is insufficient energy for the fracture to continue completely through a bone to a suture or other such structure, and the fracture will terminate in the middle of the bone. Serious complications, including intracranial hematomas, can arise from linear fractures. Therefore, even when seemingly minor and undisplaced, all such injuries should be brought to the attention of the forensic pathologist for evaluation.

Linear fractures tend to result from forces of relatively large mass. They are often found in blunt force trauma as a result of direct impact with an object, such as a weapon used in assault or a portion of an automobile frame during an accident. Linear fractures may also appear due to forces transmitted from other areas of the body, particularly through the spinal column. Blows to one portion of the head may cause linear fractures in other areas of the skull. It is more likely for blows to the upper portions of the cranial vault to produce linear fractures moving downward around the vault, than for fractures of the basicranium to transmit upwards around the top of the cranial vault. In many cases, multiple linear fractures, which have also been termed "composite" fractures (Gonzalez *et al.* 1954), produce severe comminution. For example, a blow to the right temporal may pass through the facial bones and extend posteriorly through the left frontal and parietal onto the occipital.

Compression of the skull will also produce a massive complex of linear fractures as the cranial vault ruptures, such as occurs in many train-pedestrian accidents. Tortosa and colleagues (2004) reported on 11 cases of compressive fracturing of the skull, specifically bitemporal head crush injuries. In this type of cranial crush injury, static forces are applied bilaterally to the temporal regions. In all 11 cases, basilar skull fractures resulted.

Linear fractures of the parietal bone are the most common form of skull fracture in children (Harwood-Nash *et al.* 1971, Meservy *et al.* 1987, Levinthal *et al.* 1993) although they are less common than in adults (Duncan 1993). Linear fractures are often found in victims of child abuse and careful attention needs to be paid to their identification in juvenile material. Knowledge of the normally appearing cleavages in cranial bones during the growth process is essential for distinguishing natural versus artificial separation. In young survivors of linear fractures, the fractures can enlarge in time and are known as growing skull fractures. They are most common in children under the age of three years (Naim-Ur-Rahman *et al.* 1994, de Djientchei *et al.* 2006). Fractures in children who are the victims of abusive head trauma (AHT) vary but in general are more likely to be complicated (e.g. stellate, branching, multiple, bilateral, crossing suture lines, depressed or diastatic). Albert and Drvaric (1993) found that in children fractures more complicated than simple linear fractures rarely occur from accidents, like falls.

Diastatic fractures usually are a variant of linear fractures that divert into a suture (Gurdjian 1975) (Figure 8-2). Diastatic fractures most commonly involve the coronal or lambdoidal sutures; however, these authors have seen a sagittal diastatic fracture.

Depressed fractures in the cranial vault may present with or without actual penetration of the skull (McElhaney *et al.* 1976, Heary *et al.* 1993) (Figure 8-2). Compressive forces may cause the diploë to collapse. This may be followed by failure of the outer and inner tables. Linear fractures may arise from these

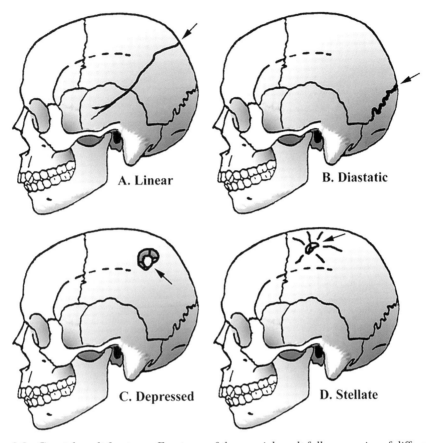

Figure 8-2. Cranial vault fractures. Fractures of the cranial vault follow a series of different patterns. A. Linear fractures can pass through a number of bones. B. Diastatic fractures are located within the suture. They may also be extensions of linear fractures. C. Depressed fractures are localized at and around areas of impact. D. Stellate fractures result from bending in the cranial vault and may be linked with depressed fractures as shown above.

defects and radiate away from the point of impact. The fracture may be limited to the outer table. Shallow depressed fractures are sometimes called *pond fractures* (Knight 1991). Pond fractures more commonly fracture only the outer table as opposed to both ecto- and endocranial surfaces. Infants sustain this kind of fractures more commonly than other children or adults.

If the force of impact and, therefore, penetration is greater, the inner table may also be involved (Gurdjian 1975, Heary *et al.* 1993). Because of the relatively localized nature of these penetrating defects, however, an approximate outline of the impacting area can be demarcated (Gonzalez *et al.* 1954, Delannoy *et al.* 2012). The internal portion of the fracture is larger due to internal beveling (Hart 2005, Delannoy *et al.* 2012). In some cases, however, the area of damage is more extensive than the size of the impacting object, and the curvature of the skull may also limit the formation of an imprint of the object (Cooper and Golfinos 2000).

The bones of cranial vault of an infant or young child respond somewhat differently because they are generally thinner and more flexible (Rogers 1992). Consequently, their cranial vaults are capable of absorbing a relatively greater impact than that of an adult without failing and fracturing. This does not mean that children are less subject to brain damage (Greenes and Schutzman 1997). The incidence of depressed fractures is 3.5 times greater in children than in adults (Zimmerman *et al.* 1981). Depressed fractures in young children, however, may never actually involve a fracture site but may be limited to a depression in the vault (Gurdjian 1975, McElhaney *et al.* 1976, Rogers 1992, Duncan 1993). These are termed *ping-pong, dishpan,* or *derby hat* fractures due to their resemblance to the depression that can be made by fingers in a ping-pong ball. Depressed fractures can occur during birth and usually involve the parietal bones (Watson Jones 1941, Dupuis *et al.* 2005, see Chapter 7).

Stellate fractures are "star-shaped" injuries that consist of multiple radiating linear fractures (Figure 8-2). These originate at the point of impact where the tensile forces become most pronounced. Heavy loads of relatively low velocity are a common cause, since they are most likely to produce the extensive in-bending that results in a stellate fracture (Gurdjian 1975, Wilkins 1997, Kroman *et al.* 2011). They tend to occur on the upper parietals although may be found somewhat lower. They are also associated in some cases with a depressed fracture at the point of impact.

Comminuted fractures of the vault result from low-velocity/heavy-impact, forces that produce fragmentation of bone (Gurdjian 1975). These types of injury are often found in crushing incidents when the skull is compacted under great force, although not necessarily with great speed. These fractures tend to form on the convexities of the skull with the central area being extensively fragmented and circular fractures extending beyond the impact point. Such fractures are often so severe that recovery of all portions and reconstruction is nearly impossible (Black *et al.*, this volume). Comminuted fractures of the occipital bone in children are often evidence that the child's skull was struck against a surface and are, therefore, suggestive of child abuse (Meservy *et al.* 1987).

Blunt force trauma requires considerable force to cause fractures in skeletal material. Linear fractures of the cranial vault usually require approximately 33–75 ft-lb of energy (Riviello 2010). Several research groups have attempted to quantify the amount of force required to induce fracture at various locations on the human skull. Their research designs vary in terms of the method used to impact the sample, whether the samples were fresh or embalmed, and the number of samples each study considered sufficient. Yoganandian and Pintar (2004) summarize the results of several experiments designed to induce temporo-parietal skull fractures. They conclude that methods and sample selection factors must be standardized if reliable and replicable results are to be achieved (Chapter 6, this volume). Verschueren and associates (2007) recognized limitations on many impact experiments that held the skull within a relatively rigid structure. Using a double pendulum arrangement, they were able to demonstrate that impacts produced skull fractures before the impact moved the cranium on its pendulum.

Cranial Morphology and Fracturing

While cranial fractures may occur in any portion of the vault, some areas are more susceptible than others. In an examination of 504 bodies, LeCount and Apfelbach (1920) revealed six regions where greater thicknesses of cranial bone form arches, which hindered the horizontal bending of bone (Figure 8-3). Normal healthy adult skull is thicker and stronger in the midfrontal, mid-occipital, parietosphenoidal, and parietopetrous buttresses. Between these arches, the bone can bend more easily in a vertical manner. It is weaker in the temporal fossa where fractures can lead to epidural hematoma and laceration of the middle meningeal artery, especially at pterion (Adelson 1974).

Since LeCount and Apfelbach's study, the work of Gurdjian and colleagues (Gurdjian and Lissner 1947, Gurdjian *et al.* 1953) examined fracture patterns

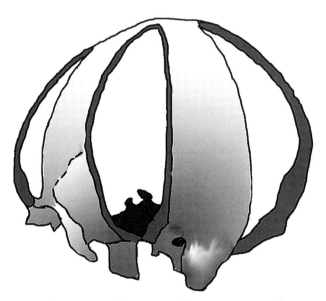

Figure 8-3. Le Count buttresses. The system of buttresses or reinforcing arches proposed by Le Count is shown. These areas help limit and redirect linear fractures of the cranial vault. Within these struts are located some of the thickest regions of the skull.

in experimental conditions. Deformation from direct impact by a striking object was more pronounced in areas of weaker buttressing, particularly the frontal bone, areas around the foramen magnum and the parietotemporal area. Linear fractures can pass through the bony buttresses of the cranial vault, but usually this happens when the direction of travel is close to perpendicular to the long axis of the buttress.

Fractures that encounter the buttresses at an oblique angle tend to be diverted toward structurally weaker areas. Blows that land on the top of the skull, between the parietal bones, tend to travel inferiorly through the side of the skull. Blows to the frontal region produce more vertically-oriented fractures whereas blows to the sides and back of the skull lead to more horizontal defects. Linear fractures usually involve the cranial base (Gurdjian *et al.* 1953, Gurdjian 1975), especially with impacts on the frontal and occipital bones. This process may involve a continuation of the initial linear fracture but also may be an indirect result of compression between the impact site and the spine.

The cranial vault, in many respects a closed structure, must allow for the passage of blood vessels and nerves. The bulk of the foramina are located in the basilar region, but smaller foramina are found in most of the major bones. These foramina serve as focal points of fractures, as stress mounts rapidly in these areas where the integrity of the bone structure is already weakened. In particular, the foramen magnum and the foramina of the frontal bone are frequently involved in fractures (Katzen *et al.* 2003).

Basilar Fractures

Basilar fractures by definition involve fracture(s) to any of the following: the cribiform plate of the ethmoid bone, the orbital plate of the frontal bone, the petrous and squamous portions of the temporal bone, the sphenoid, and the occipital bone (Golfinos and Cooper 2000). Basilar fractures may be due to blows to the front of the head or may result indirectly through compression of the spine against the base of the skull (Rogers 1992). Typically, they run across the vault base from side to side, anterior/posteriorly, or through portions of the temporal bone. Basilar skull fractures are often accompanied by extensive brain stem contusions, brain injury from intruding bone fragments (Hardt and Kuttenberger 2009), loss of cerebrospinal fluid, and tearing of major blood vessels that results in a high mortality rate (Sun *et al.* 2011). Meningeal infections also play a role in the death rate.

Longitudinal fractures often extend into the anterior cranial fossa while, posteriorly, they appear to jump the foramen magnum and continue into the occipital. They may also pass lateral to the foramen magnum.

Basilar fractures are often confined to the frontal areas of the vault where they fall into the category of frontobasal fractures. They frequently begin in the area of the frontal sinus (see below) or in the mid-third of the superior orbital border (Manson *et al.* 2009). They will continue through the naso-ethmoid region, the cribriform plate, and sphenoid anterior to the sella turcica. If they continue, they will typically pass into the temporal bone and move upward, following the line of the petrous portion. Studies on cadavers and comparisons with trauma seen in hospitalized patients revealed three cate-gories of such fractures. Type I are isolated linear fractures of the base, which originate in the cribriform plate or superior orbital roof. Type II are vertical linear fractures through the frontal bone and are often accompanied by linear fractures through the base as described above. Type III are comminuted frac-tures in which many of the bony elements have collapsed due to the impact.

Manson and associates (2009) also assessed how impacts could lead to the production of the different types of frontobasal fractures. Fractures in the mid-central forehead caused frontal sinus fractures, but the fractures then moved into all three of the fracture patterns he had identified. Impacts higher on the frontal bone typically produced Manson Type 1 fractures, although Manson Type II fractures were also seen. When the impact was lower on the frontal bone, in the area of the nasofrontal suture or laterally along the orbital rim, the fractures were usually confined to the frontal sinus or orbit, respectively (see below for these fracture patterns). These three types of fractures often co-occur with facial and nasoethmoidal fractures.

The classification system of Escher (1969, 1970, 1973; Hardt and Kutten-berger 2009), which divides frontobasal fractures into four categories, is perhaps more widely used within the medical community. Type 1 fractures result from impact on the upper frontal bone and consist of extensive comminuted frac-tures of the frontal bone and may extend into the paranasal sinuses. Type II fractures include depressed fractures or localized comminution in the frontal sinus and ethmoid regions. Type III fractures include shearing fractures of the midface from the cranial base. The final kind, Type IV, groups together fractures in the lateral orbital/temporal regions through to the frontal sinus.

Transverse or *hinge* fractures can divide the cranial vault anteroposteriorly, usually running anterior to the petrous portion and through the sella turcica. These fractures may also pass through the areas adjacent to the basilar syn-chondrosis. Longitudinal compressing loads produce this kind of fracture (Oehmichen *et al.* 2005). More forceful transverse blunt impacts can produce transverse burst fractures, although they are not reliable indicators of lateral blows to the head (Harvey and Jones 1980).

Fractures of the temporal bone may also occur in the inferior portions where it forms a critical portion of the cranial base. Temporal fractures form at least some component of about 75% of basilar fractures (Gladwell and Viozzi 2008). These temporal fractures are classified as either longitudinal or trans-verse. Longitudinal fracture lines typically begin in the squamous portion of the bone, pass along the external auditory meatus and canal and then turn anteriorly towards foramen lacerum. Longitudinal temporal fractures are the more likely to occur, forming about 80% of the temporal fractures (Nichol and Johnstone 1994, Gladwell and Viozzi 2008) and are typically linked to blows to the side of the head at the parietal level.

Transverse temporal fractures usually run from the foramen magnum anteriorly through the central portion of the petrous portion at about the level of the middle ear and terminate anteriorly, again close to foramen lacerum. Transverse fractures have been linked to blows to the frontal or occipital areas of the vault. As with any fracture pattern, comminution or fracture complexes may occur in which both elements are present. These patterns are generally referred to as "mixed."

Ring fractures of the cranial base are also found and are particularly common in falls from heights (Spitz and Fisher 1985, Spitz 2005). The skull base separates with the rim of the foramen magnum and detaches from the vault. Ring fractures are generally the result of the force of impact being transmitted through the spine when an individual lands on the feet or buttocks.

Fractures in Processes, Sinuses, Fossa and Condyles

Blunt force trauma in the form of blows to the head may result in fracturing of the temporal bone in the mastoid portion (Rogers 1992). Longitudinal fractures are more common than transverse fractures in the mastoid portion, but the courses of fracture in this area tend to be highly variable.

Frontal sinus injuries have been reported in motor vehicle accidents and assaults, although the former appear to be decreasing with increased protective equipment in automobiles (Montovani *et al.* 2006, Strong *et al.* 2006). These fractures can be classified as (1) through to the anterior cranial fossa, (2) anterior and posterior tables, (3) anterior table, (4) posterior table, or (5) frontal recess only (Strong *et al.* 2006). In a study of children whose frontal sinuses are under development, frontal sinus fractures, although rare, were always associated with orbital fractures (Whatley *et al.* 2005). When large, the frontal sinus may only be broken through the anterior wall (Gruss 1982, Strong *et al.* 2006). If the sinus is small, then intracranial extension is more likely. Often the frontal sinus is involved due to continuation of linear fractures originating elsewhere on the frontal.

Occipital condylar fractures occur, although at low frequencies, in patients who have suffered cervical fractures or who have been involved in motor vehicle accidents (Leone *et al.* 2000). Because of the ligamentous attachments around the condylar-cervical joint, there is little ability for rotation at this joint, and flexion and extension are only possible within limited ranges. Unfortunately, if the ligaments are damaged, the joint itself loses stability, and dislocation may occur. Anderson and Montesano (1988) identified three forms of occipital condyle fracture: (1) comminution due to impaction, (2) fracture as part of more extensive basilar fracture, and (3) avulsion near the alar ligament attachment due to forced rotation, often with lateral bending. A later classification by Tuli and associates (1997) is less useful as it depends on computed tomography (CT) to identify displacement of fragments.

FRACTURES OF FACIAL BONES

The face consists of a number of relatively friable bones supported on braces of more rigid bone. These latter structures, often spared during fracturing, include the alveolar process of the maxilla, the malar eminence of the zygomatics, and the nasofrontal process of the maxilla (Rogers 1992). The face can be visualized as a series of horizontal and vertical struts (Gentry *et al.* 1983, Cruz and Eichenberger 2004, Lo Castro *et al.* 2012) (Figure 8-4). Horizontal struts pass above and below the eye and at the roof of the mouth, while vertical struts pass midsagittally, along the side of the nose and diagonally from the lateral edge of the hard palate to the lateral edge of the orbit and then vertically along the orbit. Two additional struts can be visualized in the coronal plane: one formed by the anterior maxillary sinus and a second formed by the posterior wall of the sinus and associated bones. These struts provide resistance to fracture while the remaining bone tends to crumple with impact.

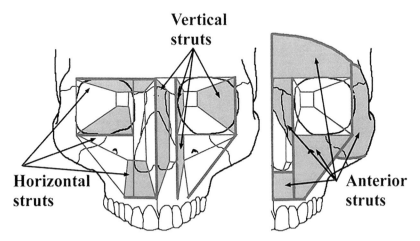

Figure 8-4. System of facial "struts." Gentry and associates visualize the face as consisting of a series of horizontal struts, vertical struts which lie in the sagittal plane, and the anterior struts form the outer surface of the face. Modified from Rogers *Radiology of Skeletal Trauma* (2nd ed.). New York: Churchill Livingstone, 1992.

In general, the facial bones can withstand considerable force if the loading is distributed widely over the face thanks to the supporting struts. Forces can also be accommodated if the impact is directed vertically onto the forehead although frontobasal fractures are a risk (Manson *et al.* 2009). Impacts that hit vertically but lower on the face, along with lateral blows, can produce a shear effect, dislocating many of the facial bones (Hardt and Kuttenberger 2009). Horizontally-directed blows, those that hit the breadth of the face, will crumple many of the facial bones, particularly around the nose and orbits, displacing the face inward and downward. If the force is greater, these fractures will continue into a frontobasal fracture (see above) as the superior orbital plates and sphenoid also fragment.

In this section, the overall incidence of facial trauma is discussed in terms of general mechanisms. Following this is a discussion by area within the face: zygomatico-orbital, orbital, nasal, and maxillary/Le Fort fractures. Obviously, these fracture complexes overlap considerably and often co-occur in a single individual after a traumatic event.

Direct trauma to the face is usually focused on the central portion in the frontonasal region or lateral to the frontozygomatic region (Gruss 1982). Most

TABLE 8-1 EXPERIMENTAL 50% FRACTURE FAILURE RATES MEASURED IN NEWTONS*		
Bone	*Applied Force for Fracture Risk*	*References*
Frontal	1885-2405N	Cormier *et al.* 2011
Maxilla	970-1223N	Cormier *et al.* 2011
Zygoma	489-2401N	Nyqvist *et al.*1986 Hodgson 1967 Gadd *et al.* 1968 Allsop *et al.* 1988
Zygomatic Arch	890-1779N	Schneider and Nahum 1972 Nahum 1976
Nose	450-850N	Cormier *et al.* 2010
Mandible Body	685-1779N	Nyqvist *et al.*1986 Gadd *et al.* 1968
Mandible Angle	300-750N	Hardt and Kuttenberger 2009
Vault	2095N	Raymond *et al.* 2009
*The force required to accelerate a 1 kilogram of mass at the rate of one meter per second squared.		

facial fractures result from one segment of the facial skeleton being sheared off from the rest of the skull. In addition, there may be depressed fractures from impacts with objects of small mass and higher force, as in the cranial vault (Rogers 1992). Fractures of the face are rarely fatal (Bone 1985, Wyatt *et al.* 2011) but are often associated with damage to other areas of the body such as the thorax or cranial vault. Fractures in the upper third of the face usually involve the frontal sinuses and ethmoid labyrinth (Bone 1985). Midfacial fractures are often of the tripod or trimalar form, followed by fractures of the zygomatic arch and alveolar process of the maxilla (Rogers 1992).

The face is frequently involved in trauma as the result of motor vehicle accidents and other forms of blunt force trauma (Rogers 1992, Brasiliero and Passeri 2006, Shahim *et al.* 2006). The combination of airbags and seatbelt use has considerably lessened the incidence of these fractures in recent years in jurisdictions where they are used (Simoni *et al.* 2003). Motorcycle and all-terrain vehicles accidents are common causes as well (Kraus *et al.* 2003, Holmes *et al.* 2004, Shults *et al.* 2005). Accidents associated with sports like football, baseball, and hockey are to blame for facial fractures in adolescents and young adults (Perkins *et al.* 2000, Marshall *et al.* 2003, Reehal 2010). Facial fractures can also be the result of interpersonal and domestic violence (Bakardjiev and Pechalova 2007, Erdmann *et al.* 2008, Arosarena *et al.* 2009, Lee 2009, Juarez and Hughes, this volume). As people age, falls become the more common cause of fracture (Iida *et al.* 2003).

Zygomatic Fractures

Zygomatic fractures usually result from a blow or impact over the malar eminence (Tadj and Kimble 2003). Zygomatic fractures normally occur at the zygomatic arch, at the zygomaticofrontal suture, and at the inferior orbital rim medial to the zygomaticomaxillary suture (Rogers 1992, Hwang and Kim 2011).

Zygomatic fractures have been classified into three basic categories (Zingg *et al.* 1992). The first involves only isolated fractures of one of the processes (frontal, temporal or maxillary) of the zygomatic bone. Zygomatic arch fractures are frequently on the temporal process but may involve the temporal portions of the arch. These fractures tend to be the product of relatively low-energy impacts as the zygomatic arch will break under only 130 to 780 psi (McElhaney *et al.* 1976; Mackey 1984). This first category also includes separation of the superior portion of the frontal process, causing a fracture of the lateral orbital border, or a small fracture at the medial end of the zygoma, causing a fracture of the inferior orbital border (Zingg *et al.* 1992). The second category involves fractures of all three processes. The term *tripod* fracture has often been used to denote this separation of the zygomatic bone (Figure 8-5).

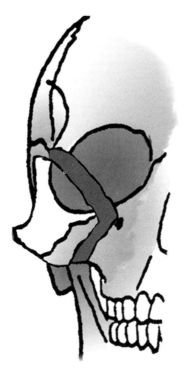

Figure 8-5. Fracture of the zygomatic bone. Frequent fracture patterns in the zygomatic include fracture of the zygomatic arch, fracture at the zygomaticofrontal suture, and fracture medial to the zygomaticomaxillary suture to form a three-legged structure known as a tripod fragment.

However, there is a fourth attachment through the frontal process to the sphenoid, which breaks to form complete separation, so the term *tripod* has fallen into disfavor. Because of the placement of this attachment, this type of zygomatic fracture also involves the orbital floor. The final category includes additional comminution of the zygomatic bone itself in addition to the complete fracturing of the processes.

Zygomatic arch or zygomatico-orbital complex fractures are usually unilateral and are dependent upon direct impact during falls, assaults, or vehicular accidents (Gomes *et al.* 2006, Bogusiak and Arkeszewski 2010, Hwang and Kim 2011, Trivellato *et al.* 2011). These fractures are among the most common due to the prominence of the malars in the face. Zygomatico-orbital fractures involve the zygoma and adjacent bones of the lateral and/or inferior orbit. Zygomatic fractures also tend to be associated with mandibular, maxillary, and nasal fractures but can occur in isolation (Eski *et al.* 2006, Gomes *et al.* 2006, Hwang and Kim 2011).

Bilateral zygomatic arch fractures are found and there is an increased likelihood of an associated basal skull fracture (Kelamis *et al.* 2011). These bilateral fractures are also often found in the absence of facial fractures, indicating that the force was directed at the cranial vault. Kelamis and associates (2011) postulate that the mechanism is not impact to the arch, rather the zygomatic arch fractures occur secondary to rotational movement of the posterior portion of the base of the skull, placing a strain on the temporal portions of the zygomatic arch.

Orbital Fractures

The orbit consists of a funnel-shaped set of bones. Fractures may occur in the rim, roof, floor, or on the medial or lateral walls and may be associated with marked displacement of bone (Gruss 1982, Manolidis *et al.* 2002). Direct blows to the rim of the eye may result in isolated fractures of the rim, especially on the superior or supero-lateral margin (Rogers 1992). Some orbital fractures occur in isolation, but many are parts of complex fracture patterns as seen in the above discussion of the zygomatico-orbital fractures. Epidemiological studies suggest that the division between isolated and complex is about 50:50 (Hwang *et al.* 2009). Among both isolated and complex fractures, fractures of the orbital floor are the most frequent and may occur as part of a LeFort or zygomatico-orbital fracture (Brant and Helmes 2007). Roof and lateral fractures are infrequent. Roof fractures are typically associated, in adults, with high-energy impacts and the victims usually suffer from multiple facial injuries (Haug *et al.* 2002). Fractures of the apex of the orbit are almost always part of a larger fracture complex (Bryant and Helmes 2007).

The most common causes of orbital fracture are assault, motor vehicle accidents, falls, and sports (Cruz and Eichenberger 2004, Hwang *et al.* 2009). These fractures are often associated with other head and neck injuries. Predominant causes vary since the use of vehicles, intoxication rates, and participation in sports also vary between and within populations. The use of airbags has lowered the rate and severity of orbital fracture for front-seat occupants (Duma and Jernigan 2003). Among pediatric patients, sports injuries predominate and orbital roof fracture prevalence is increased due to the incomplete development of the frontal sinus (Hatton *et al.* 2001).

Orbital blowout fractures are a complex of fractures that form within the orbit itself, usually on the medial or inferior wall. By definition, these are confined to the internal aspects of the orbit (Cruz and Eichenberger 2004) and appear on CT scans of fleshed individuals as extrusion of the orbital contents through the orbital wall (Chi *et al.* 2010). There are four categories (McCord *et al.* 1995): (1) linear fractures that parallel on the medial aspect the inferior orbital groove, (2) "trapdoor" fractures near the groove that will show little displacement in the skeletonized case, (3) fractures that produce a flap of bone along the inferior orbital groove and open into the maxillary sinus, and (4) comminuted fractures of the inferior wall. These fractures are typically unilateral, although in rare instances, can be bilateral (Chi *et al.* 2010). While traffic accidents and falls may produce these injuries, the bulk of the fractures are due to physical assault. The typical cause is a blow from a fist or similar sized object (e.g., a baseball) to the eye. Biomechanically, they can be produced either by buckling produced by impacts to the orbital rim or by compression of the orbital contents forcing displacement of the globe through the wall (Jatla 2004, Ahmad *et al.* 2006). The former typically produces fractures on the anterior orbital floor. The latter requires less force and directs fracturing over a larger amount of the floor and the medial wall.

Nasal Fractures

The paired nasal bones are particularly vulnerable due to their prominence on the face and the fragile nature of the supporting complex. The nasal bones articulate with the perpendicular plate of the ethmoid. The ethmoid articulates with the vomer. The ethmoid and vomer form the nasal septum, an area of bone where deviation is often found due to a prior healed fracture.

The nasal bones are more likely to fracture distally, where they are broader and thinner (Mondin *et al.* 2005, Higuera *et al.* 2007). They also fail at the junction of the nasal bone with the frontal bone (Gonzalez *et al.* 1954). Nasal fractures are often associated with fractures of the ethmoid and frontal sinuses, especially when they result from blows striking the head at nasion (Rogers 1992). Fractures in this portion of the skull are usually produced by an impact that drives the nasal complex backwards between the orbits (Gruss 1982). In these fractures, the thin medial orbital wall and nasal bones are rapidly fragmented.

Punches, kicks, and automobile accidents may all produce nasal fractures, the most common of all facial fractures (Erdmann *et al.* 2008). Nasal bones are often broken in falls, including those from a standing height. Due to the fragile nature of the associated bones, these fractures are often comminuted and impacted (Watson Jones 1941). A broken nose from typical assault usually involves a low-energy lateral impact while frontal impacts more commonly result from higher-energy incidents such as motor vehicle accidents. These events tend to result in greater comminution of the bone and septal injury. In a survey of the incidence, a bimodal pattern of the ages at which individuals experienced nasal fractures was seen with an early peak in males, usually between 20 and 40 years of age and a second peak among the elderly (Bremke *et al.* 2009).

Nasal fractures have been classified by whether they have been produced by lateral or frontal impacts (Stranc and Robertson 1979). Laterally displaced fractures can be further differentiated based on the extent of involvement of the tips of the nasal bones, more extensive nasal bone fracture, or injuries that also involve the adjacent orbital rim.

Murray and Maran (1986) developed a more elaborate seven-part classification system for frontal and lateral impact fractures based on experimental data. The first four categories involve fractures that are predominantly one-sided but extend into the nasals; nasals and ethmoid; or nasals, ethmoid, and vomer. These categories tend to occur with lateral blows although heavier frontal blows may also be involved. As the frontal impacts increase in power, both nasal bones in which the central portions are driven inward with fractures at the nasomaxillary sutures and in the ethmoid. The remaining categories reflect fractures of the nasal cartilage.

Other classifications systems also exist. Gruss (1982) classified nasal fractures into five types based on the extent of damage, with the first representing the most limited and the fifth the most extensive. Watson Jones (1941) simply grouped them into two groups based on the point of impact. Lateral impaction fractures occur when a blow to the side of the nose produces three vertical fracture lines that separate two fragments, with the one under the point of impact being driven under that of the contralateral side. Vertical impaction fractures result from blows at or close to the bridge of the nose. Central fragments are driven backwards often with four or more fracture lines and there is severe comminution. In both situations, the septum is severely deformed or crushed.

For the anthropologist, documentation of the extent of damage by charting and photographs is more useful than determining a classification, although some assessment of the direction of force is helpful. The distinction of lateral versus frontal may be determined by the presence of a central fragment, although high degrees of comminution may make identifying a central fragment difficult. Because of the vulnerability of these bones, they are frequently broken postmortem, and fracture margins should be closely examined to determine the probable time of fracture.

Maxillary and Le Fort Fractures

Maxillary fractures are one of the most common fracture complexes. The maxilla is one of the most easily broken of all the facial bones due to the thinness of the bones. Maxillary fractures constitute 10 to 20% of all facial fractures (Doerr and Mathog 2009). While the fractures tend to be depressed and comminuted (Schneider 1985), the majority of maxillary fractures are complex and difficult to classify accurately. Some facial fractures are so complex that they can only be termed small injuries.

Maxillary fractures tend to occur in motor vehicle accidents and falls or from interpersonal violence (Hogg *et al.* 2000). Motorcycle accidents are also a major cause of such fractures, especially when helmets are not used (Oginni *et al.* 2006). The most common victim is male.

Resistance to fracture by the maxilla is partly dependent upon the status of the dentition. Maxillae with poor or absent dentition tend to yield more readily, often resulting in a highly comminuted fracture (Gruss 1982, Doerr and Mathog 2009). In contrast to the massive forces needed to cause fracturing in the cranial vault, the maxilla will crumble under 140 to 445 psi, based on cadaver tests (McElhaney *et al.* 1976; Mackey 1984). Fractures of the paranasal sinuses, which consist of the frontal, ethmoidal, sphenoidal, and maxillary sinuses, are relatively common in facial fractures due to the thinness of the bone in these areas.

Alveolar fractures include those that pass through the superior parts of the maxilla. However, fracture of the labial, lingual, or both portions of the alveolar bone are due to blows directed at the dentition (Andreasen 1981, DiAngelis *et al.* 2012). Often several teeth may be affected at once and sections of the alveolar bone will be simultaneously affected. Breaks may occur at any level of the root.

Maxillary sinus and palatal fractures are also found. Posterior wall fractures of the maxillary sinus can be caused by impacts to the mandible, driving the coronoid process into the maxillary sinus (Simonds *et al.* 2011). Some have postulated that these sinuses absorb much of the impact and, thereby, provide protection for the orbits (Kellman and Schmidt 2009).

Rene Le Fort (1901) devised one commonly used system of midfacial fracture classification that involves various fractures of the maxilla. Le Fort tested his classification system of maxillary fractures using human cadavers (Figure 8-6). By doing so, he was able to observe patterned pathways of facial fractures. He divided these into a set of three basic forms. A Le Fort I fracture separates the upper palate from the rest of the maxilla. These injuries usually are the result of a blow directly against the alveolar process of the maxilla on either side of the head. They have also been reported resulting from blows to the infranasal area and may be accompanied by a midsagittal split in the maxillae (Hardt and Kuttenberger 2009). A Le Fort II causes a fracture through the maxilla, into the orbits and then through the interorbital area (Le Fort 1901). Such fractures result from a blow directed more centrally. This may also be called a pyramidal fracture. A Le Fort III goes from behind the eyes, into the orbits and through the bridge of the nose. These fractures have been reported to occur with blows to the upper midface from a superior direction (Hardt and Kuttenberger 2009). There are a number of other systems for these facial fracture patterns such as the Wassmund (1934) system, but the Le Fort system is still the most widely accepted.

In reality, the majority of these Le Fort facial fractures are variations on these three basic types, with comminution and associated fractures in other bones (Rogers 1992, Doerr and Mathog 2009). Both the second and third types are rarely encountered in the ideal form but are seen as combination of the two variations. When the two forms co-occur, the Le Fort III is usually on the side of injury, while the less severe Le Fort II is on the opposite side (Gruss 1982, Doerr and Mathog 2009).

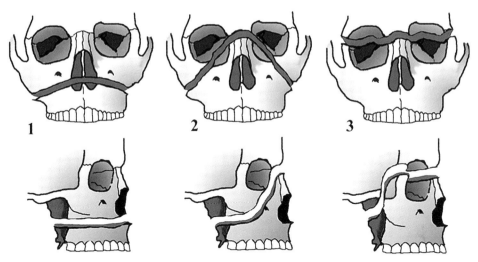

Figure 8-6. Le Fort fractures of the face. Le Fort devised a system of three different fracture patterns of the face. Type 1 passes through the maxilla and nasal aperture; Type 2 passes through maxilla, the lower portions of the orbit, and across the upper part of the nasal bones; and Type 3 extends across the upper orbits and nasal region. Actual fractures rarely follow these exact patterns, which represent guidelines rather than absolute standards and patterns that may be combined. Modified from Rogers *Radiology of Skeletal Trauma* (2nd ed.). New York: Churchill Livingstone, 1992.

Palatal fractures frequently accompany Le Fort fractures, although they can also occur in isolation (Chen *et al.* 2008). These can be divided into three categories based on the fracture location and direction. Sagittal fractures can occur along the median or in paramedian areas. Transverse fractures divide the palate coronally but may occur in transversely or obliquely. Finally, palatal fractures can be comminuted.

FRACTURES OF THE MANDIBLE

The arch shape of the mandible provides its strength, and the temporomandibular joints allow for some absorption of forces to the jaw. This architecture simultaneously makes it susceptible to multiple fractures once one section has failed. Often there is a fracture at the point of impact and another on the opposite side. Head injuries frequently accompany mandibular fractures with neck injuries also often co-occurring.

The most commonly cited location for the mandible to fracture varies by the study (Figure 8-7). Rogers (1992) reported the highest frequency for the body followed by the angle, condyle, and symphysis. In contrast, Fridrich and associates (1992) report higher frequencies for the angle, condyles with subcondylar

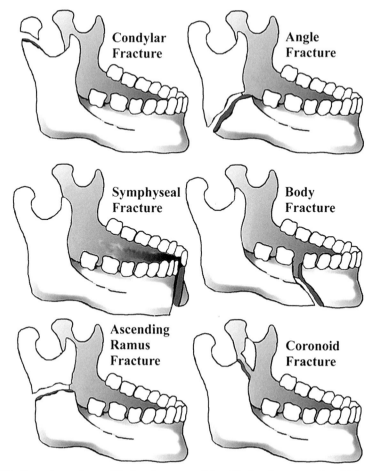

Figure 8-7. Location of mandibular fractures. Mandibular fractures should be identified by location relative to the condyles, angle, symphysis, body, ascending rami, or coronoid processes.

regions, symphysis and associated areas, with the ramus, coronoid, and alveolar fractures only rarely being noted. Another survey of mandibular fractures found that the angle is the most common site of injury, with symphyseal, condylar, and body fractures also occurring relatively frequently (Edwards *et al.* 1994, Andreas *et al.* 2011, Martins *et al.* 2011). Fractures of the coronoid process and ascending ramus are not often encountered. Fractures in adults rarely occur exactly at the midline.

Due to the prominent position of the chin, the mandible is frequently injured in fistfights, as well as in motor vehicle accidents (Fridrich *et al.* 1992; Rogers 1992). Motorcycle accidents also are a common cause of fractures along with falls, sports, and work activities. Males sustaining the majority of such fractures by a 4-5:1 ratio (Fridrich *et al.* 1992, Edwards *et al.* 1994, Sojat *et al.* 2001). The causes of mandibular fractures differ by sex. Some studies report that males most commonly sustained mandibular fractures from assaults, followed by sports and falls (Sojat *et al.* 2001, Lee 2008). Women in that same study broke their jaws in falls, assaults, and motor vehicle accidents (listed most to least frequent). Other studies suggest that traffic accidents play a more important role in fracture mechanisms (Edwards *et al.* 1994, Bormann *et al.* 2009, Sawazaki *et al.* 2010, Andreas *et al.* 2011, Anyanechi and Saheeb 2011, Chrcanovic *et al.* 2012). These differences in results may reflect local use of public transportation and personal protective gear such as seatbelts, along with differences in alcohol consumption and involvement in recreational activities.

Mandibular fractures are not common among children under five (Thoren *et al.* 1992; Cossio *et al.* 1994; Hubbard *et al.* 1995). The prevalence increases into adolescence and peaks between the ages of 16 and 20 years (Azevado *et al.* 1998). Boys of all ages appear to be more susceptible to such fractures than girls. The greater resilience of the bones in children, as well as the smaller size of the jaw in proportion to the face, may account for their lower incidence of mandibular fracture (Thaller and Mbourakh 1991). Often it is the relatively large frontal cranium that receives the impact rather than the chin, although this shifts when the children are in their early teens. In children, vehicular accidents including car passenger, car-pedestrian, and bicycle accidents cause the majority of mandibular fractures followed by falls in some studies. Other studies point to falls and sports-related injuries. In children, the condyle is the most common site of fracture. The symphysis, angle, and body are less often injured (Thaller and Mbourakh 1991, Munante-Cardenas *et al.* 2010). In infants, the primary fracture site is the symphysis (Lustman and Milhem 1994). About one-fourth of victims suffered dental fractures or avulsions.

With an intact dentition, the mandible will break at about 350–620 psi if struck centrally (McElhaney *et al.* 1976; Mackey 1984). When the mandible is struck on the side, the values for breakage drop to only 184–765 psi. If the individual is wearing dentures at the time of impact and the direction of impact has a sufficient superior-to-inferior component, the bulk of the force may be directed across the mandibular symphysis, resulting in failure of the mandibular body or symphysis (Schneider 1985). If the direction of the force, however, is approximately parallel to the denture contact line, the force will be transmitted through to the condyles, which will fail to withstand the force of the blow.

Fractures of the condyle include those superior to (high) and those somewhat inferior to (low) the mandibular notch (Inaoka *et al.* 2009). Other classifications simply refer to fractures as subcondylar or intracapsular (Marker *et al.* 2000) or to subcondylar, condylar head, and condylar neck (Lindahl 1977).

Subcondylar fractures are the most frequently found. Bilateral condylar fractures are not uncommon (Marker *et al.* 2000, Inaoka *et al.* 2009). Condylar fractures have been associated with vehicular accidents (Fridrich *et al.*1992). Automobile accidents tended to result more often in condylar fractures or symphyseal fractures. Sawazaki and colleagues (2010) confirm the frequency of condylar fractures in vehicle accidents. This cause accounted for almost 60% of their cases. This review included bicycle, pedestrian, and motorcycle accidents within the vehicle category. However, other studies have highlighted the role of physical assaults in the production condylar fractures (Ellis *et al.* 1985, Silvennoinen *et al.* 1992) or falls (Bastian 1989). Marker and associates (2000) noted that the sex differences were not distinct among those involved in road traffic accidents, however many more males were involved in physical altercations. Women were more likely to fall. Physical assault was less likely to result in bilateral condylar fractures, a condition more closely linked to higher energy impacts such as occur with motor vehicle accidents.

Angle fractures have been linked to interpersonal violence as well as to vehicular accidents (Paza *et al.* 2008, Thangevelu *et al.* 2010). In the Brazilian study, researchers also noted that the men involved tended to have a high prevalence of addiction, either to alcohol or drugs. The angle fractures tended to occur only unilaterally, regardless of the cause. However, other mandibular fractures were common, especially in the parasymphyseal area or on the body of the mandible and usually on the contralateral side.

One aspect of angle fractures that has received significant attention is the effect of the third molar. Those who have impacted third molars appear to have greater susceptibility for angle fractures and less for condylar fractures (Safdar *et al.* 1995, Hanson *et al.* 2004, Inaoka *et al.* 2009,Thangevelu *et al.* 2010, Choi *et al.* 2011). This greater risk of angle fractures appears to hold true regardless of the mechanism of injury (Duan and Zhang 2008).

Symphyseal and parasymphyseal fractures also are linked to vehicular accidents (Fridrich *et al.* 1992). In particular, motorcycle accidents resulted in higher instances of symphyseal fractures although slightly fewer condylar fractures (Fridrich *et al.* 1992). Studies by by Sawazaki and associates (2010) and Martins and colleagues (2011) derived results that support Fridrich and colleagues' (1992) work. Assaults, such as fistfights, tended to result in fractures at the mandibular angle and less frequently in condylar, symphyseal, and alveolar fractures.

Alveolar fractures are commonly associated with dental trauma and form a significant category in the classification of dental trauma. Even if the teeth themselves do not bear any fracturing, adjacent bone can be broken when the tooth is dislodged from its socket. Dental trauma classifications tend to note the degree and direction of luxation (DiAngelis *et al.* 2012). Lateral luxation, in which the tooth is displaced labially or lingually, will be accompanied by alveolar fractures. Intrusive luxation, where the bone is displaced more deeply into the alveolar bone, will probably not be evident in skeletonized material.

FRACTURES TO THE TEETH

Dental fractures are commonly noted in analyses of trauma cases. Difficulty arises in that the taphonomic processes may obscure pre-existing trauma and the distinction of antemortem must rely on observations of polishing or rounding of fracture surfaces (Schmidt 2008). Perimortem fractures and post-mortem breaks appear to have jagged fracture surfaces without any evidence of rounding. Microscopic examination is often required to identify these characteristics. Postmortem fractures are attributable to drying of the dentine, which has a higher moisture content than enamel, and subsequent strains placed on the junction between the dentine and enamel. Postmortem breakage has been shown to originate internally as opposed to traumatic fractures, which originate from the external surface (Hughes and White 2009). Unfortunately, Campbell and Fairgrieve (2011) found no means, using SEM, to examine burned teeth to distinguish between pre-existing fractures and postmortem heat-induced breaks.

Andreasen (1981) developed a classification of dental injuries, many of which would not be relevant to the forensic anthropologist. Those that are applicable to skeletonized cases include: (1) crown infraction, where there is an incomplete fracture of the enamel and loss of structure; (2) crown fracture, where there is fracture of the enamel and dentine and may expose the pulp chamber; (3) crown-root fracture; (4) tooth loss. This classification system also notes the associated fractures that can occur in the alveolar socket walls, or in the maxilla and mandible. Ellis (1970), the World Health Organization (1978), Garcia-Godoy (1981), and DiAngelis and colleagues for the International Association of Dental Traumatology (2012) use similar systems of classification. While some are more focused on treatment or prognosis, the above four categories are the most applicable to the skeletonized setting.

Epidemiological studies of dental trauma have been complicated by the various pathways victims travel in order to seek treatment. Some go directly to dental clinics but, since many suffer such fractures as the result of more complicated injuries, they may enter into the system via the hospital. Still others do not seek treatment. In one summarizing study of the Australian general population (Bastone *et al.* 2000), males clearly outnumbered females in the incidence of dental trauma, although distribution by type of injury was close. Among school-aged children, the sex ratio was close to even, but began to diverge drastically as people reached the later teen years. While falls tend to lead lists as to cause of fracture, motor vehicle accidents and fights remain significant contributors to the list. Interpersonal violence as a cause of dental fractures tends to peak in individuals who are in the late teens and early twenties (Rezende *et al.* 2007, Wright *et al.* 2007, Hecova *et al.* 2010). Bastone and colleagues' review (2000) also notes that the upper central incisors are the most frequently damaged teeth. Burden (1995) notes that the projection of the upper central dentition also plays a role as a pre-disposing factor for breakage.

Crown fractures without pulp exposure are usually the most common dental fractures seen following trauma (Laureidsen *et al.* 2012). However, these decrease in prevalence as people grow from childhood into adolescence and then adulthood. These fractures are often horizontal or angled and may involve the crown alone or portions of the root (DiAngelis *et al.* 2012). Spinas and Altana (2002) have developed a four-part classification system for crown fractures on the incisors, the most frequently affected tooth type. The first category involves only enamel at the margins or incisal edge, the second involves the enamel and dentine with loss of the mesial or distal portion along with incisal edge. The third category involves loss of up to a third of the crown including the incisal edge, while the final category includes the more extensive fractures that go into the root.

In contrast to crown fractures, crown-root fractures and root fractures increase in incidence from childhood to adolescence and to adulthood (Laureidsen *et al.* 2012). Crown-root fractures occur when the crown is broken off and the fracture line extends down into the area of the tooth root (DiAngelis *et al.* 2012). The pulp chamber may or may not be exposed.

Root fractures most commonly happen in the middle third of the tooth root and only rarely in the apical area (Caliskan and Pehlivan 1996, Malhotra *et al.* 2011). These fractures are usually horizontal or oblique and can be seen radiographically (DiAngelis *et al.* 2012). They are more likely to occur in a tooth in which root formation has been completed (Hovland 1992). Andreasen (1970) notes that the fracture angle tends to be more horizontal towards the cervical portion and more oblique towards the apical portion of the root. Because the coronal portion usually falls out with decomposition, root sockets should be checked carefully to see if remaining portions are retained. Distinguishing the timing of these fractures will likely depend on signs of infection rather than the polish/wear that is used to determine antemortem status for the rest of the tooth.

STRUCTURES OF THE THROAT

The osseous structures of the throat include the hyoid and cartilaginous components, which may ossify or calcify with age. These are subject to damage due to direct blows or compression.

Fractures of the Hyoid

The hyoid, which sits in the anterior neck posterior to the curvature of the mandible, consists of a central body with two long lateral protrusions or horns, known as the greater cornu. It serves as an anchor for musculature in the neck and tongue. This bone is usually protected from accidental violence by its position behind the mandible and anterior to the cervical vertebrae. Direct blows or compression of the lateral portions can, however, result in fracturing, especially of the greater horns. Because these structures are long and thin, they are extremely vulnerable, although breakage may not necessarily indicate any life-threatening injury occurred.

Frequently, hyoid fractures are linked to strangulation. Ligature strangulation and suicidal hanging can produce hyoid fractures, although reports place the incidence at 15–25% (DiMaio 2000, Green *et al.* 2000). Manual strangulation is the more common cause of hyoid fractures and, in these cases, males are more likely to see more damage. In the DiMaio (2000) review of data, all the male victims of manual strangulation exhibited a fractured hyoid as did half of the female victims. He notes, however, that the male victims were, on average, older than the female set. Miller and colleagues (1998) found that there are significant sex differences in hyoid shape, with females having longer distal ends of the greater cornu.

Accidental fractures have been reported (Dickenson 1991, Dalati 2005, Bux *et al.* 2006, Rash 2012). Accidental fractures are, however, usually associated with more massive damage such as mandibular fractures (DiMaio and DiMaio 1989). However, isolated hyoid fractures have been reported from falls or from sports accidents (Dalati 2005). Stress fractures have even been reported such as was the case in a man who had induced vomiting (Gupta *et al.* 1995).

Fractures associated with traumatic death including hangings are usually confined to the distal or middle portions of the greater cornu (Khokholov 1997). The body of the hyoid is usually unaffected by constriction of the neck but may be fractured in direct blows.

Care must be taken to avoid interpreting an unfused epiphysis with one that is fractured. The hyoid develops from six centers of ossification, which form the body, lesser and greater horns bilaterally. The greater horns do not fuse until late, rarely under the age of 20 years, and in a large portion of the population, as much as 25% to almost 40%, fail to ever fuse on at least one side (O'Halloran and Lundy 1987, Miller *et al.* 1998, D'Souza *et al.* 2010). The mean age of fusion appears to be between ages 35 and 45 years. Recent studies also suggest that there are no differences in fusion rate between males and females. Many individuals exhibit only unilateral fusion and this condition can persist into advanced old age. For this reason, fractures of the hyoid are rare in children and infants whose unfused bone can fold rather than fracture. Hyoid fractures increase in prevalence in the older segment of the population.

Fractures of the Thyroid and Cricoid Cartilages

Compression of the thyroid cartilages may occur when they are crushed against the vertebral column (Watson-Jones 1941, Fuhrman *et al.* 1990). This may occur with a direct blow or from hanging or strangulation. Since this region ossifies and calcifies with advancing age (Cerny 1983), fractures are more common in older individuals (Nikolik *et al.* 2003). DiMaio (2000) found thyroid fractures associated with manual and ligature strangulation while Green and associates (2000) report 38% of suicidal hanging cases exhibited thyroid fractures.

Fracture lines tend to be vertical or at a sharp oblique angle and are placed either at the midline or unilaterally across either plate (Gonzalez *et al.* 1954; Knight 1991). These fractures rarely are found extending horizontally. The superior horns may be broken preferentially with strangulation (DiMaio 2000, Nikolic *et al* 2003). While Khokholov (1997) found that hyoid fractures were often unilateral associated with hanging, the thyroid fractures were often bilateral. His careful dissections showed that not only were fractures found in the superior cornu but that they tended to focus on the base or inferior third of this portion.

Non-homicidal causes cannot be excluded, however, as two published cases of thyroid fracture were associated with falls, including from a standing height (Bux *et al.* 2006). As with the hyoid, direct blows can break this ossified cartilaginous structure, and fractures have been found in victims of automobile accidents in which the airbag was determined to be the culprit (Perdikis *et al.* 2000). Congenital absence of the superior horns of the thyroid cartilage has also been noted to occur in about 5% of one series of suicidal hangings (Green *et al.* 2000).

The signet ring-shaped cricoid cartilage is situated below the thyroid cartilage and consists of a broader posterior lamina and a narrow anterior band. This cartilage will calcify with age and may be broken in manual strangulation (Gonzalez *et al.* 1954, Knight 1991, Oh *et al.* 2007). The fracture tends to be vertical or oblique and either across the anterior midline or the sides. This type of fracture also is linked to and manual strangulation (DiMaio 2000). In hanging, Khokholov (1997) found that most of the fractures occurred in the arch.

Chapter 9

THE AXIAL SKELETON

ALISON GALLOWAY AND VICKI L. WEDEL

The axial skeleton consists of the spinal column, rib cage, and the sternum. The primary functions are enclosure of the torso, protection of the vital organs of the chest and upper abdomen, weight bearing in the spine, maintenance of mobility in both the ribs and spine, and support for the extremities. None of the axial bones have large proportions of cortical bone to prevent compressive injuries. Instead, the high mobility between skeletal elements allows for considerable absorption of energy. Impacts frequently affect multiple skeletal elements both directly and indirectly.

VERTEBRAE

The spinal column consists of vertebrae alternating with intervertebral disks. Each vertebra consists of two components: the body (centrum) and the neural arch. The centra are connected to one another ventrally via the anterior longitudinal ligament and dorsally via the posterior longitudinal ligament. The ligamentum flavum stabilizes the neural arches as it courses the length of the neural canal internally. The neural arches are also connected at the articular facets and their associated ligaments. Interspinous and transversospinal ligaments stabilize the vertebral column as does the erector spinae muscle group.

The vertebrae are grouped by type. The types reflect their function as well as critical differences in their morphology (Figure 9-1). The cervical vertebrae form the neck and consist of two units: the occipito-atlanto-axial complex (skull base-C1-2) and the lower cervical vertebrae (C3 and lower). These vertebrae are capable of high degrees of flexion and extension (White and Panjabi 1978, Standring 2008). The lower cervical vertebrae are also associated

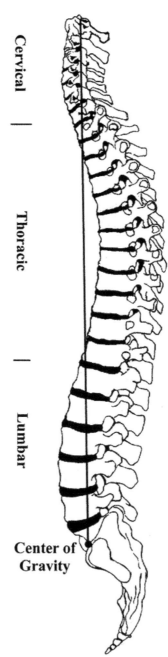

Figure 9-1. Diagram of the spine. Spinal curvature varies in relation to the line of gravity with the cervical spine showing lordosis, the thoracic spine being kyphotic and the lumbar spine returning to a lordotic curve. Since the line of gravity, extending superior to the center of gravity, indicates normal loading, the bones must resist compression and shear forces with regard to this line.

with lateral bending and rotation. The atlanto-axial joint is incapable of lateral bending but is capable of extreme rotation. The tightly bound atlanto-occipital joint is capable of some lateral bending but no axial rotation (Clark 2009). The thoracic vertebrae are largely restricted in movement by the rib cage, although axial rotation in the upper segments is possible. The lumbar vertebrae return to a flexion-extension capability but limit lateral bending and, even more severely, axial rotation.

Each vertebra develops from three centers of ossification. One forms the centrum while the others form the lateral to posterior portions of each side of the neural arch. Fractures must be distinguished from non-union of these segments, or in rare cases, non-formation of one or more of the segments (Shapiro *et al.* 1973, Bonneville *et al.* 2004). In the latter instance, there is frequently compensatory curvature or scoliosis of the spine to accommodate the angulation produced by agenesis of one portion.

In most cases, actual fractures to the spine are due to indirect trauma through excessive flexion, extension, compression, rotation, shearing action, or a combination of these movements (Rogers 1992, Bucholz 1994). Though clinically less common, direct blows to the spine may also result in fractures. They are likely to be somewhat more prevalent in the forensic material due to the nature of the events that lead to victims requiring an autopsy.

Biomechanically, the spine is often modeled as a three-column structure (Stanitski 1982, Denis 1984) with anterior and posterior portions pivoting around a fulcrum at the posterior centrum. The posterior portion is the arch and articular processes, the middle is the posterior third of the centrum and associated ligaments, while the anterior is the remainder of the centrum and associated ligaments. When the fulcrum is damaged, the entire structure loses stability. Fractures are classified as stable or unstable, depending on the degree of damage to the columns. Fractures were also grouped into compression, burst, and fracture-dislocations. The first two cervical vertebrae are regarded somewhat differently due to their structure.

Knowledge of the three-column concept and basic spinal anatomy helps in the evaluation of vertebral fractures. For example, compressive forces on the vertebral column are commonly associated with fractures. As loads exceed about 500 lbs, endplates fracture (Pennel *et al.* 1966) and the intervertebral disk, which is stronger than vertebral bone, is forced into the vertebral body (Evans 1982, Rogers 1992). This action initially results in a concave fracture of the endplate and, if the forces continue, there is often an explosive fracture into the vertebral body. In most cases compression is concentrated on the anterior column when the spine is flexed. Since the pressure on the anterior margin is 3–4 times greater than the rupture point of the posterior ligament, fracturing is concentrated anteriorly without any posterior longitudinal ligament tearing (White and Panjabi 1978, Evans 1982). This force produces a partial fracture of the vertebral body, most commonly in the form of a collapsed anterior column and is considered relatively stable. Simultaneously, there may also be fracture of the posterior portion of the vertebral centrum, which forms the middle column, to produce a complete vertebral collapse. As the fracture progresses into the middle and posterior columns, the fracture is deemed increasingly unstable.

While the three-column model is widely used to classify vertebral fractures, the medical community has not been satisfied with its usefulness in developing treatment approaches. Margerl and associates (1994), McCormack and associates (1994), and Malberg (2001) have proposed different systems. Malberg (2001) abandons the distinction often made that the first two vertebrae differ in overall anatomy from the lower ones. Each vertebra is composed of a ring of the neural arch and the centrum, while the superior articular facets and the intervertebral disk link this "ring" to the one above it. Type I injuries involve damage to the ring itself but not to the connections between vertebrae. Type II damage involves loss of the linkage between vertebrae. Type III fractures involve destruction of the ring and linked structures. Unfortunately, when only skeletal material is present, relationships between vertebrae may be less evident.

In 2010, the German *Arbeitsgemeinschaft für Osteosynthesefragen*, or AO Spine Group began a revision of the spinal classification system (Aebi 2010) initially outlined by Margerl and colleagues (1994). This revised system divides injuries into three types, each of which has three groups, which are, again, divisible into three subgroups for a total of 27 different classifications. Some of these subgroup distinctions are entirely ligamentous in nature. Type A lesions involve the anterior column injuries due to compression. This type includes superior endplate fractures, wedge fractures and vertebral collapse in Group 1, split type fractures ranging from sagittal, frontal and "pincer" fractures in Group 2, and burst fractures in Group 3. Type B lesions involve the posterior column including chance fractures. Type C injuries are largely caused by shearing forces. The strength of this system is in its prognostic value but has less applicability in forensic anthropology.

The form in which loading occurs also produces characteristic fractures. When the spine is under extension, crush fractures tend to concentrate in the neural arch. There may be little or no tension developed in the anterior ligament. Distraction, which is the opposite of compression, occurs when the spine is pulled simultaneously in two directions such as when the momentum of the head is distinct from that of the body (Rogers 1992). Distraction tends to result in fractures through the vertebral body and arch, although there may be ligamentous injury and displacement without significant skeletal damage. Shearing forces occur with other loading patterns but seldom alone, except under experimental conditions (Evans 1982). Such forces, which pull segments of the vertebrae out of alignment with the rest of the spine, may cause fractures of both the centrum and the neural arch.

The spine, especially in the cervical and thoracolumbar regions, is vulnerable to rotation (Evans 1982). Rotational forces often do not result in major fracture of bone but rather dislocation with rupture of the ligaments and joint capsule. This is more common in children because of greater ligamentous laxity (El-Khoury *et al.* 1984). In adults, posterior elements, such as the articular facets and laminae, may suffer damage during rotational movement. Fractures of the spinous processes may occur as the result of rotation of the trunk relative to the head and neck (Rogers 1992). Fractures of the articular pillars, articular facets and laminae may also occur. When combined with flexion, rotational forces often produce dislocation, but without this component, the facets are in opposition to each other and are broken (Stauffer *et al.* 1984).

Spinal fractures are much less common than fractures to the extremities, but when then do occur, they tend to congregate in three main areas: occiput – C2, C7–T1 and T11–L2 (Bucholz *et al.* 2009). Each of these three sites is an area where a rigid part of the spinal column meets a more flexible one. About half of all vertebral body fractures occur at the thoracolumbar junction (Eismont *et al.* 1994). In addition to the risk of fracturing, the numerous elements of this unit are subject to dislocation, with or without skeletal damage. The pattern does change with age as osteoporosis affects the mid-thoracic region.

The rate of loading on the spine plays a major role in vertebral failure and fracture (Rockwood and Green 2009). The faster a load is applied to the vertebral column, the greater the transient displacement of failed structural elements. Rockwood and Green (2009:1284) report that "at high loading rates, bone fails first, as opposed to the ligaments or the intervertebral disc. At low loading rates and with rotational forces the vertebral column fails through the soft tissues."

The incidence and distribution of spinal fractures varies considerably by age. In young children lower cervical fractures are less common (Hegenbarth and Ebel 1976, Hubbard 1976), while mid-thoracic fractures are more common. Horal and associates (1972) reported a concentration of injuries in the spine of children between T3 and T9 with a secondary increase in boys in T1 to L2. Most of these injuries were the result of falls from heights and motor vehicle accidents. Children also are more likely to have adjacent vertebrae fracture (Hegenbarth and Ebel 1976, Henrys *et al.* 1977, El-Khoury *et al.* 1984).

Spinal fractures are extremely common in the elderly and often occur with minimal or no associated trauma (Cooper *et al.* 1993). Compression fractures occur in the highest frequency (Old and Calvert 2004). Among women, one study showed that a prevalence of 7.6% of one spinal fracture in women aged 50–54 years increased to 64.3% in those aged 90 and over (Lane and Sambrook 2006). Age-related loss of bone mass may infringe upon bone integrity and increases the likelihood of fracture. In younger adults, the more fluid-filled intervertebral disk can accommodate greater loads. In older individuals, however, dehydration of the intervertebral disk is linked to marginal plateau fracture or general vertebral collapse when the compression is asymmetrical (Evans 1982). Age-related vertebral fractures are often associated with other fractures, especially of the hip and distal forearm (Cummings and Melton 2002).

For the forensic anthropologist working with only skeletal elements that are often found in isolation from the rest of the spine, interpretation of the skeletal damage in the vertebrae can be difficult. Basic description of the fracture form, as discussed below, is the best starting place with the context of the spinal structure and its three "column" architecture kept in mind. Descriptions should note the extent of damage in the anterior and posterior centrum, for example, rather than simply noting damage to the vertebral body. Notations of column damage will assist the pathologist in interpretation of stability and the possibility of neural damage. For compression fractures, estimation of the extent of collapse may also be helpful in assessing the consequences. Evidence of direct impacts, particularly affecting the posterior elements, should also be remembered.

Particular fractures can often be linked to specific predominant movements, but few spinal injuries are attributable to a single type of movement. More commonly, one form is the overriding type but has been modified by other factors, such as flexion-compression versus flexion-distraction. Location of all injuries should be carefully documented and recorded with illustrations and photographs. Reference to drawings that indicate the normal spinal curvature may be helpful, although significant deviations are obviously possible when the victim is hunched over or hyperextended at impact. While indirect forces account for most clinical injuries to the spine, this may not be so in the forensic population or in the individual being examined.

CERVICAL VERTEBRAE

The cervical vertebrae are particularly vulnerable to injury because they are situated between the larger masses of the torso and head. Indirect trauma is more common than direct loading in causing neck injuries (Goldsmith 1984). Hyperflexion, hyperextension, rotation, lateral bending, or a combination of forces causes fractures.

The uniqueness of the occipito-atlanto-axial complex makes this portion of the neck vulnerable to a specific pattern of injuries from indirect forces (Sherk and Nicholson 1970, Evans 1982). The atlas consists of a ring of bone and two lateral masses, which house the articular facets. The atlas has no centrum.

The atlas is weakest where the arch joins the lateral masses (Landells and van Peteghem 1988). The axis has a large process, the odontoid process or dens epistrophei, positioned above its centrum, which extends superiorly where it is held tightly against the atlas by the transverse ligament of the dens. The atlas-axis joint allows for extensive rotation but at the cost of stability (Shapiro *et al.* 1973).

The degree of permissible flexion and extension varies through the neck (Evans 1982). At the atlas-axis junction, flexion and extension are severely limited to about 10° (Shapiro *et al.* 1973). In the lower cervical spine, there is greater movement during extension than flexion, which makes this region more vulnerable to injury during flexion. The upper neck is more prone to injury during extension or extension/flexion. This difference may explain the different distribution of fractures. The most frequently injured neck vertebra is C2 followed by C5 and C6 (Ryan and Henderson 1992). Lower cervical vertebral fractures are more common in young individuals and appear to decline in prevalence with age, whereas fractures of C1 and C2 gradually increase in prevalence with age. Young children are more likely to suffer sub-luxation and dislocation without fracture, while bony injury is more common after about eleven years of age (McGrory *et al.* 1993). Fracture of the odontoid process of C2 is much more common in elderly individuals and is the neck injury most often found in isolation. Traumatic spondylolisthesis of C2 may also be found without associated injuries.

The atlanto-axial complex is also subject to a number of congenital defects, which may mimic fracture patterns when viewed radiographically (Pratt *et al.* 2008). Clefts in the posterior and even anterior midline of C1 are not uncommon. In addition, there may be cleft in the posterior of C2, additional ossicles, or fusion of C1 to either the occiput or to C2. The odontoid process may consist of a separate bone, *os odontoideum*, which may resemble a fracture of this process. Clefts are more likely to occur at the midline and both clefts and ossicles show smooth, rounded margins.

Direct injuries in the occipito-atlanto-axial complex are difficult to produce due to the depth of the overlying soft tissues at the top of the neck and base of the skull. During acceleration-deceleration situations, however, the neck undergoes violent movement. This mechanism is evident in the primary causes of fractures of the atlas. Most fractures are due to motor vehicle accidents, followed by falls and motorcycle accidents (Norton 1962, Hadley *et al.* 1988). For example, in a front-end motor vehicle collision, the head swings into hyperflexion then rebounds into hyperextension (Knight 1991). In rear-end collisions, the victim often suffers injuries of hyperextension. Typically these sequences can produce fractures in any of a number of locations including (1) the arch of C1 or C2, (2) the pedicles of C2 or (3) spondylolisthesis of the axis (Evans 1982).

Blows to the vertex of the head also may produce fractures to the atlas and axis due to compression. Diving headfirst into shallow water is a common cause of such injuries. Cervical injuries may also occur lower in the neck from impacts on the head. The power of interpersonal impact and its correlation to cervical spine injuries is seen in football players, in whom head-butts are part of the repertoire (Drakos *et al.* 2011), and in rugby players (MacLean and Hutchison 2012). These sports-related injuries tend to occur in the lower cervical spine. Assaults are less often linked to cervical spine injuries (Rhee *et al.* 2006). Spinal injuries may occur, particularly if the person has fallen as a result of the assault (Kulvatunyou *et al.* 2012).

Atlas (C1)

Because C1 is ring-shaped, fractures of the first cervical vertebra typically come in pairs or more. Gehweiler and coworkers (1976) have classified these fractures into five categories. These include fractures of (a) the posterior arch, (b) the anterior arch, (c) the lateral mass, (d) the transverse process, and (e) a burst or *Jefferson* fracture.

The most common fracture to the first cervical vertebra is a bilateral one through the posterior neural arch (Sherk and Nicholson 1970, Shapiro *et al.* 1973, Hadley *et al.* 1988, Landells and Van Peteghem 1988, Pratt *et al.* 2008) (Figure 9-2). This is caused by hyperextension of the head and neck that results in compression of the posterior portion of C1 between the occipital and the neural arch of C2. Fractures occur at the weakest point where the foramina for the vertebral arteries pass vertically through and then under the bone. About two-thirds of atlantal fractures follow this basic pattern. Bilateral fractures are more common than unilateral ones.

A similar situation, but with the fracture moved anteriorly, occurs when there are anterior arch fractures produced by hyperextension (Levine and Edwards 1989, Jarrett and Whitesides 1994, Pratt *et al.* 2008) (Figure 9-2). In these cases, the atlantoaxial joint is fixed leaving the anterior arch of Cl abutting the dens. Such fractures are relatively rare.

Fractures of the lateral masses of Cl are also possible (Landells and Van Peteghem 1988) (Figure 9-2). These fractures extend through only one arch without passing "through" the center of the vertebra. This type of fracture is less common than either of the other two forms. Blows to the neck or vertical compression can cause lateral mass fractures. It is probable that the head is out of a midline position, which drives the force through the lateral mass rather than bilaterally.

A *Jefferson* fracture is a comminuted fracture of Cl that involves both anterior and posterior portions of the ring (Jefferson 1920, Watson Jones 1941, Norton 1962, Shapiro *et al.* 1973, O'Brien *et al.* 1977, Evans 1982, Landells and Van

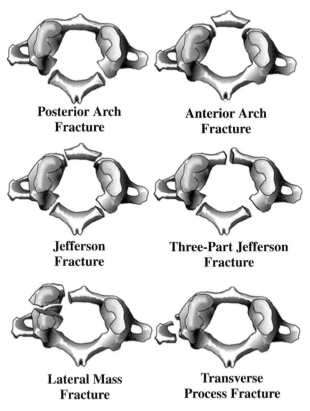

Posterior Arch Fracture

Anterior Arch Fracture

Jefferson Fracture

Three-Part Jefferson Fracture

Lateral Mass Fracture

Transverse Process Fracture

Figure 9-2. Fractures of the atlas. Fractures of the atlas include fractures of the posterior and anterior arches as well as Jefferson fractures (four or three part), which result from compression, which bursts the integrity of the atlantal ring. Asymmetrical placement of the head combined with vertical compression may produce fracture of the lateral mass while smaller fractures may include those of the transverse process.

Peteghem 1988, Jarrett and Whitesides 1994, Pratt *et al.* 2008) (Figure 9-2). In these cases, usually the result of blows to the top of the head, compression of the bone causes the segments of Cl to burst outward, which explains the alternate *burst* fracture designation (Sherk and Nicholson 1970). The laterally sloping superior articular facets of C2 form the wedge, driving apart the compacted Cl. The result is disruption of the ring of the atlas into an anterior, a posterior, and two lateral portions. These are fairly common in traffic accidents.

A variant on the Jefferson fracture is a three-part fracture with a bilateral fracture of the neural arch and a midline anterior arch fracture (Hays and Bernhang 1992) (Figure 9-2). This type of fracture is extremely rare but has reportedly been linked to hyperextension during falls from a height. There may also be a "plough" fracture in which there are bilateral breaks immediately posterior to the articular facets (Mohit *et al.* 2003).

Other fractures of Cl are less common but may occur (Figure 9-2). The transverse processes may be fractured (Levine and Edwards 1989, Jarrett and Whitesides 1994). Aside from their role in accommodating the vertebral artery, these processes form the attachment site for the deep cervical musculature. These fractures may occur bilaterally (Clyburn *et al.* 1982). Small avulsion fractures occur on the internal aspect of the lateral masses at the attachment site for the transverse ligament (Transfeldt and Aebi 1992). Anterior movement of the Cl relative to the odontoid process produces this defect. This same movement is also responsible for odontoid process fractures or simply a rupture of the transverse ligament. The inferior tubercle may also be avulsed, probably due to tension on the *longus colli* muscle during hyperextension of the neck (Levine and Edwards 1989, Jarrett and Whitesides 1994).

Axis (C2)

Odontoid process fractures are the most common fracture of C2 (Shapiro *et al.* 1973, Rogers 1992, Sasso 2001, Pratt *et al.* 2008) (Figure 9-3), although fractures of the body may also occur. They are quite rare in children because the process does not fuse to the body of C2 until between ages three to seven years (Schippers *et al.* 1995). These fractures increase in frequency in younger adults due to high-energy impacts such as motor vehicle accidents (Sasso 2001). Odontoid process fractures are also relatively common among older adults and are usually oriented in the transverse direction and occur at the base of the dens. In the elderly, they are usually attributable to simple falls and represent an additional risk associated with osteoporosis (Sasso 2001, Golob *et al.* 2008, White *et al.* 2010).

Odontoid process injuries commonly result from sudden hyperflexion or hyperextension and are seen in motor vehicle accidents and falls from heights (Shapiro *et al.* 1973, Rogers 1992). Hyperflexion produces anterior displacement of the fragment with the atlas, while hyperextension is linked to posterior displacement of both dens and atlas. They may also be produced by a combination of rotational forces with shearing aspects (Pratt *et al.* 2008). Odontoid process fractures in the elderly are usually due to hyperextension with posterior displacement (Sasso 2001).

Anderson and D'Alonzon (1974) have classified odontoid process fractures into three categories: (1) oblique avulsion fractures of the odontoid tip, (2) fractures of the process with the break occurring around its base, and (3) fractures that extend into the C2 body. The most common of these are those of the base (Pratt *et al* 2008). Avulsion fractures through the tip of the odontoid process are due to tension on the attachment for the apical ligament and are relatively rare (Sasso 2001). They may be associated with occipitoatlantal dislocations. Fractures of the odontoid process at the isthmus or waist are caused

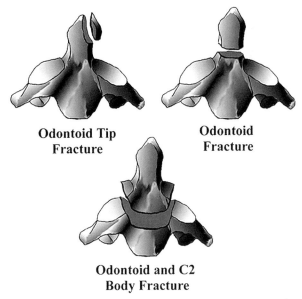

Odontoid Tip Fracture

Odontoid Fracture

Odontoid and C2 Body Fracture

Figure 9-3. Fractures of the odontoid. The classification system of Anderson and D'Alonzo (1974) divides the odontoid fractures into three groups including avulsion fractures of the odontoid tip, fractures at the odontoid waist, and fractures of the odontoid and the C2 body.

by displacement of Cl anteriorly or posteriorly (Anderson and D'Alonzo 1974). When flexion or extension is involved, the fractures are often angled from a superior-posterior to an inferior-anterior location. Benzel and associates (1994) point out that the Anderson-D'Alonzo system includes more than just odontoid process fractures and combines multiple mechanisms of injury. Hadley (1988) proposed an additional subcategory within Type II in which there is marked comminution of the odontoid process's base.

Fractures of the C2 body may be oblique, horizontal or vertical (Figure 9–4). Vertical fractures may be oriented in the coronal or sagittal plane (Benzel *et al.* 1994). Coronally-oriented fractures appear to be produced by extension with axial loading in which there is a shift of the fault line anteriorly from the *pars interarticularis,* as would occur in spondylolisthesis. Hyperextension will mimic this pattern but adds a small fracture on the anterior inferior surface of the vertebral body caused by tension extending along the anterior surface. Fracture of the posterior elements and fractures involving the transverse foramen are also found in hyperextension. There may even be a two-point arch fracture of Cl. Coronal fractures may also be produced by flexion-compressive loading and flexion-distraction. Sagittally-oriented centrum fractures are produced by axial loading usually applied to the vertex of the head and are often comminuted. The fracture line begins in the pedicle as the superior articular facets receive the load, which cannot be fully transmitted to the inferior vertebra. Horizontal fractures of the C2 body are usually flexion injuries and are often the result of a blow to the back of the head.

Pedicle fractures of C2 have been reported in the medical literature, although this fracture is extremely rare (Cokluk *et al.* 2005). The pedicle is the short section of bone immediately lateral to the odontoid and body of C2. Fractures in this area are presumed to have arisen from axial compression but with a rotational or lateral component. Reported cases are linked to traffic accidents.

"Hangman's fractures," also known as traumatic spondylolistheses of C2, involve bilateral fractures of the neural arch of the axis. This fracture pattern is the aim of the executioner in judicial hangings (Wood-Jones 1913, Lachman 1972, Shapiro *et al.* 1973, Spitz and Fisher 1980, and Spitz 2005, see Chapter 7) (Figure 9-4). Such fractures are usually found at the weakest point in the neural arch, through or posterior to the superior facets. During hyperextension of the upper neck, the fracture line itself may be vertical, horizontal, or oblique. The presence of the transverse foramen substantially weakens the bone at this point (Evans 1982). Traumatic spondylolisthesis of C2 may be found without associated injuries. Medical classification systems for traumatic spondylolistheses of C2, such as the one by Effendi and colleagues (1981), rely on the degree of dislocation, and, therefore, are not appropriate for forensic anthropology.

Judicial hangings may also result in fracture of the pedicles or lamina of C3 or C4 (DiMaio and DiMaio 1989). Frequently, however, hangman's fractures and odontoid process fractures will not occur in such circumstances and the damage may be primarily to soft tissue. In addition to hanging, traumatic spondylolisthesis of C2 may also be found in victims of automobile accidents when head movement is terminated by contact with a dashboard or other object while the body is still in motion. This subjects the bone to vertical compression and extension (Shapiro *et al.* 1973). While the ligamentous injuries are different, the skeletal trauma is quite similar (Jarrett and Whitesides 1994). These C2 injuries may also be associated with fractures at the C6/C7 level (Ryan and Henderson 1992). Extension fractures of Cl and C2 are often simultaneously inflicted by hyperextension of the neck, usually as the result of acceleration or violent movement of the head and producing fractures lower in the neck as well as in the C1/C2 complex. In these cases, the arches of both Cl and C2 fracture.

Fractures may also occur at the anterior inferior margin of C2, in the form of a tear-drop fragment (Shapiro *et al.* 1973, Pratt *et al.* 2008) (Figure 9-4). These are usually produced by hyperextension of the neck, which squeezes the spinous and articular processes together and ruptures the anterior longitudinal ligament. This movement produces a triangular fragment that is usually as tall or taller than it is wide. A similar type of fracture can be produced, less commonly, through hyperflexion accompanied by axial compression.

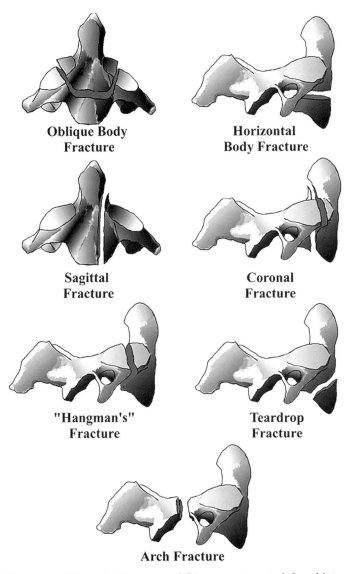

Oblique Body Fracture

Horizontal Body Fracture

Sagittal Fracture

Coronal Fracture

"Hangman's" Fracture

Teardrop Fracture

Arch Fracture

Figure 9-4. Fractures of the axis. Fractures of C2 are quite varied. In addition to those of the odontoid and C2 body, the body can also be fractured in a number of planes. Hangman's fractures rupture the ring of the vertebra. Hyperextension of the neck can produce teardrop fractures due to tension on the anterior longitudinal ligament and fractures of the posterior arch.

Finally, there may be fractures of the spinous process. These are relatively rare but may be associated with coronally-oriented fractures of the body of the axis (Iizuka *et al.* 2001). It is presumed that these originate as a flexion event associated with some rotation when this occurs unilaterally.

Cervical Vertebrae 3–7

In the lower cervical vertebrae, below the Cl–C2 region, a variety of fractures may form (Figure 9-5). Lower cervical vertebral fractures differ from C1–C2 due to the rather unique configuration of these uppermost vertebrae. Most flexion and extension in the neck occurs in the lower cervical region, with the range peaking at the C5–C6 level (Bucholz 1994). In a study on mortality in relation to cervical fractures, damage to the 4th cervical vertebra as well as the presence of lamina and facet fractures were associated with a poor prognosis (Pull ter Gunne *et al.* 2010). Fractures due to overrotation and lateral bending are also relatively high in number in the neck and peak at the C4-C5 level.

Compression in the mid to lower neck (C3–C7) may produce a burst fracture of the vertebral body with severe comminution. This pattern is similar to what may occur in the thoracic and lumbar region. Most often these burst cervical fractures occur in C5–C6 (Evans 1982) and are the most common fracture in this region (Norton 1962). These fractures are seen in football players as the result of impacts to the head (Bucholz 1994, Drakos *et al.* 2011, MacLean and Hutchison 2012).

Vertical or oblique fractures of the vertebral body have also been reported and are produced by vertical forces applied to the spine. Vertical fractures are due to massive, abrupt compressive forces and are usually in the sagittal plane. In diving accidents where the top of the head bears the brunt of impact, C5 is the most often fractured cervical vertebra (Stauffer *et al.* 1984). The anterior portion of the body may be displaced as a large teardrop fracture while the posterior portion is split sagittally. Complete and incomplete split fractures are often associated with flexion (Transfeldt and Aebi 1992). Complete fractures in the coronal plane are sometimes called *pincer fractures.*

Acute flexion of the neck may produce a *teardrop* type fracture: dislocation in the lower cervical spine that results in the production of a triangular or rectangular fragment (Schneider and Kahn 1956, Rogers 1992) (Figure 9-5). This is characterized by the crushing of the centrum by the superior vertebra, so that the anterior portion of the superior centrum is often separated by a coronally-oriented fracture line. This failure is attributable to the lipped morphology of the cervical vertebrae, which allows sufficient leverage under the vertebrae that is not possible in the lower vertebrae, which have flattened end plates. Anterior inferior margin fractures may also be linked to sagittal fractures in the posterior half of the vertebral body (Bucholz 1994, Korres *et al.* 1994). They are found following motor vehicle accidents, falls from heights and diving accidents.

The centrum may be anteriorly compressed if hyperflexion of the neck is involved. The anterior cortex may buckle and the cancellous bone will collapse. This is similar to the pattern of hyperflexion injury seen in the lower vertebrae and is called an anterior wedge fracture.

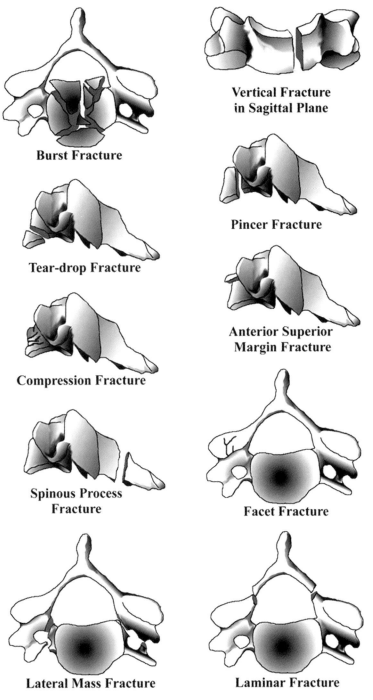

Figure 9-5. Fractures of the lower cervical vertebrae. Fractures of the lower cervical vertebrae include fractures of the body, spinous process, and laminae.

The anterior superior margin or even the entire anterior surface of the vertebra may become displaced (Norton 1962, Stauffer *et al.* 1984) (Figure 9-5). This may result from avulsion by the anterior longitudinal ligament or the annulus fibrosis or both. Shearing results from stresses induced during hyperflexion, hyperextension, or chipping from the vertebral margin of the superior vertebra. Anterior superior margin fractures, while less frequent than compression fractures, are still relatively common and account for about 10% of cervical fractures in one series (Norton 1962).

When the neck is both flexed and rotated, or when there is severe rotation, unilateral or bilateral fracturing of the facets may occur (Evans 1982, Hadley *et al.* 1992, Bucholz 1994) (Figure 9-5). Bilateral facet fracturing suggests that there was anterior dislocation of the vertebra above while the cervical spine was under distraction. This may be associated with fracture of the anterior vertebral body. In some cases, the articular facets may also be involved in fracturing due to hyperextension. In some extreme situations there may be separation of the articular mass (Transfeldt and Aebi 1992). This injury is more common unilaterally and is attributed to rotation. Facet fractures are relatively rare and appear predominantly linked to motor vehicle accidents and diving accidents (Hadley *et al.* 1992). The C6–C7 level is the area most often adversely affected by rotation but is also vulnerable to bilateral injury.

If rotation is associated with extension, the spinous process tends to become the focus of the force and consequently fractures near its base (Figure 9-5). An injury similar in appearance, the *clay-shoveler's* fracture, can result from avulsion by the ligamentous and tendinous attachments (Watson-Jones 1941, Norton 1962). In these cases, the rhomboid muscles cause avulsion of the spinous process during the upward thrust of the shoveling movement. Direct blows to the back of the neck can also induce spinous process fractures.

Fractures of the vertebral laminae occur in about one-quarter of unifacet or bifacet dislocations (Lukhele 1994) (Figure 9-5). These injuries are the result of abrupt forces and are most often seen in motor vehicle accidents. These injuries may be produced by a number of mechanisms. The initial fracture may be due to flexion, which produces an avulsion fracture by the interspinous ligament prior to dislocation. An alternate process is that the fracture is a rebound defect following flexion-distraction forces that produced the dislocation. If combined with rotation, this would explain the unilateral injuries. Plezbert and Oestreich (1994) suggest that about half of the laminar fractures are due to hyperextension in which the posterior elements are forced together. In support for this theory, they note that teardrop fragments may be present due to avulsion of the anterior longitudinal ligament. Stuaffer and associates (1984) suggest these are due to hyperextension and associated chip fractures of the anterior superior vertebral body. Fractures of the cervical laminae most often occur in the lowest parts of the cervical spine (C5–C6 or C6–C7) (Beyer and Cabanela 1992). Plezbert and Oestreich (1994) cite a number of cases in which these fractures are associated with thoracic or lumbar fractures.

THORACIC AND LUMBAR VERTEBRAE

The thoracic vertebrae have articular facets that are flat and approximately oriented in the coronal plane. While this allows for considerable movement, the degree of flexion and extension is reduced in comparison to the neck. The ribs act to stabilize the spinal column and are important in restricting flexion and extension. The amount of rotation in the thoracic region is high. The increasing size of the centrum accommodates more weight bearing.

Lumbar vertebrae tend to have great stability and resistance to loading due to their greater size. They also have greater flexion-extension mobility compared to the other portions of the spine (Levine and Edwards 1992). There is a progressive increase from L1 to L5 in the flexion-extension capability. There is also a decrease in rotation with descent down the lumbar spine. The centra are massive, and the curved and interlocking orientation of the articular facets greatly restrict the range of movement. The posterior elements support about 30% of the weight in the lumbar region due to their lordotic orientation, which eases the stress on the vertebral body. The bulky spinous processes prevent hyperextension and the predominant movements are those of flexion.

The mechanisms of injury in this region are axial compression, flexion, lateral compression, flexion-rotation, shear, flexion-distraction, and extension (Eismont *et al.* 1994). While these are the normal movements of the spine, the spine can be forced beyond its normal range. The transition areas are particularly prone to injury as they also mark changes in the curvature of the spine as well as the ranges of movement. The kyphotic thoracic vertebrae make a transition into the lordotic lumbar spine. The last lumbar vertebra, which is associated with a severely sloped intervertebral disk, also marks a transition to the sacrum. Hence, compressive loading may produce flexion injuries in the thoracic region but may produce extension injuries in the lumbar region (Stauffer *et al.* 1984).

The breaking load of the thoracic and lumbar vertebrae varies by element and by age. Load-bearing is greatest in the lumbar vertebrae and declines slightly in the lower thoracics (Sonoda 1962). Mid-thoracic vertebrae have breaking loads about two-thirds that of the lumbar vertebrae while the upper thoracics, like the lower cervicals, are relatively weak with breaking loads of only about three-fifths that of the lumbar vertebrae.

In the lower spine, most fractures occur between the last thoracic and the second lumbar vertebrae (Jefferson 1927-28, Nicoll 1949, Young 1973, Evans 1982). This is the area of transition between the thoracic and lumbar vertebrae, which differ in their form, function and range of movement.

Flexion-compression injuries peak in the thoracolumbar region, especially at T12–L1 (Kricun and Kricun 1992).

Age-related loss of cancellous bone, which may be particularly extreme in women, is responsible for much of the incidence of vertebral fractures. As trabecular cross-struts are lost within the centra, the remaining trabeculae often thicken in an effort to withstand normal weight bearing, but the thoracolumbar spine becomes ill-equipped to resist any additional loading. When the spine fails due to osteoporosis, fractures concentrate at the mid-thoracic region (T7–T8) and the thoracolumbar junction (T11–L1) (Christiansen and Bouxsein 2010). The upper area coincides with the maximum thoracic kyphosis. The lower area coincides with the spinal curvature transition from kyphosis to lordosis and the loss of support from the rib cage. The number of fractures associated with only mild to moderate trauma skyrocket in the elderly of both sexes (Cooper *et al.* 1993).

The most common thoracolumbar injuries are due to high- or moderate-speed impact motor crashes or to falls averaging about three meters in height (Cooper *et al.* 1993, Meldon and Moettus 1995, Hsu *et al.* 2003, O'Connor and Walsham 2009). These fractures are those associated with some flexion that usually occurs when a person falls from a height into a sitting or hunched position, when a weight falls onto the hunched-over back of a person or when a person is struck from behind by a moving object (Watson Jones 1941). Auto accidents, in which the movement of the vehicle is arrested while that of the occupants is not, are the most common means of achieving acute flexion. These accidents may also be involved in the production of distraction injuries when the body is thrown forward while the vehicle decelerates. The angle of the body, the amount of weight bearing on the legs at the time of impact and the force involved will all affect the degree of compression or distraction. Compression fractures, whether vertical or combined with flexion, are identified by the presence of a shortening of the anterior vertebral height, while lengthening indicates some degree of distraction (Ferguson and Allen 1984).

Fractures in the thoracolumbar spine can be grouped by the forces and motions involved in producing them. These include (1) flexion fractures with varying levels of compression, which are primarily wedge fractures, but also may form a burst fracture; (2) vertical compression; (3) lateral flexion; (4) flexion-distraction injuries, which include the Chance fractures; (5) torsion flexion; (6) translational or shear; and (7) distractive-extension injuries (Ferguson and Allen 1984).

The majority of the thoracic and lumbar fractures are simple wedge-shaped compression fractures (Denis 1984, Ferguson and Allen 1984, Kricun and Kricun 1992, Levine and Edwards 1992, Rogers 1992, Eismont *et al.* 1994) (Figure 9-6). These defects result from compression with a degree of flexion. Wedge fractures are usually defined as those with less than 50% anterior compression. These fractures can involve (1) the fracture of both endplates, (2) only the superior surface, (3) only the inferior surface, or (4) buckling of the anterior cortex (Denis 1982, Eismont *et al.* 1994). Under flexion and compression, the anterior body of the vertebra is severely compressed and anterior wedging dissipates the energy (Evans 1982). This preserves the posterior portions of the vertebrae, which, therefore, usually remain intact. The fracture dissipates the energy, relaxing the tensile forces on the posterior ligaments. Posterior avulsion fractures may, however, also be found (Eismont *et al.* 1994). Wedge fractures are less frequent in the lower spine because anterior compression is usually less in the lumbar vertebrae than in the thoracics or at the thoracolumbar junction (Kricun and Kricun 1992, Levine and Edwards 1992).

Wedge fractures often affect more than one vertebra. Multiple fractures may reflect an osteoporotic condition, and the wedges may have formed on different occasions. In younger adults or children, the traumatic nature of an accident may produce loading on multiple vertebrae, which causes fracturing. These fractures may be found in cases of child abuse and may be accompanied by the presence of small bony fragments along the antero-superior aspect, which penetrate the end plate (Kleinman and Marks 1992). Such injuries in the lower thoracic and upper lumbar region are probably the result of violent shaking of the child.

As the level of forces applied to the centrum increases, so too does the destruction. About 10–15% of vertebral body fractures are comminuted.

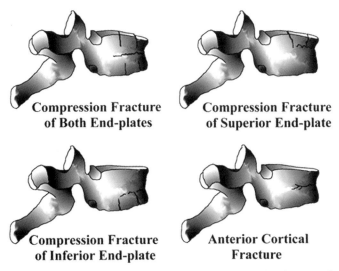

Figure 9-6. Flexion-compression fractures of the thoracic and lumbar vertebrae. Flexion-compression fractures in the thoracic and lumbar vertebrae produce damage to the end plates as well as partial collapse of the centrum. Denis (1982) divided these fractures into four classes based on end-plate involvement.

These are produced by more localized acute flexion of the spine, such as occurs when a person falls and lands on the shoulders (Watson-Jones 1941). These involve some degree of vertical compression, which distinguishes them from the flexion-distraction injuries described below. When compressive forces on the vertebral body are extremely high during trauma, as in vertical compression, fractures of both the anterior and posterior elements commonly occur (Ferguson and Allen 1984, Kricun and Kricun 1992, Levine and Edwards 1992, Rogers 1992). Acute fracture of the posterior portion of the centrum, a form of *burst* fracture, causes spreading of the posterior element (Figure 9-7). These usually involve horizontal fractures of the laminae, spinous processes, pedicles, and facets of the margins. Bone may be retropulsed into the spinal canal. In such cases, the anterior centrum is usually severely comminuted. A sagittal or Y-shaped fracture may be present in the lower half of the vertebral body. The spinous process may be split sagittally. This tends to occur in the thoracolumbar junction and upper lumbar region where the normal curvature tends to align the spine with the line of gravity (Levine and Edwards 1992, Eismont *et al.* 1994). These fractures most often affect L4 and L5 and are usually found in young adult patients. Anecdotal data also indicate that the extreme muscle tetany associated with tonic-clonic (*grand mal*) seizures can cause thoracic and lumbar burst fractures (Rockwood and Green 2009).

Denis (1984) classified burst fractures into five different types (Figure 9-7). While this system has been commonly used, alternate systems have been devised (Malberg 2001, Aebi 2010). However, the system for burst fracture classification by Denis is useful for forensic anthropologists because it is based on skeletal anatomy rather than dislocation or soft tissue damage. Denis' Type A involves fracture of both end plates due to pure axial loading. Type B is the fracture of the superior end plate and is the most common form. Type B fractures are usually the result of axial loading with flexion. Type C involves the fracture of the inferior end plate. This is very rare as the superior end plate is more vulnerable and both B and C are due to the same mechanism of injury. Type D consists of fractures similar to Type A but with a rotational component as well as axial loading. The final Type E is due to lateral flexion but differs from injuries due to simple lateral flexion with compression.

Lateral flexion combines flexion-compression with some degree of lateral bending of the spine to produce compression of the vertebral body and posterior elements unilaterally (Ferguson and Allen 1984, Eismont *et al.* 1994) (Figure 9-7). The anterior and middle portions of the vertebrae may fail with shortening of the vertebral height or there may be both compressive failure on one side with tension failure on the contralateral side. These are not common but, when they do occur, they are usually in the mid-lumbar region (Stauffer *et al.* 1984).

Compression fractures including wedge fractures, lateral fractures and, in some cases, complete collapse of the centrum may be due to simple skeletal

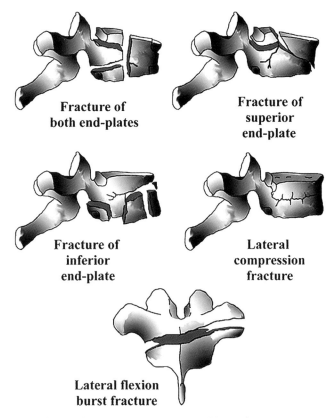

Fracture of both end-plates

Fracture of superior end-plate

Fracture of inferior end-plate

Lateral compression fracture

Lateral flexion burst fracture

Figure 9-7. Burst and lateral compression fractures. Vertical compression may produce a burst fracture, classified by Denis (1982) into three categories based on end-plate involvement, He also identified lateral flexion burst fractures which extend through the anterior and posterior elements. This fracture pattern extends the effects of lateral compression, which merely collapse the centrum.

insufficiency and they occur more often in women than men. This type of fracture is not generally seen in anyone younger than 50 (Galloway *et al.* 1990b) (Figures 9-6 and 9-7). They are more common in individuals of European and Asian ancestry than those of African ancestry. Changes in dietary and exercise patterns, among other factors, have meant that these fractures are increasing throughout the population. Unlike the traumatic compression fractures, these commonly occur in the mid to upper thoracic spine. These are linked to not only bone mineral loss but also to lack of trabecular integrity as evidenced by decreased trabecular connectivity (Recker 1993).

Flexion-distraction injuries can occur in the lumbar vertebrae when the body is thrown against a fulcrum (Figure 9-8). In these injuries, the pelvis and lower spine are secured while the remainder of the body is thrown forward. Seat belt injuries, in which the person is thrown forward over a lap-type seat

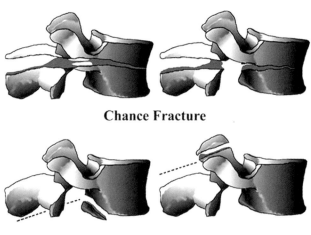

Chance Fracture

Smith Fracture with   Smith Fracture with
Posterior Centrum Avulsion Articular Facet Avulsion

Figure 9-8. Flexion-distraction fractures. Chance and Smith injuries indicate flexion-distraction of the spine, particularly in the lumbar region. Chance fractures pass through the posterior elements and may extend into the centrum. The fracture line may pass through the pedicles or into the foramina. Smith injuries are primarily ligamentous (*indicated by the dotted line*) but may include damage to the posterior centrum or superior articular facet.

belt, consist of distraction of the posterior elements and posterior intervertebral disk and are widely recognized in this category (see Chapter 7). This fracture complex can involve (1) fractures that run horizontally from posterior to anterior through the vertebra, (2) avulsion of the posterior portion of the centrum, or (3) avulsion of the articular facets (Denis 1982, 1983; Evans 1982; Levine and Edwards 1992). The first of these has been termed *Chance* fractures of the lower lumbar vertebrae (Chance 1948, Haddad and Zickel 1967, Ferguson and Allen 1984, Kricun and Kricun 1992, Levine and Edwards 1992, Eismont *et al.* 1994). Chance fractures, in which there is a horizontal fracture of the spine and neural arch, became more frequent as the use of lap-style seat belt became more widespread (Fletcher and Brognon 1967, Dehner 1971). This type of injury is less common with the use of a shoulder-harness seat belt. When the flexion-distraction is combined with rotation there may be facet dislocations and fractures. In some cases the fracture may pass through the pedicles into the centrum causing a horizontal or splitting fracture (Kricun and Kricun 1992). Smith injuries are found when the failure line passes through the ligaments and into the intervertebral disk. In some variants of this injury type, a small posterior inferior fragment is broken off the vertebra above the rupture or the superior articular facet it sheared off the vertebra below. Watson-Jones (1941) also reports on comminuted anterior centrum fractures with pure flexion as well as fractures in which the flexion results in the shearing of a wedge of the centrum that is deeper anteriorly than posteriorly. These usually occur at the level of L1–L3.

Rotational forces can produce massive disruption of the ligamentous attachments with associated avulsion fractures (Figure 9-9). This type of movement is often combined with flexion. If the force of the rotation is positioned directly through the vertebral body, a *slice fracture* may occur (Holdsworth 1963, 1970; Ferguson and Allen 1984; Kricun and Kricun 1992) in which the fracture line passes through the body to form two segments. Posterior fractures of the transverse processes and superior articular process are common and also occur in extension injuries. Rib fractures are often associated with rotational types of injury. The majority of such injuries occur between the T10 and L1 levels where the stiffness of the rib cage is lessened and the torsional stiffness of the lumbar regions has not yet been fully implemented (Stauffer *et al.* 1984).

Shearing or translational injuries often form elements within the trauma produced during flexion, compression, and distraction (Figure 9-9). When the shearing forces are directed anteriorly, fracture of the posterior arch and spinous process of the vertebra above are common co-occurrences (Kricun and Kricun 1992). There may be a "floating" posterior portion of the vertebra (Denis 1984). When the displacement is posterior, then the superior articular facets of the inferior vertebra may be damaged. These fractures usually indicate a displacement of 25% or more (Ferguson and Allen 1984). The mid to upper lumbar regions are the most often affected (Stauffer *et al.* 1984).

The last lumbar vertebra is naturally subject to high shear forces that must be counteracted to prevent subluxation (King 1984). This predilection is largely due to the approximately 45° angle at which the inferior surface articulates with the top of the sacrum (Levine and Edwards 1992). Such forces may initiate spondylolysis, the separation of the neural arch from the centrum. This condition may affect any vertebra, but it is particularly common in the last lumbar vertebra. This condition may begin as an acute incomplete fracture that appears to require hyper-lordosis to initiate failure such that the inferior facets of L4 make contact with the neural arch of L5 (Jacob and Suezawa 1985). This is common in athletes such as in gymnasts, broad-jumpers and football players whose activities require forced lumbar extension (Stauffer *et al.* 1984). Over time the acute fracture progresses to full separation of the two portions of the element (Merbs 1995).

End-plate avulsions are a recognized problem for adolescents because the ligamentous attachments are often stronger than the bony attachment of the endplate (Levine and Edwards 1992). This fracture can be of a unilateral portion or the entire plate fragmentation and are most common in the L4–S1 region. In the younger child, there may only be avulsion of the cartilaginous ring apophysis.

Fractures of the transverse processes are quite common and can occur as the result of direct blows (Rogers 1992, Levine and Edwards 1992) or muscular

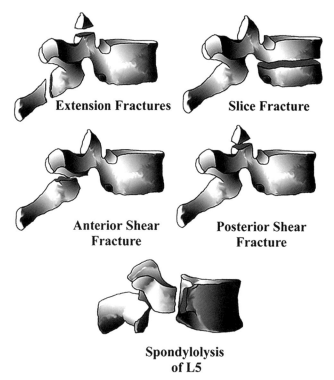

Extension Fractures

Slice Fracture

**Anterior Shear
Fracture**

**Posterior Shear
Fracture**

**Spondylolysis
of L5**

Figure 9-9. Extension, rotational and shearing fractures. Hyperextension will produce fractures of the spinous process and, occasionally, of the articular facet. Excessive rotation, when positioned through the centrum, may split the vertebral body. Shear fractures differ by the direction of movement. When the vertebra is shifted anteriorly, the spinous process may be sheared while posterior movement of the centrum may fracture the superior facets. The angle of the junction of the L5 and sacrum may induce spondylolysis, separation of the neural arch, due to shear forces possibly over a period of time.

contraction (Watson-Jones 1941). In most cases, these fractures are vertically or obliquely oriented. Falls and motor vehicle accidents are frequently the causes of transverse process fractures. Avulsion fractures are often the result of indirect muscle tension as well as direct trauma (Levine and Edwards 1992). Blows to the back can produce massive contraction of the musculature of the spine, which results in such fractures. In the lumbar region, the *psoas* muscle may be responsible (Krueger *et al.* 1996). Often a series of transverse processes are avulsed simultaneously and there may be associated rib fractures (Watson-Jones 1941). Vertical shearing fractures in the pelvic ring, when produced by superior forces, may produce fractures of the transverse processes of L5 (Meek 1992).

Of lesser occurrence are pure extension fractures. Hyperextension may produce fractures of the spinous processes or lamina and there may be some damage to the facets (Evans 1982, Eismont *et al.* 1994). The *pars interarticularis* is also vulnerable to stress fractures. Avulsion fractures of the anteroinferior portions of the vertebral body, while not diagnostic of extension fractures, are also common co-occurrences.

Facet injuries are not common in the thoracic and lumbar areas as most dislocations are usually limited to soft tissue (Levine and Edwards 1992). Facet fractures, when they occur, are often seen as severe comminution of the articular surface and may be associated with fracture of the lamina, *pars inter-articularis*, and the body. As noted above, they may be found in extension and posterior shear injuries and in some forms of Smith injuries. Avulsion of the transverse process may be associated with unilateral dislocations of the spine.

Lumbar and thoracic fractures are often associated with other skeletal damage. For individuals who have been injured in a fall, calcaneal fractures are common (Young 1973) (Chapter 11, this volume). Compression-related and shearing injuries in the pelvis and skull may also occur. Motor vehicle accidents that produce hyper-flexion lumbar injuries may produce only isolated injuries, since these may be linked to the restraint system, which may protect the individual from other skeletal harm. Thoracolumbar spinal injury in motor vehicle accidents in unrestrained individuals, however, are often associated with a pattern of severe fracturing as the person has braced for impact but then been thrown by the impact into adjacent fixed objects. The pattern of associated injuries in younger adults in falls and auto accidents contrasts with that seen in osteoporotic individuals. Falls and motor vehicle accidents are associated with simultaneous injuries to the head, chest, and extremities. For older individuals, other skeletal injuries may have occurred at other times, undergone degrees of healing and reflect the specific suite of fractures associated with diminished bone mass: hip fractures, Colles' fracture of the wrist, fracture of the proximal humerus.

SACRUM

The sacrum plays a critical role in both the spine and the pelvic ring, transferring weight between the two structures and forming the posterior segment of the pelvis. It often is fractured in conjunction with compression or shearing of the pelvic ring but also may fail under axial loading of the spine. Structurally, the sacrum normally resists compression well, but is ill suited to tension, rotation, and shear such as are commonly produced in pelvic ring disruption (Bonnin 1945). The sacral foramina weaken the connection between the spine and the pelvic ring. Fractures in the area between the first and second anterior and posterior sacral foramina are most common (Kane 1984). Sacral injuries, usually vertical paralleling the sacroiliac junction, may also occur in the elderly due to pathological bone loss (Peh and Evans 1993, Blake and Connors 2004).

    Isolated sacral injuries are rare. Forces transmitted either through the spine or
the pelvic ring usually cause them (Bonin 1945, Boachie-Adjei 1992, Levine and
Edwards 1992, Gotis-Grahham *et al.* 1994). A majority of sacral fractures result
from indirect forces linked to disruption of the pelvic ring. This is particularly
true in the upper portion of the sacrum where it articulates with the innominates
and where the bone is wedged between the ilia. Because of this, approximately
45–90% of all pelvic fracture involves generation of some defect within the
sacrum (Bonin 1945, Schmidek *et al.* 1984). Anteroposterior compression, lateral
compression, and vertical shearing can all transmit sufficient energy to produce
sacral fracturing (Boachie-Adjei 1992, Meek 1992). Forces applied to the
anterior of the pelvis usually cause disruption of the sacroiliac joint while those
applied directly to the posterior cause more massive damage to the sacral bone
as well as to the ligaments. Lateral compression of the pelvic ring can produce
anterior compression fractures of the sacrum. In vertical shearing, sacral fractures are usually lateral to or between the foramina and only rarely occur
medial to the sacral foramina. Isolated sacral injuries may result from direct
blows in the region of the sacroiliac joint (Kane 1984). In the lower segment,
direct violence is the most common mechanism of injury, although these may
result from falls onto the buttocks as well as blows (Levine and Edwards 1992).
    Sacral fractures tend to follow one of three patterns: (1) vertical, usually
through the sacral foramina; (2) oblique, passing from one side to the other but
with shifting levels of fracture; or (3) transverse, often passing through the sacral
foramina at one level (Levine and Edwards 1992) (Figure 9-10). The vertical
pattern is the most common. Transverse fractures are relatively uncommon,
accounting for only 5–10% of sacral fractures (Boachie-Adjei 1992, Kim *et al.*
2001). They may also be classified into lower and upper segment fractures.
    Vertical fractures have been classified by Schmidek and colleagues (1984)
and Denis and associates (1988) (Figure 9-11). Schmidek and associates devised
a system with four patterns: (1) lateral mass fracture, (2) juxta-articular fracture,
(3) cleaving fracture, and (4) avulsion fracture. The Denis system relies upon
zones of fracture with the emphasis on the probability of neural involvement.
The first zone is the alar region and includes sacrotuberous ligament avulsions.
Defects in this region are often associated with lateral compression of the
pelvic ring. Zone 2 includes the foramina and these often result in some vertical
shear component in the trauma. The final zone is that of the central sacral
canal. Some transverse fractures would also pass through Zone 3. For the
anthropologist, a combination of the initial orientation (vertical, oblique, transverse) classification and, if appropriate, the Schmidek system seems most useful.
    High-energy trauma is more likely to result in transverse fractures, with the
S1–S2 region being most vulnerable. There is often some comminution of the
alar regions, and the transverse processes of the last lumbar may also be fractured (Bucknill and Blackburn 1976). Direct blows to the sacrum may result

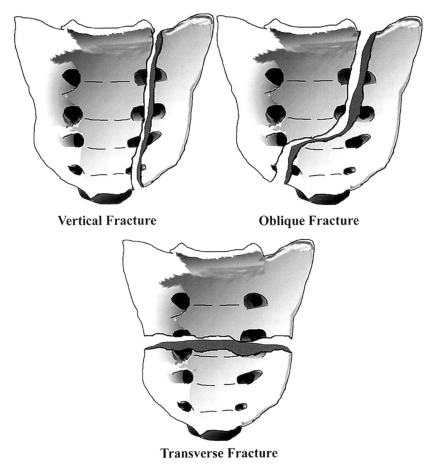

Vertical Fracture **Oblique Fracture**

Transverse Fracture

Figure 9-10. Classification of sacral fractures. Sacral fractures usually fit within one of three basic forms: vertical, oblique, and transverse. Vertical and oblique fractures usually form secondary to pressure placed on the spine or pelvis while transverse fractures are usually attributable to direct blows.

in transverse fractures in lower portions of the sacrum, often at the S3–S4 level, where alar support is lacking. In the upper segment fracture, a typical scenario involves a fall from a height, accidental or suicidal, or a motor vehicle accident (Kim *et al.* 2001). Based on experiments with cadaver material, Roy-Camile and associates (1985) grouped upper transverse fractures into three types based on the mechanism of injury: (1) flexion, (2) flexion with posterior displacement, and (3) extension. The status of the lumbar spine also influences this typology. Unfortunately, the interpretation is dependent upon the displacement of fragments relative to each other, contextual information that is usually unavailable to the forensic anthropologist working with skeletal material alone.

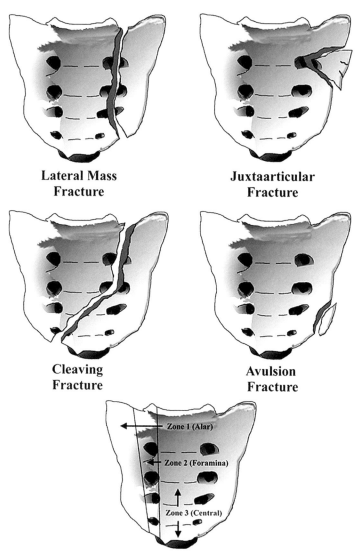

Figure 9-11. Classification of vertical sacral fractures. Vertical fractures are identified by their location on the sacrum according to the systems of Schmidek and colleagues (1984) (*upper four images*) or Denis and associates (1988) (*lower image*).

The forensic anthropologist should note the location and direction of fracture in the sacrum. If possible, the remainder of pelvic girdle should be examined for indications of the mechanism of injury and the direction of impact. In discussing these injuries and presenting them to counsel and the jury, models or laser-scanned images may be important given the three-dimensional nature of the pelvic structure and the many avenues by which the sacrum can be damaged.

COCCYX

Coccygeal fractures, uncomfortable though not life threatening, often occur when an individual lands in a sitting position (Watson Jones 1941). These fractures are more common in women than men because female pelvic morphology must accommodate childbirth. This morphology, with a relatively straight sacrum, leaves the coccyx in females more exposed to injury (Kane 1984).

Coccygeal fractures may be difficult to distinguish in skeletal cases as taphonomic factors often prevent recovery of the coccyx. The bones themselves may have been consumed by carnivores or eroded by weathering prior to discovery of the remains. Further, if present, bones of the coccyx may go unrecognized by untrained personnel. Determination of peri- versus postmortem injury may be problematic as this bone is relatively thinly walled. The level and direction of fracturing should be noted.

RIBS

Ribs form semi-elastic ribbons that curve around the thorax. Each rib is elliptical in cross-section and is composed of an outer layer of cortical bone with a central zone of marrow and trabeculae. The cortical area is primarily responsible for the resistance to loading, but this ability is small when compared to other bones (Verriest 1984). Cortical bone thickness decreases progressively with age, and resistance to loading also varies by individual frame size, rib height and curvature, and skeletal robusticity. Rib morphology allows for substantial in-bending prior to fracture, which results in compaction of the viscera. For example, due to the elastic nature of their bones, children usually experience only greenstick fractures of the ribs (Blount 1955, 1977).

Rib fractures result from accidents, falls, and direct blows to the chest. Ribs differ in their vulnerability because of their differing sizes, shapes, and position in the thorax. The first and second ribs are the most protected by the pectoral girdle, and the eleventh and twelfth ribs often do not suffer from compaction such as do the third through tenth ribs (Watson-Jones 1941). The ribs most often broken are the sixth to eighth ribs, generally more often on the left than the right. Fractures of the upper ribs (ribs 1–3) tend to be associated with more extensive injuries, which are more often fatal (Bassett *et al.* 1968, Poole and Myers 1981). This may be due to their proximity to essential vasculature or could be influenced by the effects of age. In some instances, coughing has produced rib fractures (Begley *et al.* 1995). These usually affect the fourth through ninth ribs in the elderly and osteoporotic but also may occur in higher ribs or in younger, healthy people. In children, more dramatic fracturing above the greenstick level may occur with forcible compression or crushing as would occur during child abuse (Blount 1955). The chapter by Love, in this volume, provides a comprehensive review of rib fractures in abused infants and children. In neonates, injuries from child abuse must be distinguished from birth trauma because infants, especially larger babies, may suffer rib fractures during parturition (Barry and Hocking 1993). In some individuals, additional ribs are present in the cervical or lumbar regions. Fracture of the cervical ribs during a motor vehicle accident by a seat belt has been reported (Bould and Edwards 1994).

Mortality tends to be relatively high with chest wall injuries with ranges of 4–20% (Zeigler and Agarwal 1994, Quaday 1995). A meta-analysis of studies suggests that age and the presence of multiple rib fractures are significant risk factors for mortality from blunt chest wall trauma (Battle *et al.* 2011).

Compression on the rib cage rarely causes a fracture at the point at which the force is applied if the application is relatively slow (Watson-Jones 1941). Anteroposterior compression of the rib cage usually results in fractures of the ribs at the point of lateral curvature (DiMaio and DiMaio 1989). If the compaction is directed anteriorly along the spinal column, the breakage point is more likely to be near the spine. Lateral compaction will yield fractures along both the spine and sternum. CPR is a common cause of compression rib fractures, particularly among women and older individuals (Kim *et al.* 2013). Cadaver studies have shown that rib fractures begin to occur with loading causing changes of only 12–16%, significantly less than the 20-30% commonly assumed (Kemper *et al* 2011).

Rib fractures are classified as transverse or oblique (Gonzalez *et al.* 1954) (Figure 9-12). Transverse fractures are more common and are usually produced by direct blows to the chest. Depending upon the size of the impact area, one or a number of ribs may be fractured. Oblique fractures are found more frequently in motor vehicle accidents and falls from a height. Oblique fractures are concentrated on the lateral curvature of the ribs, and the sharp points produced often penetrate the overlying soft tissue.

Multiple unilateral or bilateral rib fractures may give the appearance of a "stove-in" chest (Adelson 1974) or "flail chest" (Knight 1991). Inspiration by the victim through diaphragmatic contraction causes inward movement of the thoracic wall. This fracture pattern is usually produced by frontal violence, usually in motor vehicle accidents or when the victim is stomped while in the supine position. In skeletonized remains, this can, however, be mimicked by natural decompositional changes combined with carnivore activity.

The first rib is usually well protected under the clavicle, and its robust form makes it less vulnerable to injury than other points in the rib cage. These ribs are most frequently broken due to impact in motor vehicle accidents and are usually accompanied by more significant chest injuries, although they can also occur in isolation (Richardson *et al.* 1975, Lorentzen and Movin 1976, Yee

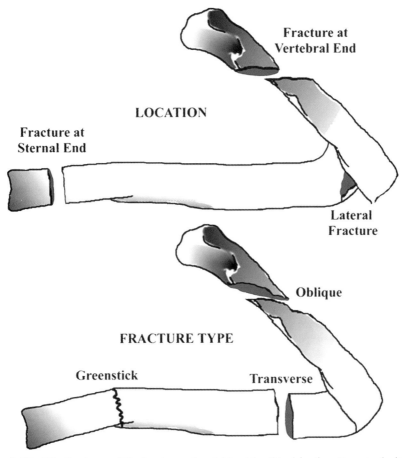

Figure 9-12. Rib fractures. Rib fractures should be identified by location, including the distance from either the vertebral or sternal end. Fracture morphology includes transverse fractures, usually due to direct blows, or oblique fractures due to a twisting motion. In some cases, the fracture is incomplete producing a greenstick fracture.

et al. 1981, Fermanis *et al.* 1985). Other causes include assault and falls. In these situations, the fractures are usually in the posterior or lateral thirds of the rib. Impacts that produce these fractures are usually in the shoulder or neck.

Fractures of the first rib may result from occupational or sport-related stresses such as lifting heavy loads or overhead use of the arms and occur more often in younger individuals (Lorentzen and Movin 1976, Pavlov and Freiberger 1978, Poole and Myers 1981, Vikramaditya and Pritty 2001, Sakellaridis *et al.* 2004). Stress-related fractures usually occur in the middle third, through the weakest part of the rib at the subclavian groove. They have been attributed to sudden contraction of the *scalenus* anterior muscle. Stress fractures are also found in those undertaking strenuous physical activity such as weight lifting. Such fractures have also been designated as "surfer's rib" due to its incidence amongst those paddling surfboards or being caught by waves while surfing (Bailey 1985) although, in vernacular usage, that term is not necessarily linked to first rib fractures. Other fractures sites are reported, including a posterior third rib break produced by shoveling snow (Chan *et al.* 1994).

Postmortem rib fractures are very common from carnivorous scavengers. Many carnivores target the internal organs and gain entry through the peritoneal and thoracic cavities. Chewing on the sternal ends of the ribs enlarges the area of access, and many such scavengers gain leverage for removal of tissue by standing on the rib cage. Fractures along the spine are common as the ribs are forced out of alignment. Anterior compression results in fractures at the mid-shaft.

For the forensic anthropologist, the rib cage is an important area to examine. Unfortunately, this often means that the entire torso must be carefully cleaned, which can be a tedious, although necessary process. After the ribs have been sorted by side and number, they must each be examined carefully for indications of fracture or other skeletal reactions. The location and nature of injuries should be documented carefully, and the possibility that multiple defects may be attributable to a single instance of violence should be considered.

STERNUM

Sternal fractures may be produced most frequently by direct violence to the chest. Less frequent mechanisms are those that are indirect including flexion of the thoracic cavity or in association with spinal hyperflexion injuries (Jones *et al.* 1989). Direct blows tend to produce transverse fractures in this bone (Fowler 1957, DiMaio and DiMaio 1989, Collins 2000). Direct trauma may involve crushing of the lower chest with transverse fracture of the sternum above the impact. Such events are often associated with high mortality in the victims, although the generalized chest injuries rather than the sternal fractures are the underlying cause. When the forces are more localized, the sternal injuries also are limited in extent. Sternal fractures can be classified by location: manubrium, upper third of the body, middle third of the body, and lower third of the body (Brookes *et al.* 1993). The presence of multiple fractures should be anticipated and noted. Isolated fractures are rare but do occur in auto accidents when an unrestrained driver hits the steering column.

About two-thirds of sternal fractures occur in women, most frequently in older individuals (Brookes *et al.* 1993). However, in motor vehicle accidents, the victim is usually male by about a 3:1 ratio (Athanassaidi *et al.* 2002, Recinos *et al.* 2009). Almost all sternal fractures are produced during motor vehicle accidents, usually when seat belts are in use or in pedestrian versus automobile accidents. When seatbelts are not involved, sternal fractures typically occur from impact with the steering wheel (Ben-Menachem 1988). The downward change in mortality associated with sternal fractures may well reflect the shift to seat belts as these injuries are increasingly isolated events in motor vehicle accidents. Specifically, shoulder-harness seat belts have been implicated in sternal fractures, which may occur without associated rib fractures (Fletcher and Brogdon 1967, Cameron 1980, Johnston and Branfoot 1992, Restifo and Kelen 1993, Peek and Firmin 1995). These fractures actually increased two- to threefold with the implementation of mandatory seat belt laws but are rarely associated with any serious direct soft tissue damage (Rutherford 1985, Purkiss and Graham 1993). More recently, airbags have been associated with sternal fractures along with rib fractures (Matthes *et al.* 2006, Monkhouse and Kelly 2008).

Sternal fractures may also result from homicidal actions, particularly stomping on the chest of a supine victim (Knight 1991). They have been associated with repeated punching in this area as may occur in some contact sports (Collins 2000). The sternum may also fracture during cardiopulmonary resuscitation (CPR) (Kim *et al.* 2013). CPR-induced sternal fractures tend to occur lower on the sternal body, usually in the inferior portion and are associated with rib fractures (Lederer *et al.* 2004).

Sternal fractures are usually transverse or close to transverse in appearance, most often in the midbody or manubrium (Athanassiadi *et al.* 2002) (Figure 9-13). The most common site is at the sternal angle (Collins 2000) while the manubrium is less frequently broken (Crestanello *et al.* 1999). Vertical, longitudinal, chip fractures or other less common fracture patterns occur. Vertical fractures can be produced by direct blows by a vertically aligned object (Gonzalez *et al.* 1954) or may be secondary to a transverse fracture. Since the cortical plates are thin, the fracture may occur at different levels on the anterior and posterior aspects by moving superiorly or inferiorly as it progresses through the depth of the bone.

When a blow is directed toward the upper portion of the sternum, the manubrium is displaced posteriorly. The upward and outward movement of the lower portion by the lower ribs, which are moved by the diaphragm and abdominal contents during breathing, causes this repositioning. The upper portion of the sternum is forced downward by the clavicle and first rib. If the blow occurs lower, the inferior portion moves posteriorly with the upper segment supported by the clavicles and first ribs. Associated fractures of the ribs may be found (Gonzalez *et al.* 1954).

Compression fractures due to hyperflexion of the chest and spine usually result in fractures at or near the joint between the manubrium and the gladiolus (Gonzalez *et al.* 1954, Fowler 1957, Cameron 1980, Dastgeer and Mikolich 1987, Purkiss 1993). These fractures tend to be oblique or have a backward angulation.

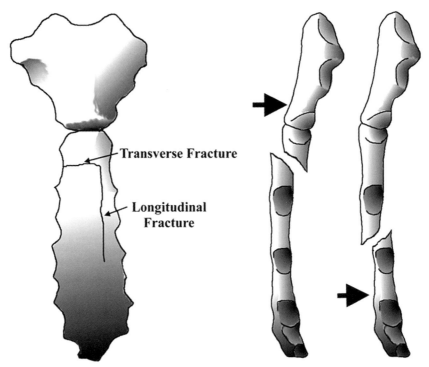

Figure 9-13. Classification of sternal fractures. Sternal fractures may be transverse or longitudinal and may affect either or both the anterior or posterior surfaces. Complete fractures to the sternum may be angled to reflect the direction of force (*large arrows*).

Indirect fractures in the sternum may also occur due to hyperflexion of the spine. One instance of sternal fracture associated with a *grand mal* seizure has also been reported (Dastgeer and Mikloich 1987). It is believed that sudden contraction of the musculature attached to the manubrium along with forced inspiration produced posterior displacement of the manubrium. Spontaneous fractures are also reported during coughing and vomiting (Itani *et al.* 1982).

Forensic anthropologists should examine both the anterior and posterior sternum for evidence of fracturing. Given the thin cortical bone, fractures may affect only one aspect yet provide valuable information on the mechanism of injury. For example, an incomplete fracture on the posterior aspect can indicate pressure placed on the anterior chest, which produced excessive tension along the posterior wall (Galloway 1999). Documentation of all fractures in this bone, as in the rest of the body, is essential. Location, extent, and direction of fracture should be noted and photographed.

Chapter 10

THE UPPER EXTREMITY

Alison Galloway

The upper limb, for the purpose of this chapter, consists of the pectoral girdle, the arm, the forearm, the wrist, and hand. While generally lighter in humans than in quadrupedal animals, the upper limb includes bones of remarkably different strengths. Following the model of our nearest relatives, the great apes, the upper arm with its associated chest and shoulder musculature is relatively stronger than the forearm. In humans, the upper limb has been modified for fine manipulation, losing much of its function for weight bearing. The differences in "typical" bone strength are often exaggerated by the effects of senile bone loss, leaving some areas particularly susceptible to fracture. The upper limb also is not well adapted for the abrupt transfer of loads between bones. Falls onto the hand focus forces into a narrow transition that centers around the scaphoid and distal radius. As forces move into the forearm, they encounter a divergence in joint stability with the proximal radius being less confined than the proximal ulna. While the humerus is relatively strong, at the shoulder there is a range of possible positions through which the loads must be transferred to the scapula, itself a bone with few skeletal articulations. Because of the high degree of mobility of the upper arm, there is a wide spectrum of possible injuries that depend upon the position of the arm at impact. All of these factors make interpretation of injuries to the skeletal elements of the upper limb difficult.

The long bones of the upper and lower extremities are very anisotrophic in that they are able to withstand loading along one axis better than others (McElhaney *et al.* 1976). The modulus of elasticity reflects the internal organization in which such structures as the Haversian canals travel along the long axis of the bone. This is characteristic of the long bones that form all of the extremities.

CLAVICLE

The clavicle is exposed to both direct and indirect trauma, but pure bending is unlikely given the relative freedom the structure retains at the sternal end (Stanley *et al.* 1988). Similarly, rotation is relatively great in this bone, which lessens the likelihood of torsion as a mechanism of fracture. Isolated, the slenderness of the clavicle appears relatively sturdy, but the S-shape and cross-sectional geometry accentuate loading and increases the risk of fracture.

In falls onto the outstretched hand, forces are transmitted through the arm to the scapula and from the acromion to the clavicle, which allow substantial dissipation of force. The position of the arm is often critical in determining the fracture pattern. When the arm is to the side upon impact, the blow is more likely to be transmitted to the clavicle. The surrounding soft structure also is important. In the midshaft region, the bone is relatively free of the strong ligamentous and muscular attachments that characterize both the sternal and acromial ends. The bone is also prone to anterior or posterior dislocation at its joint with the sternum, although the joint is strong due to the capsular ligamentous structures (Chadwick and Kyle 1992). Anterior dislocation is much more common.

The clavicle can be relatively easily broken during birth (Watson-Jones 1941, Rubin 1964, Pavlov and Freiberger 1978, Neer 1984, Roberts *et al.* 1995, Many *et al.* 1996, Lametal 2002, Moczygemba *et al.* 2010), and the incidence of such fractures increase with the birth weight of the infant (Cohen and Otto 1980, Ohel *et al.* 1993, Brown *et al.* 1994, Chez *et al.* 1994, Roberts *et al.* 1995), the length and difficulty of the labor (Many *et al.* 1996) and the mode of delivery (Moczygemba *et al.* 2010). These fractures result from the difficulties of passage through the birth canal in human births. The process requires rotation of the infant once the head is cleared so that the shoulders can be maneuvered past the ischial spines. The shoulders may fail to complete this shift or the pelvic outlet may be too small, which leaves the bony support of the shoulder abutting the pelvic outlet. Shoulder dystocia is more common among those infants whose clavicle is fractured during birth (Brown *et al.* 1994, Roberts *et al.* 1995, Many *et al.* 1996, Lam *et al.* 2002). While instrument-assisted delivery may be responsible in some cases, clavicular fractures are also reported with spontaneous vaginal delivery. Fractures decrease with Cesarean delivery, dropping from an average of 3.29/1000 to 0.25/1000 births (Moczygemba *et al.* 2010).

The clavicle becomes a more frequent site of fracturing, especially in childhood and adolescence (Blount 1955, Buhr and Cooke 1959, Rogers 1992, Thornton and Gyll 1999). About half of all clavicular fractures occur in children around age eight years (Calder *et al.* 2002), usually as the result of a fall on the shoulder (Stanley *et al.* 1988). In most cases, the mechanism of fracture is longitudinal compression from forces transmitted through the acromion process of the scapula. In very young children, the clavicular fracture is often of the greenstick or bow variety rather than complete separation of the segments (Rang 1974, Bowen 1983, Thornton and Gyll 1999). These may be seen as lines of cortical disruption along the concave side of the bone where compression is greatest. Epiphyseal fractures are quite rare and suggest non-accidental injuries (Thornton and Gyll 1999).

In adults, clavicular fractures are more common in men, who tend to suffer a slightly higher risk throughout life (Nordqvist and Petersson 1994, Postacchini *et al.* 2002). This is probably associated with greater exposure to the dangers of both recreational sports and occupational hazards (Robinson 1998). The left side is injured at a slightly higher rate (68%) compared to the right (Postacchini *et al.* 2002). Traffic accidents are the usual culprit. However, a high percentage (39%) occurs in cyclists (Robinson 1998). The frequency of injuries at the acromioclavicular joint is highest from simple falls, sports activities, and motor vehicle accidents and falls (Dias and Gregg 1991, Robinson 1998, Sigurdardottir *et al.* 2011). Midclavicular fractures often occur from motor vehicle accidents, sports, and falls from a moderate height such as from a bicycle or horse (Wurtz *et al.* 1992, Robinson 1998, Sigurdardottir *et al.* 2011). Most injuries at the sternal end are associated with falls, motor vehicle accidents, or sports injuries (Chadwick and Kyle 1992, Robinson 1988). At the sternal end, there appears to be a correlation with age where fractures increase in both males and females past about 70 years of age (Nordqvist and Petersson 1994).

In most cases, the clavicular fracture occurs in the middle third and is usually transverse and complete (Watson-Jones 1941, Rowe 1968, Pavlov and Freiberger 1978, Eskola *et al.* 1986, Stanley *et al.* 1988, Habermeyer *et al.* 2006, Nordqvist and Peterson 1994, Postacchini *et al.* 2002), about a fifth of these will be comminuted. Allman (1967) postulated that these injuries resulted from a fall on the outstretched hand. However, the mechanism in such injuries is usually difficult to reconstruct. Surviving patients often show evidence of a blow to the point of the shoulder either due to a fall with landing on the shoulder or due to an object falling and striking them on the shoulder (Stanley *et al.* 1988). Clavicular fractures also may occur from direct trauma to the bone.

Fractures of the sternal end tend to result from direct violence that drives the clavicle medially (Neer 1984, Habermeyer *et al.* 2006). Found in only about 2% of clavicular fractures, these defects are not a frequent occurrence (Postcchini *et al.* 2002) However, CT findings suggest that many more medial clavicular fractures go undetected medically: perhaps over 9% of all fractures of this bone. Lateral compression may force dislocation of the sternoclavicular joint with consequent fracture in the medial portions of the bone (Chadwick and Kyle 1992). Lateral compression will require some support of the opposite side of the body during impact. When this force is directed anteriorly, the clavicle will be displaced posteriorly while it will move anteriorly when the force is directed toward the posterior of the shoulder. The most common cause has been found to be motor vehicle accidents, especially those associated with a high mortality rate due to extensive associated injuries (Throckmorten and Kuhn 2007).

The acromial end is an infrequent location for breakage (Nordqvist and Petersson 1994), occurring in 12–15% of clavicular fractures (Habermeyer *et al.* 2006). These fractures can be associated with displacement due to the pull of the attached muscles. Acromial end fractures probably result from blows to the shoulder, which force the humerus and scapula downward (Horn 1954, Allman 1967, Hoyt 1967, Neer 1984).

The sternal end of the clavicle is often braced by the presence of the first rib and the stability of the sternoclavicular joint. If the downward forces continue, the scapula will tend to rotate away from the clavicle, eventually causing avulsion of the ligaments. Damage to the acromial end of the clavicle may be associated with rib fractures when this portion of the bone is displaced along with the scapula.

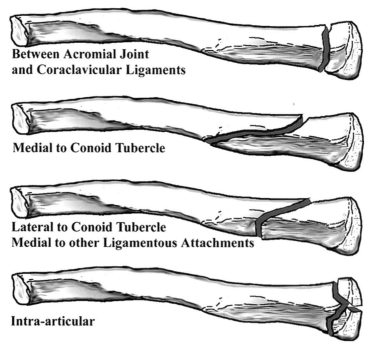

Figure 10-1. Classification of lateral fractures of the clavicle. Modification of the Neer (1984) classification of distal clavicular fracture (*shown on right clavicle*) depends on the position of the fracture with regards to the articular surface and the conoid tubercle.

A classification of lateral clavicular fractures has been proposed by Tossy (1963) and expanded by Allman (1967) and Rockwood and Matsen (1990). This established a set of six types of fractures but is distinguished entirely on the extent of ligamentous damage and displacement of the elements. The Allman system tends to be used medically and in its simplest terms, divides fractures as being in three groups numbered according to incidence: I. middle, II. distal, and III. proximal. Group I also includes a subgroup with fracture comminution and dislocated fragments. Neer (1984) proposed an alternative system (Figure 10-1). Under the Neer system, Type I injuries include those lateral to the conoid tubercle where ligaments will attach the bone to the coracoid process and are undisplaced. Type II fractures separate the clavicular shaft from the surrounding ligaments through an oblique fracture. Type III injuries are those which affect the facet for articulation with acromion. More complex classifications have been introduced, but they relate to the surgical complications, which arise from reattaching ligaments and muscle attachments and variations in outcome (Craig 1990, Robinson 1998).

Anthropologists should note the direction of fracture and its location with respect to the ligamentous attachments and proximity to the sternal or acromial ends. Biomechanical studies suggest that there is significant variability in the force required to fracture the clavicle. Cortical thickness and overall geometry are important factors (Duprey *et al.* 2008).

SCAPULA

Although it plays a role in the stability of the upper limb, the scapula in humans lacks the major weight-bearing role that is necessary in quadrupedal animals. Its broad surface and long edges provide for points of origin and insertion of the musculature of the superficial back and upper arm.

Scapular fractures are relatively uncommon, occurring most often in people ages 40 to 60 years (Neer 1984). The body of the scapula is rarely injured due to protection by the overlying group of muscles (Watson-Jones 1941, Pavlov and Freiberger 1978, Rogers 1992). Similarly, this bone is less prone to indirect trauma due to the "floating" nature of its anatomical position. The acromial and coracoid processes and the glenoid fossa are more vulnerable to both direct and indirect trauma than the body or spine (Rogers 1992). Despite this, the body of the scapula is the most frequently broken portion. Fractures of the body form about one-third of scapular breaks, while those of the scapular neck account for about one-quarter (Miller and Ada 1992). Fractures of the spine, glenoid, and acromion are approximately equal in frequency, each forming about 10% of scapular fractures. Fractures may be associated with dislocations and stress damage.

In adults, direct trauma is the most likely cause of fractures (Stanley *et al.* 1988). Severe injuries to this bone is usually indicative of extremely severe trauma (Miller and Ada 1992), frequently associated with motor vehicle accidents. In a large study of motor vehicle crash victims, Coimbra and associates (2010) found that scapular fractures result from impact with the car's side interior. Rib fractures are commonly associated, occurring in 27–54% of cases with scapular fracture (Zuckerman *et al.* 1993, Stephens *et al.* 1995) and the presence of scapular fractures tripled the odds of associated thoracic fractures and doubled the odds of spinal fractures (Coimbra *et al.* 2010). Clavicular fractures associated with scapular fracture are also a concern, occurring in 19–39% of cases. Because of the associated injuries, victims in motor vehicle accidents are significantly more likely to die than those who experience scapular fractures from other causes (Theivendran *et al.* 2008, Coimbra *et al.* 2010).

Glenoid fractures are almost always due to impact with the humeral head and are usually caused by anterior dislocations when the glenoid labrum fractures in a *Bankart* lesion (Tile 1987a). Occasionally, the glenoid labrum will be avulsed (Rogers 1992). Fractures of the glenoid fossa are most commonly on the inferior margin (Pavlov and Freiberger 1978). In more severe cases, glenoid fractures may extend into the coracoid process (Miller and Ada 1992).

Acromial fractures may have multiple causes: direct blows, forces transmitted through the humerus, avulsion, and stress or fatigue. Fractures of the acromion, which result in separation at the base, are usually the result of direct violence, whereas similar fractures on the coracoid are less frequently linked with direct blows to this area (Rogers 1992). Acromial fractures also may be produced by upward displacement of the humeral head (Neer 1984). It is important to distinguish such acromial fractures from the possibility of an *os acromiale*, a benign congenital separation of the acromion process from the scapula (Rogers 1992).

Coracoid fractures are relatively uncommon, although fractures at the base and avulsion fractures at the tip do occur (Neer 1984). These fractures can result either from a direct blow, subsequent to dislocation of the humeral head, or indirectly by the tensile forces produced by the attached ligaments to the clavicle and tendons (Goss 1996). Breakage at the coracoid base is usually due to a direct blow to the point of the shoulder. Fractures of the coracoid tip are usually avulsive in nature. Transverse fracture has also been reported in people who puts their hands down to soften the impact of falling from standing height into a sitting position (Guiral *et al.* 1996).

Fractures of the scapular neck may occur from direct blows and are often associated with fractures of the humerus at the surgical neck or clavicular fractures. The blows may be directed anteriorly, posteriorly, or directly onto the point of the shoulder (Neer 1984). Motorcycle accidents also appear to produce fractures of the scapular surgical neck (van Noort and van Kampen

2005). When associated with a fracture of the upper humerus or a clavicular injury, a clinical condition known as "floating shoulder" can be produced (Theivendran *et al.* 2008).

Scapular fractures, either in the body or in the neck, tend to be somewhat idiosyncratic, depending upon the circumstances of the trauma. Force directed on the posterior of the body may bend the scapular body over the first rib (Miller and Ada 1992). It is this type of fracture that frequently is associated with fracture of the underlying ribs. The underlying ribs may also form the fulcrum over which the scapula bends, which usually causes it to fracture along the vertebral border.

Avulsion fractures involving the inferior glenoid, the inferior angle or lateral and superior border have also been reported (Rogers 1992). Scapular fractures have also been attributed to indirect trauma from unusual circumstances. Isolated injuries have also been reported, such as a fracture of the scapular body near the glenoid in a professional boxer who missed a punch (Wyrsch *et al.* 1995). Two cases of scapular fracture due to electrical shock from normal household/office equipment have been documented (Dumas and Walker 1992, Liaw and Pollack 1996). In both cases, there were bilateral fractures of the scapular body. The mechanism may be the same as that found in scapular fractures due to convulsive seizures (Shaw 1971). It is possible for massive contraction of the shoulder muscles to drive the humeral head into the glenoid. This action was also determined to be the cause of a scapular body fracture below the glenoid found after electrical shock given during cardiopulmonary resuscitation (Kam and Kam 1994).

Scapular fractures are best described on the basis of structural anatomy (Miller and Ada 1992) (Figure 10-2). A four-category system includes: (1) Type I – fractures of the processes (acromion, spine, acromial base, and coracoid), (2) Type II – fractures of the neck, (3) Type III – glenoid fractures, and (4) Type IV – body fractures.

Since glenoid fractures provide specific information on direction of dislocation or subluxation at the shoulder joint, they are separately classified into five types (Ideberg 1984, 1987; Ideberg *et al.* 1995). Type I is avulsion of the anterior margin. Type II involves fractures that travel inferiorly from the glenoid. Type III describes fractures that exit superiorly often involving injury to the acromioclavicular joint. Type IV is a horizontal fracture of the scapular neck and body, inferior to the scapular spine, while Type V extends this to include an additional neck fractures.

For the anthropologist, descriptive designations are the most useful and provide information not muddied by various numerical classifications. The location and nature of the fracture should be noted. Scapular fractures should be carefully charted and associated rib, clavicular or humeral fractures noted, too, as all are important in documenting the magnitude and direction of the

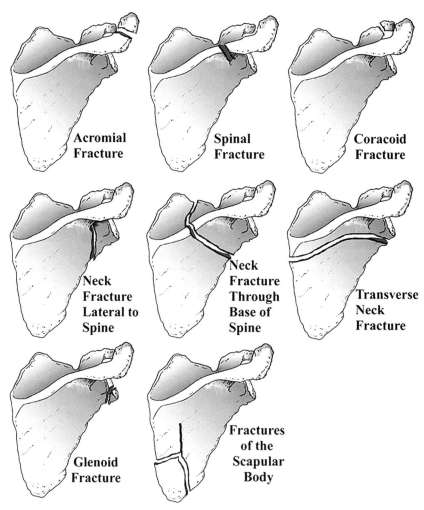

Figure 10-2. Classification of scapular fractures. Miller and Ada (1992) classifies scapular fractures: fractures of the acromial process, spine and corocoid process, neck fractures, glenoid fractures, and fractures of the body. Descriptive designations of the fracture location and direction are used in the above illustration (*right scapula*).

force. The floating nature of the scapula with respect to the ribs means that often-associated fractures are not immediately obvious simply by positioning the bones in anatomical position. Instead, the full range of movement should be considered which includes extreme positions that may occur during periods of violence. Detailed photographs and sketches are helpful in documenting these injuries and in explaining them to others. Demonstration with anatomical models may be helpful in demonstrating to counsel and to the jury how dislocation of the humerus can produce scapular fractures.

HUMERUS

The humerus is vulnerable to direct violence but is also vulnerable to the indirect effect of forces imparted through the forearm and hand. The effects of both young and old age are great in this bone: epiphyseal vulnerability is present in subadults while trabecular and cortical bone loss takes its toll in advancing years. The large muscle mass of the rotator cuff surrounding the shoulder provides some protection, but distally this protection lessens. The flexors and extensors of the wrist and hand originate in large part in the humeral epicondyles, and morphological change in the arm bone to accommodate both these sites, as well as articulation with the radius and ulna, makes the distal humerus a frequent site for fractures.

Proximal Humeral Fractures

Fractures of the proximal humerus most often occur in youngsters and adolescents as well as in older adults, particularly women (Buhr and Cooke 1959, Horak and Nilsson 1975, Norris 1992, Chu *et al.* 2004, Palvanen *et al.* 2006). This pattern is due to changes in the anatomy of the bone. The first period of humeral vulnerability is due to the possibility of separation of the epiphysis. In young children, proximal humeral fractures usually take the form of Salter-Harris Type I separations and occur before age five years (Thornton and Gyll 1999). Fractures of the proximal humerus are the second most frequent fracture during birth, resulting from rotation or hyperextension (Della-Guistina and Della-Guistina 1999). Type II forms predominate after about age 10 years. By this age, sports accidents and falls from heights cause the fractures and they tend to occur more frequently in boys (Williams 1981). Falls onto the outstretched hand are commonly cited as a cause along with direct impact to the shoulder (Carson *et al.* 2006, Shrader 2007). In addition to accidental injuries, humeral fractures at the proximal end have been associated with child abuse (Shrader 2007, Love this volume).

The second period of vulnerability coincides with the substantial bone loss associated with advancing age (Lee *et al.* 2002, Chu *et al.* 2004). The incidence increases after about 45 years of age and is three times higher in women than in men due to post-menopausal bone loss. As in many other portions of the body, there is also a shift in the mode of injury. In younger individuals, fractures are usually the result of severe trauma such as falls from a height or motor vehicle accidents. With advancing age, moderate trauma is more likely to produce proximal humeral injury. These fractures also seem to be found in women who are generally less healthy and exhibit low bone mineral density (Kelsey *et al.* 1992). Bone mineral status will affect the nature of the fracture. In individuals in whom age has led to gradual reduction of cortical bone, proximal fractures tend to be less displaced and with less associated soft tissue damage. In younger individuals, high-energy trauma is often needed to produce fractures and therefore associated with greater soft tissue damage.

Fractures in the proximal humerus usually result indirectly from falls onto the outstretched hand. This mechanism accounts for 87-93% of the proximal humeral fractures among the elderly (Court-Brown *et al.* 2001, Lee *et al.* 2002, Palvanen *et al.* 2006). Axial loading transmitted through the humerus often will exceed the ability of the bone to withstand the stress (Norris 1992). With abduction of the arm, there is lateral rotation, but, during impact in a fall, this exceeds the rotational ability of the joint (Neer 1984). In younger individuals, ligaments may be torn, but in adults, the ligamentous strength often exceeds that of bone and which leads to fracture. During dislocation, the greater tubercle may be unable to clear the acromion resulting in damage to both the humerus and the scapula (Norris 1992). Rotational forces can also cause fragmentation and subsequent displacement of pieces. Humeral fractures may coincide with fractures of the distal radius (Colles' type).

Direct blows may also cause damage to this region of the bone (Pavlov and Freiberger 1978, Neer 1984, Chadwick and Kyle 1992, Norris 1992). Comminuted fractures of the humeral head may occur as the result of a direct blow to the shoulder, which drives the humeral head into the glenoid fossa of the scapula (Rogers 1992).

Besides blows and indirect forces through the arm, bilateral shoulder fractures can also be produced during convulsive seizures and electrical shock. Convulsive activity is most likely to affect areas of insertion by internal rotators, which are about 50% stronger than external rotators and by adductors that are twice as strong as abductors (Chadwick and Kyle 1992). Proximal humeral fractures have even been reported due to shocks given during cardiopulmonary resuscitation. This is probably the result of massive muscle contractions, which drive the humeral head into the glenoid (Kam and Kam 1994).

Due to the lack of a rigid bony enclosure at its articulation with the scapula, the humerus is susceptible to dislocation at the shoulder. The muscles of the rotator cuff provide some limitation on the extent of dislocation but, nevertheless, fracturing of the bone often occurs. The combination of musculature and bony support results in a tendency for the humerus to be moved anteriorly rather than posteriorly at the shoulder. Anterior dislocation is usually associated with a compression fracture on the posterolateral aspect of the humeral head (Pavlov and Freiberger 1978) and has been called a *Hills-Sachs defect* (Neer 1984). This fracture pattern is produced by the impact of the humeral head against the anterior rim of the glenoid fossa. These breaks are often associated with fractures of the greater tubercle as well as compression fractures of the inferior lip of the glenoid fossa.

Compression fractures on the anteromedial aspect of the head of the humerus are infrequently found but occur when the bone is dislocated posteriorly. When there is severe impact of the head against the glenoid rim during posterior dislocations, large impression fractures are formed. An even more infrequent dislocation is one that is inferiorly directed and may also be associated with fractures of the greater tubercle, inferior glenoid, and acromial process. These injuries usually result from falls on an abducted arm.

In many cases, the humeral head will fail in central displacement with the result being a *head-splitting* fracture of the humeral head (Neer 1984). The articular surface will be highly fragmented and the tubercles also may be broken. The rarest form of dislocation is interthoracic in which the humeral head is thrust between or through the ribs and is probably the culmination of an extreme inferior dislocation (Brogdon *et al.* 1995). The humeral head becomes detached, remaining within the rib cage.

Specific fractures of the greater and lesser tubercles may result from avulsion, often with displacement of the fragments (Chadwick and Kyle 1992). Fractures of both tubercles produce fractures at either anatomical or surgical neck. Those of the lesser tubercle occur with posterior dislocation at the shoulder while greater tubercle fractures are linked to rotator cuff injuries and anterior dislocation (Tile 1987a). The most common is avulsion of the greater tubercle by the *supraspinatus* tendon, but other rotator muscles may be involved (Watson-Jones 1941). Fracture of the lesser tubercle often is associated with such dislocations due to tension of the *subscapularis* tendon and the anterior capsule (Neer 1984). Direct blows or falls onto the side of the shoulder may also cause massive comminuted fractures of the greater tubercle.

Proximal humeral fractures account for about 5% of all fractures receiving medical attention (Chadwick and Kyle 1992). A portion of these fractures consists of those associated with dislocation and avulsion as described above. Fractures in the proximal humerus are often more extensive, however, and they usually involve a combination of the surgical neck, anatomical neck, or greater or lesser tubercle (Neer 1970, Seeman *et al.* 1986). Fractures of the anatomical neck are extremely rare while those of the surgical neck distal to the tubercles are relatively common (Chadwick and Kyle 1992). Because the bone in this area is often quite thin, the fractures are of a crumbling nature. Since the surrounding muscles are dense, there is rarely loss of bone fragments until full skeletonization occurs.

Proximal humeral fractures are clinically classified by the number of resultant fragments (Codman 1934). These fragments usually consist of the head, lesser tubercle, greater tubercle, and the shaft, reflecting the old epiphyseal plate scars (Norris 1992). Most proximal fractures show no displacement of the fragments and are classed as *one-part fractures*. Next most frequent are those in which a single portion has been detached resulting in a *two-part fracture*. *Three-part fractures* involve displacement of two fragments, while *four-part fractures* involve displacement of the lesser and greater tubercles in addition to fracture of the anatomical neck of the humerus.

Neer (1970) revised this classification based on the locations, displacement, and relationships among fragments, and his system is widely used. Group I includes those with minimum displacement. Group II consists of fractures at the anatomical neck. Group III includes fractures distal to the tubercles at the surgical neck, and epiphyseal fractures are subsumed into this category. Groups IV and V consist of greater and lesser tubercle fractures, respectively, while Group VI includes fracture-dislocations. Neer's groups are then cross-tabulated with Codman's classification based on fragment number. The articular surface is usually the first segment, and this may be split as well as detached. The greater tubercle is usually the second segment and is often comminuted, probably, in part, because it is the attachment site for a number of the muscles of the rotator cuff. The third segment is the lesser tubercle, which leaves the fourth segment as the shaft.

The Neer classification system has subsequently been modified in line with the AO classification system to include 25 variables in nine groups based on displacement and capsular containment of the segments (Jakob *et al.* 1984, Norris 1992). Type A fractures are single line fractures with subtype 1 involving either tubercle, subtype 2 an impacted metaphyseal fracture, and subtype 3 a non-impacted metaphyseal fracture. Type B fractures encompass extra-articular fractures and have two fracture lines. Subtype B1 is a tubercle with an impacted metaphyseal fracture, subtype B2 is similar but with a non-impacted fracture, and B3 involves tubercle and metaphyseal fractures with glenohumeral dislocation. Type C injuries to the proximal humerus include fractures of the articular surface itself. These fractures are divided into C1 – fractures with slight displacement, C2 – impacted with significant displacement, and C3 – with associated displacement. Analysis of inter- and intraobserver reliability also showed that agreement on classification was relatively low (Siebenrock and Gerber 1993).

This is a rather confusing arrangement and not useful for the anthropologist for whom the extent of displacement may be produced by taphonomic processes. Figure 10-3 presents the descriptive terminology based on the anatomical features (head, anatomical and surgical neck, and lesser and greater tubercles), which are the most useful in anthropological analysis. Age assessment of the individual should also be taken into account when discussing the magnitude of the forces that produced the injury. Radiographic observations on bone density and trabecular integrity may be helpful if possible, but a qualitative assessment should be attempted in all such fractures.

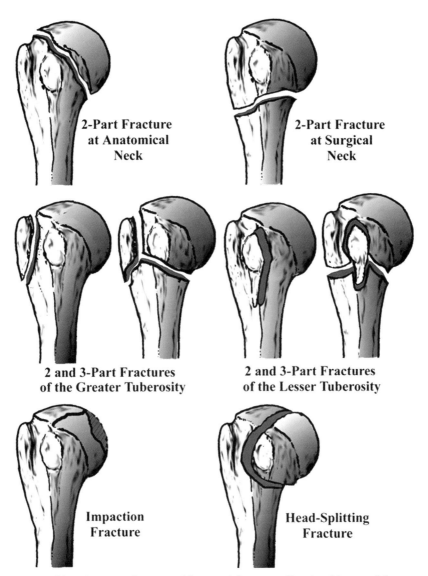

Figure 10-3. Classification of proximal humeral fractures. Proximal humeral fractures are classified by the number of parts and the location of the fractures (*right humerus shown*). Neer's classification emphasizes displacement and dislocation. The above system is modified from Neer (1970).

Humeral Shaft Fractures

Fractures of the humeral shaft are commonly the result of accident or directed violence. Most fractures occur at about midshaft with relatively few in the proximal or distal shaft sections. Falls and motor vehicle accidents are the most common causes. Humeral shaft fractures are usually transverse or spiral in nature. Severe bending of the bone results in transverse fracture while rotation of the arm during the blow yields a spiral or oblique fracture (Epps 1984, Rogers 1992). Humeral shaft fractures have also been caused by birth trauma (Watson-Jones 1941, Blount 1955), often associated with breech births or impaction of the shoulders. In older children and adults, spontaneous fractures may occur from torsional stress during periods of muscular contraction (Gregersen 1971, Branch *et al.* 1992), including pitching (Ogawa and Yoshida 1998). Also, seemingly innocent pastimes such as arm wrestling have been implicated in spiral fractures (de Barros and Oliveira 1995). Like proximal fractures, shaft fractures cluster in the younger and older age ranges and are least common in individuals between about 30 to 50 years of age (Swanson and Gustilo 1993). They increase in frequency among older individuals as bone mineral decreases and usually result from simple falls (Ekholm *et al.* 2006).

Humeral shaft fractures may form part of a complex of elbow injuries. *Sideswipe* fractures, in which the distal humerus is severely fragmented, occur when people are struck by a motor vehicle – usually when they have their elbow out the window (Rogers 1992). These may also be called *traffic elbow* or *car window elbow* injuries (DeLee *et al.* 1984, Morrey 1993). In most instances, the left arm of the driver is involved – except, of course, in those countries where cars are driven on the left side of the road. With increasing force of impact, the distal humerus may be broken and the humeral shaft may be thrust against the doorpost, which induces a fracture in the proximal region. In the less severe cases, olecranon fractures are common. When the arm protrudes further, both bones of the forearm are involved. Incidence has decreased with the introduction of air conditioning and turn signals in cars.

Epps (1984) classifies humeral shaft fractures in relation to the insertion points for *pectoralis major* and the deltoid muscles. Skeletally, the crest of the greater tubercle and the deltoid tuberosity, respectively, indicate these points. The character of the break is also noted as being longitudinal, transverse, oblique, spiral, segmental, or comminuted. The AO classification for the humeral shaft is similar to that for the shafts of the femur, tibia, and fibula. Simple fractures, type A, are divided into (1) spiral, (2) oblique, and (3) transverse. The wedge fractures, type B, are classifiable into (1) spiral wedges, (2) bending wedges, and (3) fragmented wedges. The final group of fractures, type C, are the complex fractures and are grouped into (1) those of spiral generation, (2) those that are primarily segmental, and (3) those that are highly irregular and comminuted. For the anthropologist, location of the fracture with respect to anatomical landmarks, type, direction, and extent of fracture are important in reconstructing a profile of the forces and movements involved.

Condylar and Supracondylar Fractures

The distal humerus is relatively fragile and the pattern of fractures may often be complex, traveling from articular and condylar regions into the supracondylar portions of the bone. Condylar fractures occur lower on the bone than supracondylar fractures and, clinically, are characterized by adhesion of the flexor or extensor muscle masses. In the lateral condyle, fractures are produced in the sagittal plane, which serves to distinguish these from the fractures of the articular surface alone that tend to occur in the coronal plane (Morrey 1993). Supracondylar fractures include all fractures through the distal part of the humerus above the condyles (DeLee *et al.* 1984). They pass through the medial and lateral columns and the bony separation of the olecranon and coronoid fossae. These fractures often include bony defects in the areas of the condyles and articular surfaces but extend more proximally than the condylar fractures. The collateral ligaments enhance the forces that will produce fractures above the epicondyles.

Fractures of the distal portion of the humerus are more frequent in youngsters but are relatively rare in adults and older individuals (Buhr and Cooke 1959). Fractures of the lateral condyle are found in children, as are avulsive fractures of the medial epicondyle (Blount 1955, Salter and Harris 1963). True supracondylar fractures are quite common in children, and account for 30–50% of elbow fractures in children (Bensahel *et al.* 1986). The injuries tend to be more common in boys except for the first three years of life when they are occur slightly more frequently in girls (Henrikson 1966). These injuries peak in boys between seven and nine years of age and about two years earlier in girls. In children, ligamentous laxity may increase the chances for such fractures during a fall (Green *et al.* 1994). The fracture pattern appears to change with the changes in skeletal growth. Frequencies decrease once epiphyseal fusion occurs. Injuries tend to shift distally, and frequencies of epicondylar fractures increase.

In adults, distal humeral fractures occur most often in middle- to older women (Miller 1964). The elderly are prone to fractures low on the columns that are designated *transcolumnar fractures*. These breaks are most common in those suffering from osteoporosis (Morrey 1993). Y- or T-shaped fractures often result from falls from a standing height in the elderly (Miller 1964). Among condylar fractures in adults, those of the lateral condyle are much more common than those of the medial condyle (DeLee *et al.* 1984).

Supracondylar fractures occur, in most instances, indirectly as a result of a fall in which the forearms and hand bear the weight of the body or blow (Rogers 1992). The circumstances of injury include traffic injuries, climbing, stumbling, and sports activities. Of these injuries, the most common cause seems to be falls while climbing. Apparently, the height of the fall seems to be a critical determinant for the extent of injury. As the fall's height increases above about five meters, injuries to the elbow are more extensive with fracturing appearing in the ulna as well as in the humerus. Industrial accidents are also cited as a common cause of distal humeral fractures (Kaushal *et al.* 1994).

Supracondylar fractures are a relatively common childhood injury, particularly between ages five and 10 years (Kasser and Beaty 2001). Within the first decade of life, supracondylar fractures can occur with either extension or flexion of the elbow (DeLee *et al.* 1984, Green *an.* 1994); however, forced hyperextension is the most common mechanism of supracondylar fracture (Morrey 1993). Fractures of the distal humerus in children are often associated with forearm fractures or dislocations. Hyperextension of the arm occurs as the ulnar olecranon process applies force onto the distal humerus (Rogers *et al.* 1978). Rang (1974) postulates that these fractures are produced as the olecranon acts as the fulcrum over which the humerus breaks.

Many supracondylar fractures in children are incomplete and are actually transcondylar (Rogers *et al.* 1978). The incomplete fractures include greenstick fractures, fractures involving only a single cortex, torus fractures, cortical buckling, and plastic bowing. Complex fractures are found to a lesser extent in children where the fractures tend to be limited to the supracondylar region (Blount 1955, 1977; Henrikson 1966).

A small number of fractures are produced by falls directly onto the olecranon process while the elbow is flexed. Single-column fractures appear to derive from direct blows to the olecranon process in younger individuals. They are relatively common in children (Kuhn *et al.* 1995), usually beginning in the trochlea, bifurcating the olecranon fossa and passing out through either the medial or lateral column. This single-column fracture pattern appears to be associated with the presence of a large fossa or septal aperture between the olecranon and coronoid fossae.

In adults, the most likely cause of a supracondylar fractures is a direct blow on the elbow as may occur with a fall onto the joint (Miller 1964, Morrey 1993). Blows force the olecranon process into the intercondylar space producing the fracture.

Like supracondylar fractures, condylar fractures are caused by transmission of forces from the forearm but may also be due to forces brought to bear indirectly from the collateral ligaments (Morrey 1993). Both condyles are subject to fracture during falls. Lateral condylar fracture is usually attributable to axial loading with valgus stress resulting in shearing stress. Avulsion fractures may occur with axial loading and varus stress and can produce a relatively large fragment.

Medial condylar fractures are produced by shearing stresses and may involve a large portion of the trochlea when combined with inward or varus stress (Morrey 1993). Valgus or outward stress may result in avulsion of the condyle.

The fractures originate in the depths of the trochlea and angle up to the end of the supracondylar ridge (DeLee *et al.* 1984). Falls onto the outstretched hand are implicated with the elbow being forced into varus position. In some cases, direct blows to the point of the flexed elbow may produce these fractures.

The classification of condylar and supracondylar fractures is relatively complex due to the lack of clear definition between these fractures and the extensive nature of the damage often found in the distal humerus. Designation of condylar fractures may be more straightforward in that they do not involve the extent of damage often seen in supracondylar fractures (Figure 10-4). Type I or low condylar fractures involve either the capitulum or the medial aspect of the trochlea depending on whether the lateral or medial condyles are affected (De Lee *et al.* 1984, Morrey 1993). Type II or high condylar fractures involve more articular surface with lateral Type II fractures showing breaks through the capitulum and lateral trochlea while the medial form involves both sides of the trochlea.

Supracondylar fractures can be grouped into extension or flexion injuries. With extension fractures, the break usually extends from the distal anterior to the proximal posterior and anterior displacement is common. There may be

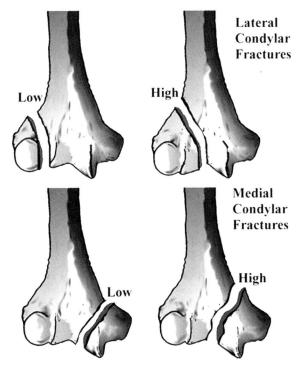

Figure 10-4. Condylar fractures of the distal humerus. Condylar fractures are classified by location and height of the fracture (De Lee *et al.* 1984, Morrey 1993).

some lateral or medial angulation as well that has been attributed to adduction or abduction (Kocher 1896), but this claim has not been validated.

Extent of the fracturing and the proportions of the various segments are the characteristics used to classify supracondylar fractures (Miller 1964). Many systems, including the AO classification, combine supracondylar, condylar, and epicondylar fractures, despite distinct differences in the causal mechanisms from which each result (Schatzker 1987a). Some, such as the classification of intra-articular fractures by Riseborough and Radin (1969), distinguish fractures on the basis of displacement, rotation, and comminution.

Jupiter and Belsky (1992a) proposed a more systematic classification system, which includes fractures traditionally considered condylar fractures. This system incorporates an anatomic concept of the distal humerus as being composed of a medial and a lateral column. Using these columns as location guides, Jupiter and Belsky (1992a) proposes three broad groups of fractures using a "high" and "low" designation (Figure 10-5). High fractures are those that include the majority of the trochlea while low fractures originate well to either side of the center of the trochlea. Jupiter's first category involves intra-articular fractures that are subdivided into single- or bicolumn fractures, capitulum fractures, and trochlear fractures. Single-column fractures are relatively rare, although lateral column fractures outnumber those of the medial column. Essentially, these fracture are those traditionally considered condylar fractures (Figure 10-4). The bicolumn fractures, the most common distal humeral fracture, may take the T, Y, H, or A patterns (Figure 10-4). These have long been considered to be due to the wedging action of the olecranon, but cadaver studies have shown that these fractures will only occur if the elbow is flexed to an angle less than 90°. At 90°, the olecranon process itself breaks, but when the angle is less, the body is displaced anteriorly moving the bending point into the supracondylar area. Capitulum and trochlear fractures included in Jupiter's first category are discussed separately below.

Jupiter and Belsky (1992a) second broad category includes the extra-articular or transcolumn fractures that pass through the medial and lateral supracondylar columns (Figure 10-5). These are subdivided based not only on the height of fracture but on the mechanism of injury. Those produced under extension usually are angled more proximally on the posterior to more distally on the anterior surface. Those produced under flexion reverse this pattern. Adduction produces angulation from the proximal portion medially to the distal portion laterally and this is reversed in abduction (Figure 10-5). They usually transect the olecranon fossa, although may occasionally appear above this line. Extension fractures tend to result from falls. Flexion fractures are attributed to blows to the lower back of the arm or other loading forces in this region. Adduction and abduction fractures result from axial loading while the arm is in a varus

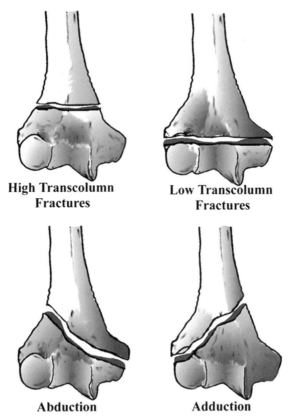

High Transcolumn Fractures   **Low Transcolumn Fractures**

Abduction   **Adduction**

Figure 10-5. Transcolumnar fractures. Extra-articular or transcolumnar fractures may be designated as high or low, and distinctions are made as to whether they occur during abduction or adduction of the forearm (Jupiter 1992).

or valgus (inward or outward) orientation. A distinguishing feature of these fractures is that, viewed laterally, the fracture appears to be transverse (Morrey 1993). The final group consists of extracapsular or epicondylar fractures (Jupiter 1992), which will be discussed in the following section.

Anthropologists should find some form of the Jupiter system most useful (Figure 10-6). The configuration of the fracture, angle of the break as viewed frontally and laterally, and the age of the individual are important in determining the mechanism of injury.

In some individuals there is a supracondylar process on the anteromedial aspect of the distal humerus that arches over the median nerve and brachial artery. It is usually located 5-7 cm above the medial epicondyle and may be 2-20 mm in length (Morrey 1993). This may be fractured by direct trauma to the area (DeLee *et al.* 1984). The larger the process, the more vulnerable it is to fracturing (Morrey 1993).

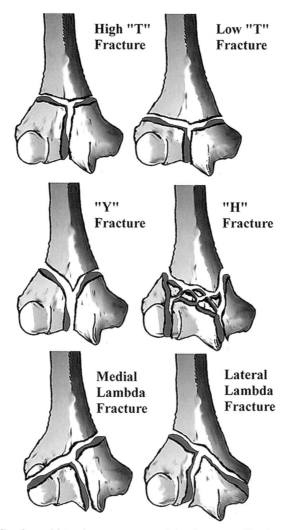

Figure 10-6. Single and bi-column supracondylar fractures. Single and bi-column supra-condylar fractures may be classified by the fracture shape and height of the fractures (Jupiter 1992).

Epicondylar Fractures

Epicondylar fractures are relatively rare and usually avulsive in nature (DeLee *et al.* 1984, Morrey 1993). Epicondylar fractures can be produced by either tension on the collateral ligaments or by direct blows. Collateral ligaments provide tension around the elbow joint and can produce avulsion fractures. Since the medial epicondyle is more prominent, medial fractures are more common than those of the lateral epicondyle. Both regions, however, are most often broken in association with other injuries.

In children, these fractures may occur as separation of the epiphysis from the bone. In adults, the incorporation of the epicondyle into the bone is solid and fracturing is the consequence. Epicondylar fractures are most common in the early teens and approximately equal in frequency in boys and girls (Henrikson 1966) and at higher frequencies in boys in some studies (Beaty and Kasser 2006). These fractures account for about 10–20% of the elbow fractures in children (Bensahel *et al.* 1986, Beaty and Kasser 2006).

Fractures of the medial epicondyle are more common in boys and often result from direct trauma, usually from the victim falling onto the elbow (Bensahel *et al.* 1986). Indirect trauma has also been implicated in these cases, primarily falls onto the extended forearm or sudden valgus strain. Overall these fractures are quite rare in children. They are also relatively rare in adults, possibly because direct blows are absorbed by failure of the medial condyle rather than being confined to the epicondyle (DeLee *et al.* 1984). The mechanisms of injury are similar to those seen in children, usually attributable to blows directly to the epicondyle. Scharplatz and Allgower (1976) consider sudden abduction another mechanism of injury.

Fractures of the lateral epicondyle due to avulsion are extremely rare in adults and uncommon in children (De Lee *et al.* 1984, Schatzker 1987a). Such fractures are usually produced by hyperextension combined with angulation. This may be induced by direct and indirect trauma, resulting in a fracture from the lateral epicondyle into the trochlea. They also may be induced by posterior or posterolateral elbow dislocation. With posterior dislocations, associated medial epicondylar fractures may be found. Adduction can lead to avulsion while abduction usually produces fracture of both the lateral epicondyle and the capitulum (Scharplatz and Allgower 1976).

Transphyseal fractures are relatively uncommon in children and have been associated with child abuse (DeLee *et al* 1980; Akbarnia *et al.* 1986). The mechanism of injury is believed to be rotational forces along with hyperextension (Shrader 2008). Fracture is typically through the growth plate and skeletal damage may not be clearly visible in the dry bone.

Distal Articular Fractures

Articular fractures tend to occur parallel to the anterior surface of the distal humerus (DeLee *et al.* 1984). Usually these will involve both the capitulum and the trochlea and are produced by shearing forces and, sometimes, by compressive wedging. Such fractures are confined to the articular areas and do not extend up onto the epicondylar region. Forces are also transmitted from axial loading of the radius and ulna.

Capitulum fractures are often called *Kocher fractures* and are rare (DeLee *et al.* 1984). When seen, they are associated with radial head injuries, usually

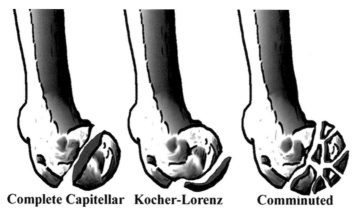

Complete Capitellar   Kocher-Lorenz   Comminuted

Figure 10-7. Fractures of the distal humerus. Articular fractures of the distal humerus (*right shown*) include the Hahn-Steinthal type, which is a complete capitular fracture; the Kocher-Lorenz type of the surface; and a comminuted fracture of the articular portion (Wilson 1933, DeLee *et al.* 1984).

resulting from shearing action. Two to three separate forms are recognized (DeLee *et al.* 1984, Bryan and Morrey 1985, Morrey 1993) (Figure 10-7). The Hahn-Steinthal type or Type I involves much of the capitulum and often includes part of the adjacent lip of the trochlea. The Kocher-Lorenz form or Type II usually has only minor bony involvement, focusing on the articular cartilage and is relatively uncommon. Wilson (1933) also described a form where the articular surface is compacted proximally and this is given the designation Type III (Morrey 1993).

Kocher (1896) advocated the view that hyperextension of the elbow produced avulsion fractures but this does not adequately explain those fractures that occur in areas where there is no attachment to the joint capsule. Fractures of the capitulum may result from forces through the radial head while the elbow is flexed. This fracture often occurs with falls onto the flexed arm and may be associated with radial head fractures (DeLee *et al.* 1984, Morrey 1993). Bryan (1981), however, argued that the Hahn-Steinthal type of fracture is due to shearing forces produced by falls while the elbow is extended. Alternately, they may be formed by direct blows to the lateral aspect of the elbow while the elbow is flexed such as would occur when a person falls, landing on the elbow (Morrey 1993). Type II injuries may be due to the shearing motion produced by blows to the radial head when the elbow is flexed. The location of the fracture may help determine the position of the elbow at the time of injury. Milch (1931) argued that the anterior surface is involved when the elbow is extended, while the posterior aspect is fractured when the elbow is flexed. A possible scenario includes fractures occurring when the arm is being used in a hammering activity where strong movement is abruptly halted.

Type III fractures are found in falls on the outstretched hand. Experimental data show that, in pronation, greater force is transmitted across from the radial head than in supination, and a "screw home" mechanism is also involved with pronation (Morrey and Stormont 1988). This movement effectively drives the radial head into the capitulum.

Isolated trochlear fractures, sometimes called *Laugier's fractures*, are exceedingly rare. This region is well protected by the olecranon from direct blows, and the forces from falls onto the arm are usually transmitted through the radius to the capitulum (DeLee *et al.* 1984, Morrey 1993). The distal humerus is more vulnerable higher up the diaphysis and is more likely to absorb any energy that might fracture the trochlea.

For the anthropologist, careful examination of the distal humerus is required. Taphonomic factors often preclude assessment of this area as the elbow is a frequent site for scavenging activity. Injuries to this area are important in determining the victim's behavior during the fatal event, as most, though not all, such injuries are due to defensive maneuvers by the victim, usually during a fall. Documentation of the presence or absence of such injuries may shed light on how the victim responded, and this information might assist the coroner or medical examiner in determining the manner of death.

RADIUS

Biomechanically, the radius combines high mobility and maximal load transmission. In some respects, the morphology of the elbow joint, which predisposes the radius to dislocation, saves it from fractures. However, since loading from the hand is transmitted through the scaphoid and lunate to the distal radius, this lower region is highly vulnerable, especially since bipedality increased the height from which we fall, and our focus on fine motor skills lightened the bones and musculature of the hand.

The mechanism of radial fracture has been debated. Some argue that it almost always is due to a direct blow (Hughston 1957), while Mikić (1975) and Chung and Spilson (2001) argue that, like many other upper limb injuries, fractures are again due to falls on the outstretched arm. In direct blows, the ulna is usually more susceptible than the radius, especially if the forearm is being used defensively to deflect a blow. In these cases, the forearm is pronated, moving the radius toward the body and leaving the ulna to bear the blow. Both bones, though, are subject to breakage during falls. Isolated fractures of the radius due to direct blows are relatively rare.

Forearm fractures are extremely common in children, accounting for about 45% of all childhood fractures (Gandhi *et al.* 1963). These injuries are most common when children reach school age and become involved in sports and independent or minimally supervised activities (Lawson *et al.* 1995). As with the elderly, the most frequent location of radial fractures is the distal third of the diaphysis, and fractures decrease in frequency toward the proximal end of the forearm. In children, fractures of both bones in the forearm are common and single fractures are unusual. Single fractures are more likely attributable to direct blows (Armstrong *et al.* 1994). As the child ages, the diaphyses of the forearm bones become more resistant to fracture and breakage is found more often in the metaphysis.

Fractures among the elderly occur primarily at the distal end (Bauer 1960). In younger adults, males exhibit slightly more fractures, wherease after age 45, the prevalence in women rises rapidly. The degree of trauma needed to produce fracture also plummets with advancing age, particularly in women.

Radial Head and Neck Fractures

Fractures of the radial head and neck are very common in elbow injuries (Rogers 1992, Teasdall *et al.* 1993). The transmission of forces during a fall is responsible for most proximal radial fractures. Sometimes they are associated with fractures of the capitulum (Rieth 1948, DeLee *et al.* 1984, Karlsson *et al.* 2010). Proximal radial fractures vary by age (Green and Swiontkowski 1994) and are more common in women than men (Johnston 1962). The incidence of radial head fractures peaks at 30-40 years of age (Conn and Wade 1961, Morrey 1993). However, microarchitectural studies show that the radial head is highly susceptible to age-related osteoporotic changes, increasing its vulnerability in older women (Gebauer *et al.* 2010).

In the radius, childhood fractures usually occur in the radial neck, whereas, in adults, the radial head itself is involved (Alffram and Bauer 1962). The childhood fractures are characterized by displacement of the head and cleavage of a metaphyseal flake (Blount 1955). These fractures usually involve dislocation at the elbow with the radius being injured by the distal humerus. In children, however, fractures of the radial neck or head tend not to be associated with interosseous ligament damage as is more common in adults (Armstrong *et al.* 1994). This probably reflects changes in the nature of the growth plate. As the epiphyseal line closes, there is a shift from neck fractures toward those of the radial head (Henrikson 1966).

Radial head fractures (Figure 10-8) are common injuries and, like many upper limb injuries, result from indirect forces applied during falls onto the outstretched hand when the forearm is pronated and the elbow partially flexed (DeLee *et al.* 1984). The radial head is driven into the capitulum, which may also be damaged. If a valgus force is involved, olecranon fractures may accompany the injury (Schatzker 1987b). Experiments show that the normal impact site in pronation is the posterolateral portion of the radial head, which

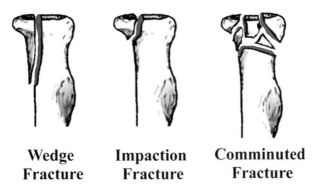

Wedge Fracture   **Impaction Fracture**   **Comminuted Fracture**

Figure 10-8. Fractures of the radial head. Fractures of the radial head are divided by the direction of fracture and magnitude of damage. Wedge fractures include an extension down the neck while impaction or marginal fractures are confined to the radial head. Comminuted fractures consist of a complex of fractures that disrupt the radial head. Bakalim (1970) also recognized transverse fractures. Illustration modified from Bakalim (1970), Schatzker (1987), and Teasdall *et al.* (1993)

is weaker due to its lack of subchondral bone and its eccentric placement respective to the long axis of the radius (Thomas 1905).

Essex-Lopresti dislocations are usually considered the mechanism in which the radioulnar joint was challenged and the interosseous ligaments disrupted. Alternately, Leung and associates (2005) suggest that the most common mechanism for injury of the radial head is a "criss-cross" injury. In studying both a clinical review and a cadaveric experiment, they found that, in pronation, pressure on one end of the forearm could produce dislocation at the other end, involving either the ulnar or radial heads.

Scharplatz and Allgower (1976) grouped radial head fractures among the elbow injuries produced by axial loading. Bakalim (1970) and Mason (1954) both identified three groups of fractures that include vertical fractures through the head, horizontal fractures separating the head from the neck, and comminuted fractures. Johnston (1962) added a category for fractures associated with elbow dislocation. Schatzker (1987b) identifies (1) wedge fractures in which part of the head remains intact, (2) impaction fractures that are similar to wedge fractures but involve crushing and impaction of bone along with some comminution, and (3) severely comminuted fractures (Figure 10-8). The medical community further classifies fractures based on the degree of separation and displacement of the fragments. In many cases, these fractures also extend into the radial neck. Generally, more severe forces result in higher degrees of comminution. Associated fractures may be found in the humeral capitulum, ulna, and wrist bones. In fact, severe dislocation of the radial head without injury to the ulna is unusual, and radial head fractures at the anterior margin are the typical associated fracture for the posterior *Monteggia* fracture of the ulna (Pavel *et al.* 1965). Radial head fractures may accompany an *Essex-Lopresti fracture dislocation* of the forearm (Putnam and Fischer 1993). In these injuries, forces driving the forearm into the distal humerus are responsible for longitudinal rupture of the interosseous membrane. Marginal fractures may result from abduction with contusion (Scharplatz and Allgower 1976).

Radial Shaft Fractures

Fractures of the radial shaft are common in children who, in some studies, account for four-fifths of all shaft fractures of the forearm. These fractures in children can be produced by both direct and indirect trauma (Blount 1955). Often both of the bones of the forearm are broken with direct impact, although these tend to be greenstick fractures. Diaphyseal fractures tend to occur more frequently in children at beginning school age, whereas the incidence of more distal fractures in the juxtaepiphyseal area increases by about age 10 (Thomas *et al.* 1974). Distal shaft fractures in children are four to 10 times more frequent than are middle diaphysis fractures (Gandhi *et al.* 1963, Tredwell *et al.* 1984).

Complete fractures are more likely in adults, although spiral fractures of the forearm occur but are quite rare (Müller *et al.* 1991). As with the humerus, the majority of radial shaft fractures occurs at the middle third of the shaft and these are usually oblique. The most common cause of adult fractures is motor vehicle accidents with direct trauma (Anderson 1984). Other high-energy trauma such as industrial accidents and assaults are also to blame (Putnam and Fischer 1993).

The primary fracture forms found in the forearm are simple fractures of the transverse or oblique nature (Müller *et al.* 1991). Butterfly or fragmented wedge fractures also are common, forming about 12–15% of forearm fractures. More complex fractures are also found and are indicative of severe trauma.

Galeazzi fractures involve the radial shaft, usually the distal or middle third, with disruption of the distal radioulnar joint (Cooper 1822, Galaezzi 1934). These have also been called reverse *Monteggia* fractures, *Piedmont* or *Darrach-Hughston-Milch* fractures (Anderson 1984, Kellam and Jupiter 1992). These fractures are relatively uncommon and are believed to result from axial loading on the hyperpronated forearm. The fracture pattern is usually transverse (Walsh *et al.* 1987) or short oblique and angulated dorsally (Kellam and Jupiter 1992). Like most forearm injuries, these fractures occur with falls on the hands under extreme pronation, often from a height or in motor vehicle accidents, although falling while running or during sports has also been implicated. Occasionally, direct blows may be involved (Hughston 1957). In children, these fractures are relatively rare, although the distal portion is more vulnerable than in adults (Gandhi *et al.* 1963). Children will usually experience radial fracture accompanied by separation of the distal ulnar epiphysis (Mikić 1975).

Diaphyseal fractures are not classified according to any widely recognized system (Kellam and Jupiter 1992). The OTA classification (Gustilo 1990) simply places them by morphology into transverse, oblique, spiral, butterfly, comminuted segmental, or with bone loss. Other systems place them only by simple, wedge, or complex fractures, often linking both the radius and ulna together in descriptions of forearm fractures. Anthropologists should note pattern and location of fracture and pay special attention to associated injuries. Examination of the associated ulna, scaphoid and humerus, if available, should be done with care to help distinguish injuries from falls versus those from direct blows.

Distal Radial Fractures

The distal radius is a frequent site of fracturing, primarily from falling, and fractures are usually accompanied by dislocation of adjacent bones (Rogers 1992). Alffram and Bauer (1962) found that about three-quarters of all forearm fractures were located on the distal radius or ulna. While men are more likely to break the distal radius in adolescence and early adulthood, the rates for women dramatically surpass those for men at about age 45–50 years and remain consistently high (Buhr and Cooke 1959, Alffram and Bauer 1962, Vogt *et al.* 2002). The mechanism of injury tends to be low-energy trauma in the majority of cases, although more severe trauma is often involved in forearm fractures of younger adults of both sexes and in adult men until about age 60. Extreme trauma resulting in distal forearm breaks is more common in younger women while mild to moderate trauma, such as falls from standing height, is responsible for distal forearm breaks in older women. Risk factors include osteoporosis; problems with balance; and a history of frequent falls, diabetes, and dementia (Vogt *et al.* 2002).

Distal forearm fractures are also common in children where both boys and girls are afflicted with these injuries (Alffram and Bauer 1962). Epiphyseal fracture of the radius in children is usually encountered (Blount 1955), frequently of the Salter-Harris Type II form (Rogers 1992). These occur in older children, usually after age 10 and are produced by the child falling on an outstretched hand. In young children, there is more often a greenstick fracture close to the wrist. These may be combined with greenstick ulnar fractures (Blount 1955) or torus fractures. When there is marked displacement of the epiphysis, direct trauma is usually indicated.

Distal radial fractures may be found in association with other, more distant, fractures. Alffram and Bauer (1962) found that associated long bone and skull fractures in adult men were more common than in women. In older women, distal forearm fractures may occur along with simultaneous fracture of the proximal end of the femur.

Distal radial fractures usually occur in one of three major groups (Figure 10-9). The *Cones'* fracture of the wrist, also known as *Pouteau's* fracture, is more accurately a bending fracture of the distal radius within about 1.5 inches (4 cm) above the articulation with the carpals. This injury occurs primarily in older women with the incidence increasing after about age 45 years (Alffram and Bauer 1962; Dóczi and Renner 1994). Kelsey and associates suggest that these often occur in women who are relatively active for their age yet exhibit decreased bone mineral density. During a fall onto the outstretched pronated arm, the dorsal surface of the arm is placed under compression while the ventral surface is under tension. The tensile forces cause a transverse fracture and there is subsequent crumbling of the posterior surface. There is often a shear stress line of about 45°. The amount of force required is relatively small, ranging from 230 to 970 pounds (105 to 440 kg), with a mean of only 430 pounds (195 kg) for women (Dobyns and Linscheid 1983).

A *Smith's* fracture of the distal radius is also known as a *reverse Colles'* fracture in that the fracture line is angled so that the ventral side is more proximally located. This, like the Colles' fracture, is a bending fracture. According to one scenario, the mechanism of injury is simply the reverse of that seen in a

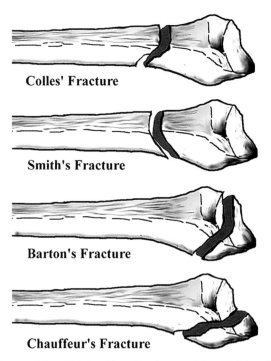

Figure 10-9. Fractures of the distal radius. Fractures of the distal radius (*right shown*) include extra-articular (Colles' and Smith) and articular fractures (Barton's and chauffeur's).

Colles' fracture or falling onto the back of the hand (Dobyns and Linscheid 1983). Alternatively, it has been suggested that falling on the forearm in supination but rotating into pronation with a fixed dorsiflexed hand may be more consistent with the mechanism of injury (Thomas 1957, Ellis 1965). It may also be due to a direct blow to the back of the hand or knuckles, particularly in motor vehicle accidents. This fracture is more common in older women (Dóczi and Renner 1994). It may be associated with fracture of the styloid process of the radius (Dobyns and Linscheid 1984).

Barton's fracture is the third major type of distal radial fracture. It is produced by dorsiflexion and pronation of the forearm over the wrist with fractures beginning in the articular surface and extending to the dorsal surface of the arm. As well as elderly individuals who have fallen, this type of fracture is also found in motorcycle accidents. Technically this is a shearing fracture of the joint surface. A *volar Barton's* fracture begins at the articular surface and extends to the ventral surface of the arm (Putnam 1993).

In addition to the above more commonly occurring set, there are a number of other specific fractures. "*Die-punch*" fractures are breaks in the joint surface due to impaction of subchondral and metaphyseal bone (McMurtry and Jupiter 1992). *Chauffeur's* fractures, also known as *Hutchinson's* fractures, are fractures of the radial styloid process due to blows or other forces, which drive the scaphoid into the process. The primary mechanism of injury is impact along with avulsion of the radiocarpal ligaments or radial collateral ligament. The name derives from the use of cranks to start engines, which often backfired, abruptly reversing the crank (Dobyns and Linscheid 1984). In adults, these fractures are more often found in men and are usually associated with severe trauma. The fracture generally runs from the articular surface for the scaphoid laterally to the radial metaphysis. It may also originate at the junction of the articular surfaces for the scaphoid and lunate (Watson-Jones 1941).

In addition to these impact fractures, avulsion fractures may occur in the radial styloid (Watson-Jones1941). These are derived from the attachment of the external lateral ligament and may occur with dislocation of the wrist.

Minor marginal fractures may also occur during wrist dislocations or forced dorsiflexion. Posterior marginal fracture is one such break and may be associated with a comminuted Colles' fracture or be an isolated occurrence (Watson-Jones 1941). Anterior marginal fractures merge into the Smith's fracture classification.

In lieu of the system of named fractures, McMurtry and Jupiter (1992) devised an alternate system of distal radial fracture based on anatomic type, local factors, and patient considerations. The anatomic type is divided between extra-articular and intra-articular and the latter subdivided into two-, three-, four-, and five- or more part fractures. The two-part fractures include the *Barton's fractures*, radial styloid fractures, and "die-punch" fractures. Three-part fractures involve the lunate and scaphoid facets of the radius. Four-part fractures extend the fractures of the three-part classification by dividing the lunate facet into dorsal and volar fragments.

Forensically, the anthropologist needs to record the extent of damage to the articular surfaces, direction of fracture, and angulation. Involvement of other bones as well as the age and general health of the individual may be critical for interpretation of the severity of the force applied. As with many forearm and humeral fractures, many injuries are attributable to defensive moves by the victim during falls. However, this cannot be assumed, nor can direct blows be automatically eliminated in distal radial fractures.

ULNA

The ulna is vulnerable to breakage due to two factors: the stability of its hinge joint with the humerus, which restricts movement, and the fact that it is usually the first bone encountered when the forearm is used to ward off blows. However, its lack of direct articulation with the carpals frees it to some extent from the problems of axial loading seen in the radius during falls. Instead, dislocations of the radius become a primary cause of ulnar fracture as the radius can be dramatically displaced.

Olecranon Fractures

Because there is little soft tissue overlying the olecranon process, it is particularly vulnerable. Fractures of the olecranon process may occur in children but rarely as an isolated injury (Blount 1955). Avulsion fractures are more common in the elderly (DeLee *et al.* 1984).

Fractures to the proximal ulna occur both as the result of falls when the arm is flexed and also through direct blows to the olecranon (Rogers 1992). Falls combined with strong contraction of the triceps muscle may also be involved, resulting in transverse or oblique fractures (DeLee *et al.* 1984). Direct blows to this area of the bone tend to result in greater fragmentation but are less frequent. Direct blows to the extended elbow may produce forward displacement with transverse or comminuted fracture of the olecranon. Contraction of the biceps at the time of impact would prevent extension of the joint in compensation and transverse fractures can be produced (Scharplatz and Allgower 1976).

Most fractures in this area are transverse, originating at the trochlear or semi-lunar notch. Schatzker (1987b) presented a classification of olecranon fractures (Figure 10-10). These include transverse fractures that occur at the deepest point of the trochlear notch. This form is primarily an avulsion fracture

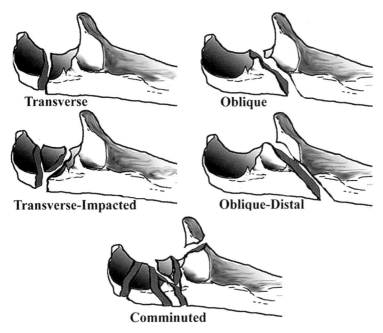

Figure 10-10. Olecranon fracture classification. Olecranon fractures of the ulna (*right shown*) have been classified by Schatzker (1987) based on the morphology of the injury.

caused by the sudden pull of the triceps and *brachialis* muscles. It may also be produced by a fall directly on the olecranon. These simple fracture forms may become more complex when there is more severe trauma, producing comminution and depression of the articular surface. In some cases, smaller transverse fractures are seen at the tip of the olecranon and are avulsion fractures produced by the triceps tendon. Simple oblique fractures usually result from hyperextension of the elbow with the fracture line beginning at the midpoint of the trochlear notch and traveling distally. Comminuted fractures are the result of high velocity direct trauma and have variable fracture lines. These usually include fractures of the coronoid process. Associated fracture or dislocation of the radial head is frequently found. This system is roughly equivalent to that of DeLee and associates (1984) but does not rely on displacement. A separate recognition is given to oblique fractures, which occur distal to the midpoint of the trochlear notch (Schatzker 1987b). Location, angulation, and magnitude of injury are important to document skeletally.

Coronoid Process Fractures

Fracture of the coronoid process may occur with posterior fracture dislocations of the elbow (Regan and Morrey 1989, Jupiter and Belsky 1992).

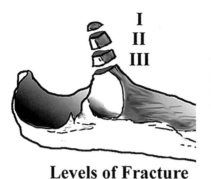

Levels of Fracture

Figure 10-11. Classification of coronoid fractures. Coronoid fractures are classified by the height of the injury from primarily an avulsion of the tip (I) to over half of the process (III) (Regan and Morrey 1989).

Impact along the long axis of the arm may be one mechanism of injury (Scharplatz and Allgower 1976) as the radius is displaced, pulling the ulna along with it. The coronoid process will then be driven against the trochlea. This small protrusion of bone also serves as an attachment site for anterior ligaments of the elbow and such is vulnerable to avulsion. The *brachialis* muscle provides the mechanism of injury, especially when the elbow is hyperextended (DeLee *et al.* 1984). These avulsive fractures form Type I of the Regan and Morrey (1989) classification system for this region of the bone (Figure 10-11, above). Type II consists of single or comminuted fractures encompassing up to half of the process while Type III involves over half of the coronoid. Recovery of the fragment may be difficult in skeletal cases, but the extent of bone loss should be assessed to help distinguish avulsive and impact injuries.

Ulnar Shaft Fractures

The ulnar shaft is relatively thin compared to the strength of the proximal portion. Since the elbow joint tends to be strong for this bone, the shaft is left absorbing much of the bending forces generated during loading. For this reason, shaft fractures are often a component of a complex of injuries to the forearm. Direct blows also play a role in some fractures. Age will alter the possibility of fracture. Falls onto the outstretched arm in children are partly ameliorated by the greater deformation potential in the forearm prior to fracturing. The bones of young children should be carefully examined for indication of plastic deformation.

Monteggia fracture was originally a term applied to fractures of the proximal third of the ulna and anterior or posterior dislocation of the proximal radius (Monteggia 1814). The definition has been expanded to include ulnar shaft fracture with dislocation at the elbow. These are relatively uncommon (Kellam and Jupiter 1992). The fractures are usually transverse or somewhat oblique and may be accompanied by a butterfly fragment. The most frequent site of injury is the junction of the proximal and middle thirds of the ulnar shaft. These fractures are unusual occurrences in children (Gandhi *et al.* 1963).

Classification of *Monteggia fractures* relies heavily on the direction of dislocation as well as mechanisms of injury and fracture patterns (Bado 1967) (Figure 10-12). Type I with anterior dislocation at the elbow is the most frequent form of this injury. This fracture-dislocation complex is due to hyperextension or hyperpronation of this joint (Reckling 1982), often from a fall on the outstretched arm while the forearm was maximally pronated (Evans 1949a). In addition to the impact, the body is often rotating during the fall, resulting in rotation of the arm and forearm, which cannot be transmitted to the already planted hand. Bending due to longitudinal compression and rotation produces this anterior fracturing. The radius is extremely pronated and the upper end provides a fulcrum against which the ulna will fracture. The ulnar shaft fracture may occur at any level but usually in the proximal or middle third (Bado 1967). In children, a more proximal fracture of the radius is common. Type II with posterior dislocation occurs when the forearm is supinated, while Type III is associated with lateral dislocation and is usually due to acute adduction of the forearm (Kellam and Jupiter 1992; Armstrong *et al.* 1994). Penrose (1951) provided an alternate explanation for the production of posterior dislocation. In cadaver studies, blows to the wrist when the elbow was flexed and the forearm was in either a moderately pronated or a relatively neutral position, neither fully pronated nor supinated, could produce *Monteggia fractures.* Excessive rotation did not appear to be involved. Pavel and colleagues (1965) reported that the majority of posterior Monteggia fractures in their study were due to direct trauma, although they cautioned that since most occurred in falls, people might have extended their arms behind them to break the fall. *Monteggia* fractures appear to be more common in middle age and particularly in women (Penrose 1951).

Skeletally, Type II occurs in the shaft of the ulna and is indicative of posterior angulation (Bado 1967) with a comminuted fracture of the proximal ulna, usually at the level of the coronoid process (Pavel *et al.* 1965). A separate triangular or quadrilateral fragment from the area inferior to the coronoid may be displaced anteriorly (Penrose 1951). Chip fractures of the radial head are a typical accompanying fracture in posterior dislocations due to the pressure against the capitulum (Pavel *et al.* 1965). Other associated injuries are fracture of the distal radius, distal humerus, or olecranon. Type III usually involves the ulnar metaphysis (Bado 1967). This injury appears to occur almost exclusively in children, presumably due to falls onto an outstretched hand (Putnam and Fischer 1993). Adduction leads to varus angulation focused on the proximal ulna while the radius tends to move laterally. In many instances, the ulnar

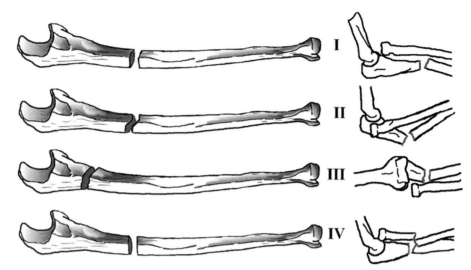

Figure 10-12. Monteggia fracture classification. Four types of Monteggia fractures have been identified based on the mechanism of fracture. Skeletally the easiest distinction will be for type III in which the fracture is located more proximally. Associated injuries in the radius become important in distinguishing other forms.

fracture is limited to an incomplete greenstick fracture (Mullich 1977). Type IV in which both bones are fractured is due to forced pronation (Armstrong *et al.* 1994). In this category, the radius is usually broken at the same level as the ulnar shaft (Bado 1967). These fractures are almost always found in adults. While these define the majority of cases, there are many variations of these fracture patterns.

The *pulled elbow syndrome* in many ways mimics an anterior *Monteggia*-fracture complex. These injuries occur when someone suddenly lifts a child under about five years of age by the hand (Bado 1967). The forearm is pronated and supination is not possible given the roughness of the pull. Since skeletally, the injuries are virtually identical whether produced by sudden traction or by a fall onto the arm, mechanisms cannot be reliably attributed.

As previously stated, direct blows also may cause ulnar damage as pronation of the forearm places the ulna outermost, away from the body. Such resulting fractures to the shaft region are called "nightstick," "fending," "pool cue," or "parrying" variety (Rogers 1992, Brogden 1998). In these, the victim raises an arm to shield the body against a blow from a club or other object. These cluster in the distal third of the bone. These fractures tend to be transverse or short oblique. They have been reported archaeologically and are often taken as indicators of a heightened level of interpersonal violence.

As with radial fractures, the anthropologist should focus on the entire arm when attempting to interpret injuries to the ulnar shaft. Since both *Monteggia* and parrying fractures can be transverse in form, associated injuries may be critical in distinguishing between injuries from a fall and defensive injuries. One feature, which may differ between the two forms, is the location where *Monteggia fractures* occur at the junction of the proximal and middle thirds of the shaft, while parrying fractures are usually placed in the distal third.

Distal Ulnar Fractures

Fractures of the distal ulna often center on fractures of the styloid process, since there is little contact between the distal ulna and the carpals except in extreme loading. Such fractures usually indicate considerable force such as in motor vehicle accidents or falls from heights. Leung and associates (2005) noted that criss-cross fractures, which occur when people fall on an outstretched pronated hand, can produce dislocation of the ulnar head. This dislocation may be associated with styloid process fractures.

CARPALS

The carpals form the transition from the long bones of the forearm to the hand. As such they are frequently subject to extreme loading forces when a person attempts to ease the impact during a fall. Many of these forces are transmitted to the radius since it directly articulates with the carpals. Two theories have been proposed for how forces are passed through the carpals. In the row theory, the scaphoid forms a bridge between the proximal and distal rows. Compressive forces would then be transmitted from distal to proximal rows and then to the long bones of the forearm. The majority would go through the trapezoid and capitate, then scaphoid and lunate and to the radius. In the competing columnar theory, forces from the distal row are passed to the lunate (Taleisnik 1980). The scaphoid forms the radial column while the triquetrum forms the ulnar column. Deviation of the hand will shift the column of support. These theoretical frames become important in interpreting the impact point and hand position during a fall.

Carpal fractures can be classified by bone and location in the distal, middle or proximal third of the element (Amadio 1992, Ruby 1992). The vast majority involves only the scaphoid. A small number involve the triquetrum with the remaining scattered amongst the remaining bones of the wrist. They may be associated with distal radial fractures or fractures at the elbow (Amadio 1992). Fractures of the carpals, however, are generally less common than breaks in the distal radius and are particularly rare in children. Garcia-Elias (2001) discusses the relative incidence of carpal bone fractures. The most common are those of the scaphoid (68.2%), followed by the triquetrum (18.3%), trapezium (4.3%), lunate (3.9%), capitate (1.9%), hamate (1.7%), pisiform (1.3%), and trapezoid (0.4%).

Scaphoid Fractures

Scaphoid fractures are the most common carpal breakage, comprising about 70% of such fractures (Borgeskov *et al.* 1966; Botte and Gelberman 1987, Garcia-Elias 2001). This is primarily due to the quadrupling of the forces that pass from the palmar surface of the hand and into the articulation with the radius (Weber and Chao 1978). These fractures are relatively rare in children and in the elderly. They generally are more common in men than women and approximately equally distributed between the right and left wrists (Brondum *et al.* 1992). This bone is the carpal most frequently fractured in children despite any such fracture being quite uncommon (Blount 1955, Armstrong *et al.* 1994, Stanciu and Dumont 1994).

The most common causes of scaphoid fracture are falls or blows to the palm of the hand (Watson-Jones 1941, Borgeskov *et al.* 1966, Dobyns *et al.* 1982, Amadio 1992, Larsen *et al.* 1992). As a result of falls, the scaphoid is often compacted between the distal radius and the capitate. This will result in failure on the palmar surface due to tension while the dorsal surface is under compression (Weber and Chao 1978, Ruby 1992). Rupture of the waist or proximal pole of the scaphoid may be produced.

Scaphoid fractures as the result of punching have also been reported (Horii *et al.* 1994). In these instances, the fractures are almost always confined to the dominant hand. The hand was in a neutral or slightly palmar-flexed position with the forces unevenly distributed across the knuckles, focusing particularly on the second metacarpal. None of the reported injuries occurred in professional boxers, rather the fractures were observed in people hitting a punching bag. Horii and associates (1994) noted that most of their reviewed cases of fracture due to punching were transverse waist fractures. No horizontal or distal fractures were seen in their case sample.

In adults, scaphoid fractures are usually located in the middle third, and are about evenly split between transverse and oblique fractures. The latter may be horizontal or vertical. In children, scaphoid fracture tends to occur more distally than in adults (Brondum *et al.* 1992). This distal placement probably reflects the buffering provided by the greater cartilagenous coating and the relative weakness of the distal radius (Albert and Barre 1989). Some of these fractures are actually avulsion fractures (Stanciu and Dumont 1994).

Most classification systems divide the fracture by location to proximal third, middle third, and distal third (Dobyns and Linscheid 1984) (Figure 10-13). In some cases the distal third is subdivided into those of the distal body, distal

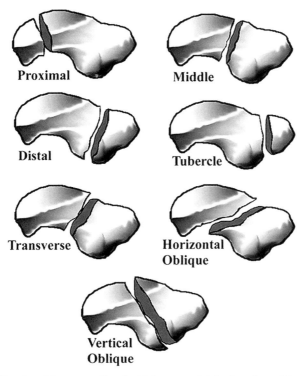

Figure 10-13. Scaphoid fractures. Scaphoid fractures (*right shown*) are identified by location of the break as well as direction. Upper illustrations show the approximate regions while the subsequent illustrations show specific fracture of the tuberosity and directional information on fracture pattern.

articular surface, and the tuberosity. Additional distinctions include the direction of the fracture and the amount of comminution.

Lunate Fractures

In some studies, lunate fractures follow the scaphoid in frequency of fractures among the carpal bones (Botte and Gelberman 1987), but more recent data places them at much lower frequencies (Garcia-Elias 2001). Lunate fractures are often subject to dislocation (Fisk 1984). Most frequently these injuries are of the avulsion or chip nature, although fractures of the lunate body may also occur (Teisen and Hjarbaek 1988). These fractures are classified by the plane of the axis of the fracture. Those in line with the plane of axis are called transverse or frontal (Beckenbaugh *et al.* 1980, Dobyns 1990) (Figure 10-14). The mechanism of injury is usually a fall on the extended hand. Chip fractures on the dorsal margin have been attributed to impacts to the heel of the hand (Cooney *et al.* 1996).

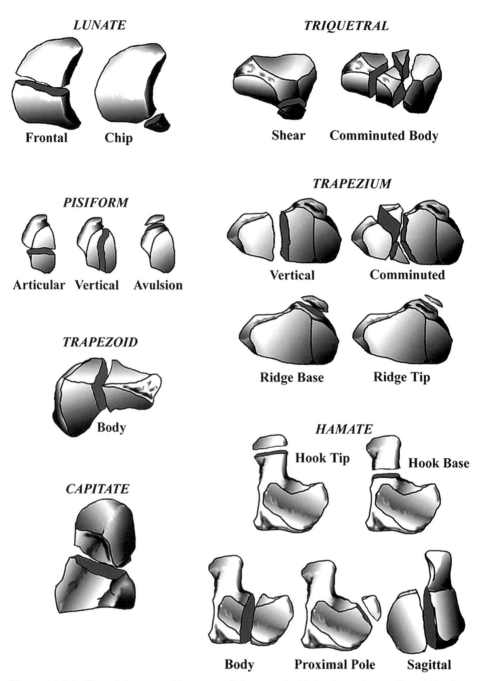

Figure 10-14. Carpal fractures. Fractures of the carpals (right shown) are often difficult to classify. Many are produced by compression or impaction while others are attributable to avulsion or shearing actions. Location and the plane of fracture are useful in describing these injuries.

Triquetral Fractures

The third most common fracture of the wrist is a fracture of the triquetrum (Ruby 1992). These fractures are most often produced by a shearing force or by a chisel effect produced by the ulnar styloid during dorsiflexion. This is most often produced by falls onto an outstretched hand (Smith and Murray 1996). Specifically, the falls involve extreme palmar flexion with radial deviation (Bonnin and Greening 1944). Less frequent are fractures due to high-energy direct blows to the wrist (Marchessault *et al.* 2009).

These fractures are classified by the location and severity of the injuries (Levy *et al.* 1979, Bryan and Dobyns 1980, Dobyns and Linscheid 1984) (Figure 10-14). Type 1 includes isolated avulsion and shear fractures involving the dorsal cortex and ridge. These are the most common and are produced during hyperextension and ulnar deviation. The hamate shears the postero-radial projection of the triquetral. A second mechanism of injury is avulsion due to the dorsal radiotriquetral ligaments. These fractures are also grouped together as "chip" fractures (Hocker and Menschik 1994, Papp 2010). The size of the ulnar styloid may also play a role because those who experience dorsal fractures often also have enlongated styloids (Garcia-Ellis 1987).

Type 2 or midbody fractures are comminuted fractures of the triquetral body and are much less commonly found. When they occur, it is usually in conjunction with a number of associated wrist dislocations and fractures as part of a "greater arc" injury (Papp 2010).

Pisiform Fractures

The small pisiform is rarely fractured. When it occurs, it is usually associated with other fractures in the wrist, particularly the distal radius, hamate, or triquetral. It may be injured during a fall onto the dorsiflexed, outstretched hand or by a direct blow while the pisiform is suspended in the tensed *flexor carpi ulnaris* and held against the triquetral (Vasilas *et al.* 1960, Dobyns and Linscheid 1984, Fleege *et al.* 1991). This can produce avulsion of the distal portion, vertical cracking or fracturing of the articular surface (Figure 10-14).

Trapezium Fractures

Isolated fractures of the trapezium are quite rare. Fractures in the body of the element are either oriented vertically or severely comminuted (Ruby 1992) (Figure 10-14). These are produced by loading from the base of the first metacarpal onto the articular surface with the trapezium while the thumb is in adduction. Walker and associates (1988) classified these as Type 1 (transverse fracture), Type 2 (distolateral fractures), Type 3 (proximolateral fracture), Type

4 (distomedial fracture), Type 5 (sagittal fracture), and Type 6 (comminuted fracture). Of these, Type 5 is the most common.

A second form of trapezium fracture may be located in the trapezeal ridge that has been classified into Type 1 consisting of fractures of the base of the ridge and Type 2 that are avulsions of the tip (Palmer 1981). Direct blows tend to produce Type 1 fractures, while avulsion of the flexor retinaculum is more frequently confined to the tip. Ridge fractures may also be caused by stress (Botte *et al.* 1992).

About 15% of all trapezium fractures are associated with ipsilateral Bennett's fracture of the first metacarpal (Garcia-Ellis *et al.* 1993). Loading onto the out-stretched hand can rotate the adjacent bones in a manner that increases the vulnerability of the trapezium (Walker *et al.* 1988). Often resulting from motor vehicle accidents, it appears the mechanism of injury is leverage to the dorsum of the first metacarpal with axial loading. This movement produces a metacarpal fracture along with increased force on the ligaments, which then produce an avulsion fracture of the trapezium.

Trapezoid Fractures

Trapezoidal fractures are rare due to the relatively protected position of this bone in the wrist. However, forces applied to the second metacarpal may cause injuries to this bone (Dobyns and Linscheid 1984). Less common than these are trapezoidal fractures due to direct impact on the dorsal wrist (Seitz and Papandrea 2002).

Capitate Fractures

Fractures of the capitate are relatively rare (Guiral *et al.* 1993, Papp 2010) despite the fact that this bone acts as the center for movement in the wrist (Fisk 1984). These fractures may be isolated or associated with scaphoid frac-tures. Scaphocapitate syndrome is produced through the same hyperdorsi-flexion that produces scaphoid waist fractures (Ruby 1992, Guiral *et al.* 1993, Seitz and Panandrea 2002). The usual point of breakage is in the neck of the capitate and probably is due to pressure from the distal radius (Figure 10-14). Direct blows to the wrist may also be involved (Hokan *et al.* 1993). Falling onto a clenched fist has been associated with fractures at the midbody of the capitate (Volk 1995).

Hamate Fractures

The hamate can be fractured in the body, at the hook, in the distal articular surface, at the triquetral facet or at the proximal pole (Milch 1934, Dobyns and Linscheid 1984) (Figure 10-14). Fractures of the body are relatively rare while the fractures of the hook are much more likely to occur (Ruby 1992, Chase *et al.* 1997). Hirano and Inoue (2005) classified hamate fractures as Type 1 (fractures of the hook), Type 2A (coronal split fractures), Type 2B (transverse fractures). Type 2A fractures are the most common.

Body fractures usually occur in association with dislocations of the fourth and fifth carpometacarpal joint and often also fractures at these locations (Papp 2010). Thomas and Birch (1983) suggested that these occur when there is ulnar deviation of the wrist so that the hamate is wedged against the triquetral bone. Forces passed along the metacarpals then split the hamate coronally. If the wrist were in radial deviation, it is likely that the fracture would pass sagittally. Longitudinal fractures are even more rare. Striking an object with the fist can cause such fracture-producing forces.

Fractures of the hook are due to direct pressure on the anterior wrist either as the result of direct violence or a fall on the dorsiflexed wrist (Kerr 1992). It is a common sports-related injury (Dobyns and Linscheid 1984) and can occur when a forceful swing of a bat/club traps the hook of the hamate against the handle of the equipment (Papp 2010). The fractures are more likely to be located at the tip of the hook rather than closer to the base.

A "die-punch" fracture of the distal articular facet has been reported due to flexion injury during a fall or blow while the hand is ulnarly deviated (Dobyns and Linscheid 1984, Jones and Kutty 1993). Forces applied from the fifth metacarpal are the probable cause. Fractures at the proximal pole and the articular surface with the triquetrum are usually due to impaction against the articular surface of the lunate during dorsiflexion and ulnar deviation (Dobyns and Linscheid 1984). Wrenching movements may also produce these injuries.

METACARPALS

The bones of the hands and fingers are particularly vulnerable in humans. The emphasis on fine manipulation of tools not only exposes the hands to a number of risks from the objects being handled but also means the muscle mass around the bones is reduced in comparison to other primates. Human anatomy emphasizes fine motor control rather than force. In addition, the hands are used in thwarting impacts to the body as well as catching ourselves when we fall. The curved shape of the metacarpals focuses the stress on the weakest portion of the bone, which is located just proximal and dorsal to the head (Kaplan 1965).

Fractures of the metacarpals are fairly common, especially for the first and fifth metacarpals (Rogers 1992), accounting for about 20–40% of all hand fractures (Hunter and Cowan 1970, Ashkenaze and Ruby 1992). Metacarpal fractures are particularly common in young adult men (Buhr and Cooke 1959). These fractures can be classified by the location of fracture: base, shaft, neck, and head (Jupiter and Belsky 1992). Dobyns and associates (1983) found that about a quarter of their sample of metacarpal fractures were located in the neck, a quarter in the articular regions of the base and head. Almost 40% were in the shaft and the remainder in the base.

McElfresh and Dobyns 1983 argue that the second metacarpal is the most often broken. In the second and fifth metacarpal, fractures are usually located in the distal shaft or neck, whereas fractures in the third and fourth metacarpal are usually midshaft. Often the third and fourth metacarpals will break simultaneously. This uneven distribution of injuries and locations of the fractures results from differences in morphology, placement in the hand with regards to the impact, and angulation of the long axis with respect to the base.

Injuries at the carpometacarpal joint often result in fractures at the base of the metacarpals (Jupiter and Belsky 1992). A combination of forces produces these injuries. Forces along the axis of the metacarpals tend to produce the more comminuted fractures. Direct blows or torque may also be involved. These fractures can be grouped into four categories (Figure 10-15). Epibasal injuries segment the bone through the metaphysis so that the articular end becomes a separate unit. These fractures tend to be oblique, although they are often transverse in the first metacarpal (Jupiter and Belsky 1992). Two-part injuries include fracture of the lateral or medial portion, while a three-part fracture usually is a Y fracture of the base. The final group includes the comminuted fractures. Both three-part and comminuted injuries tend to be associated with high-energy trauma. Avulsive fractures at the base of the second and third digits can result from the strains on *extensor carpi radialis longus* and *extensor carpi radialis brevis* tendons (Ashkenaze and Ruby 1992).

Metacarpal shaft fractures include those of the spiral or oblique, transverse, longitudinal, and comminuted forms. Dobyns and associates (1983) suggest that most fractures are transverse, followed by spiral/oblique fractures. The other forms are relatively uncommon. Direct blows commonly produce transverse, short oblique, or comminuted fractures in this area while indirect or rotational forces produce more spiraling or long oblique fractures (Green and Rowland 1984, Bowman and Simon 1993). Fractures by direct blows may be found in cases of child abuse, particularly in children after infancy (Swischuk 1992). Falls onto the ulnar border of the hand followed by rolling on the back of the hand may be linked to spiral fractures of the third through fifth metacarpal shafts (Watson-Jones 1941). When these fractures are present with overall bone loss, they are often found to be only one part of a complex of skeletal injuries (Jupiter and Belsky 1992).

Fractures of the metacarpal neck are the most common. These usually result from direct impact – often due to hitting with the hand in a clenched

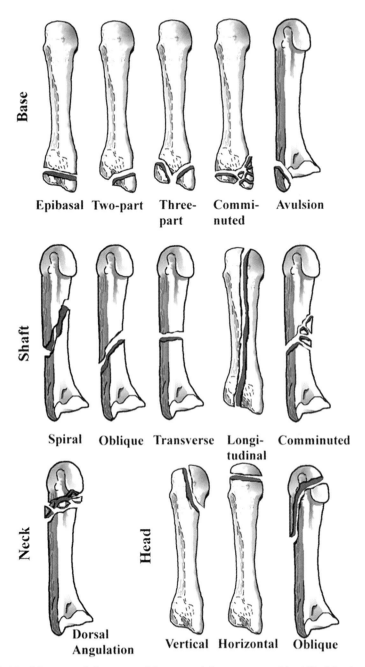

Figure 10-15. Metacarpal fractures. Metacarpal fractures are identified by location and fracture morphology. Jupiter and Belsky (1992) have identified the principal forms of basal fractures. Dobyns and associates have classified shaft fractures. Neck and head fractures may be less variable with neck fractures usually showing dorsal angulation. Metacarpal head fractures are classified by the plane of failure (McElfresh and Dobyns 1983).

fist (Ashkenaze and Ruby 1992, Jupiter and Belsky 1992, Bowman and Simon 1993). The fracture is usually angled dorsally and comminution is present. While these fractures are often referred to as a *Boxer's* fractures, they are exceptionally rare in professional fighters. Instead, they appear most often in those whose punches are poorly directed (Walsh 2004, Bloom *et al.* 2012).

Fractures of the metacarpal head are relatively rare (Jupiter and Belsky 1992). They usually occur with direct blows or from a missile or crushing injury (Bowman and Simon 1993). Fractures usually form distal to the collateral ligament insertion. Fractures at the head of the metacarpals are extremely variable in form. While the most common form is comminuted, two-part fractures are also represented. These may take the form of vertical fractures (anteroposterior), horizontal fractures (transverse across the articular surface), or oblique fractures, which extend into longitudinal fractures of the shaft (McElfresh and Dobyns 1983).

The first metatarsal tends to have a specific suite of injuries due to both structural differences in the bone as well as its anatomical location in the hand. Fractures of this bone rank second in frequency among metacarpal fractures, surpassed only by the fifth metacarpals (Gedda 1954). Fractures of the first metacarpal tend to occur with punches, falls, and blows (Watson-Jones 1941, Lowdon 1986, Rogers 1992). Extra-articular fractures of the base and the shaft are more frequent than those involving the articular surfaces (Bowman and Simon 1993). These are usually oblique, transverse, or, in children, epiphyseal. Fractures are usually produced by direct blows, axial loading from the distal phalanx, or impaction. Both hyperabduction and direct blows can also cause fracture of the sesamoid at the base of the thumb (Jones and Leach 1980, Clarke *et al.* 1983).

About one-third of first metacarpal fractures are termed *Bennett's* fractures. They involve the base of the first metacarpal. This is the most common location for fractures in this bone (Figure 10-16). Specifically, these involve the proximal articular surface and are characterized by cleavage of the inner side of the proximal base adjacent to the articulation with the wrist bones (Rider 1937, Green and Rowland 1984, Jupiter and Belsky 1992). The mechanism of fracture is hyperextenstion or hyperabduction of the thumb secondary to a person striking a rigid surface with a closed fist. They are not seen in young children (Blount 1955). Males predominate by 10:1 in these fractures and they usually occur on the dominant hand (Pelligrini 1988). *Reverse Bennett's* fractures involve the separation of a medial or lateral portion at the base along the sagittal rather than coronal plane. These fractures may also be known as "mirrored Bennett's fractures (Goedkoop *et al.* 2000).

Another fracture specific to the first metacarpal is the *Rolando's* fracture, which consists of an uncommon three-part fracture (Jupiter and Belsky 1992). These may take a T or Y form in either the frontal or lateral aspect

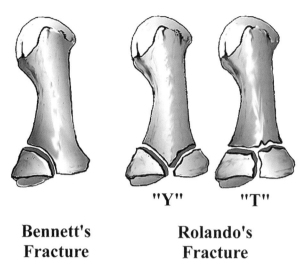

"Y"   "T"

Bennett's   **Rolando's**
Fracture   **Fracture**

Figure 10-16. Bennett's and Rolando's fractures of the metacarpal of the thumb. Fractures of the base of the first metacarpal include those assigned to Bennett's fractures and Rolando's fractures. The latter can be distinguished by its three part configuration and characteristic T or Y pattern.

and essentially form an expansion of the *Bennett's* fracture (Figure 10-16). The mechanism of injury appears similar as well.

Similarly, the fifth metacarpal is also vulnerable to fracture in ways that are less common in the other metacarpals. Fractures in this bone are relatively common. The most vulnerable portions appear to be the head and neck, accounting for 60% of fractures in this bone in one study (Hunter and Cowen 1970). About one-third consisted of basilar fractures with the remainder occurring in the shaft. A Boxer's fracture, consisting of a transverse fracture of the neck of the fifth metacarpal and sometimes also the fourth, are most frequently caused by a blow struck with the fist but also occur in motor vehicle accidents, sports, and catching the hand in a closing door (Rider 1937, Hunter and Cowen 1970, Dobyns *et al.* 1978, McCue *et al.* 1979, Lowdon 1986, McKerrell *et al.* 1987). Jupiter and Belsky (1992) point out that professional boxers are much more likely to fracture the second or third metacarpal than the fifth, so the so-called *Boxer's* fracture usually indicates amateur status. These fractures result from axial loading of the flexed metacarpophalangeal joint. There is frequently comminution of the palmer cortex (Siegel 1995).

Skeletal examination of the metacarpals is often essential in determining whether the decedent was attempting to withstand an assault. The hands may block direct blows, producing fracture of the metacarpals. These defensive injuries may be important in reconstructing both victim and perpetrator behavior at the crime scene. Location and characteristics of the injuries should be recorded. Charts and detailed photographs may be important in presentation of the case involving possible defensive injuries.

PHALANGES OF THE HAND

As with metacarpal fractures, phalangeal fractures are more common in young men. De Jonge and associates (1994) concluded that, until age 60 years and older, men exceed women in rates of phalangeal fractures by about 2:1, peaking at 5.4:1 in the 40-49 year age group. Sports injuries account for many of these breaks, although crushing injuries were also very common, especially in young children. A study by Gedda and Moberg (1953) showed that more than half occur in the proximal or middle phalanges, although in another study, the distal phalanges were found to sustain over half the phalangeal fractures (Butt 1962). Thomine (1975) recorded most fractures in the second digit. The phalanges often do not undergo the more simple transverse or longitudinal fractures but, instead, are subject to comminuted and avulsion fractures. Due to the danger of fingers getting trapped in machinery or between colliding objects, severe crushing is common among the injuries to the phalanges.

Proximal Phalangeal Fractures

In addition to direct impact, fractures of the proximal phalanx may also result from falls. The more proximal regions of the bone are the most frequently affected (Watson-Jones 1941). Proximal fractures are usually transverse or oblique or, more rarely, nearly longitudinal (Rider 1937). Frequently there is more serious comminution, which involves more extensive soft tissue damage. In some cases, indirect forces that twist the finger can produce spiral fractures of the phalangeal shaft (Bowman and Simon 1993). Fractures in the proximal phalanx of the thumb tend to be transverse more often than of other forms. Fractures of the phalangeal neck and head are not common (Thomine 1975).

Intra-articular fractures involve either or both the head and base. Clinically, they can be divided by the degree of displacement and location. The head fractures may involve one or both condyles (Jupiter and Belsky 1992). Those involving only one condyle tend to result from exposure to shearing forces while those involving both condyles usually result from compressive forces. Small chip fractures may occur on the volar lip in dorsal dislocation. Impaction fractures may be confined to a depression of 1–4 mm of around 30% of the articular surface into the metaphysis leaving a portion of the articular rim intact (Wolfe and Katz 1995). These fractures often appear as if the rim is being separated leaving the more central portions of the articular surface to bear the load. Usually these depression injuries lie lateral to the midline of the bone, reflecting both axial loading and angulation. Avulsion fractures produced by the collateral ligament may be found (Jupiter and Belsky 1992, Bowman and Simon 1993). This situation is particularly true for the ulnar collateral in the thumb. Avulsion of the extensor tendon may also produce a small fracture in the bone on the dorsal surface (Green and Rowland 1984).

Middle Phalangeal Fractures

Fractures of the middle phalanges are particularly rare, accounting for as low as 6% of phalangeal fractures (Rider 1937). Fractures to the middle phalanx are usually due to direct blows while blows to the whole digit often lead to failure of the base of the proximal phalanx (Armstrong *et al.* 1994). The "jammed finger" tends to lead to fractures on the palmer surface of the base of the middle phalanx and are relatively more common (Jupiter and Belsky 1992). When the loading is asymmetrical, fracturing of only a portion of the phalangeal base may occur. The twisting, which produces a spiral fracture on the proximal phalanx, is rarely seen in the middle phalanx where dislocation of the proximal interphalangeal joint is much more common (Bowman and Simon 1993). Avulsion fractures on the dorsal surface of these bones may result at the attachment site of the central slip of the extensor mechanism as the finger is forced into flexion from rigid extension. These fractures are usually produced by forced hyperflexion, hyperextension, or radial or ulnar traction (Bowman and Simon 1993). Similar fractures on the palmar surface of the phalanx base are produced during dorsal subluxation or dislocation at the adjacent joint. These may be called *Wilson's fractures*. Ulnar or radially directed forces may produce tension on the collateral ligaments producing avulsion fractures along the medial or lateral sides of the base. As with the proximal phalanges, comminuted fractures are common in high-energy or crushing injuries.

Distal Phalangeal Fractures

Distal phalangeal fractures are most common on the third or first digits (Jobe 1993). The distal phalanx may be fractured in a number of ways, which can be grouped into three to four categories (Rider 1937, Kaplan 1940) (Figure 10-17). Splitting or longitudinal fractures divide the bone along the long axis and are commonly caused by blows at the end of the finger. Transverse fractures may occur in any portion of the phalanx but are most common in the midsection. Chip fractures can be caused by blows but usually occur when the finger becomes trapped between two solid surfaces. These fractures most frequently are comminuted (Jupiter and Belsky 1992) and may be called "crushed eggshell"-type fractures (Rider 1937), providing a good image of the extent of the damage. All these can be considered extra-articular.

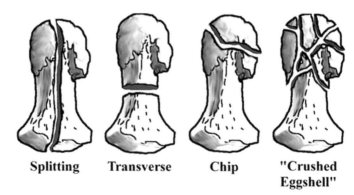

Figure 10-17. Classification of distal phalanx fractures. Distal phalanx fractures can be classified by direction of fracture and severity of injury (Rider 1937, Kaplan 1940).

Intra-articular fractures include the baseball or mallet fractures, which are avulsive fractures of the distal phalanx (Rider 1937, Watson-Jones 1941, McMinn 1981, Wehbe and Schneider 1984, Jupiter and Belsky 1992, Rogers 1992; Bowman and Simon 1993). These fractures are characterized by a finger that may drop toward the palmar surface resembling a mallet. In this fracture, the force is directed at the extended distal phalanx rapidly forcing it into a flexed position. As a result, the extensor tendon causes avulsion of the proximal dorsal margin of the phalanx. This defect is generally rather small, although, when the fractured area is wider, it may be caused by compression of the finger and compaction of the distal phalanx against the head of the middle phalanx. In children, avulsion of the whole epiphysis may occur. A third mechanism is sudden hyperextension, again impacting the base of the distal phalanx against the head of the middle phalanx. About half of the injuries are reportedly due to falls or blunt trauma in which the victim reported "jamming" the finger (Wehbe and Schneider 1984).

Mallet fractures have been classified according to the extent of subluxation (Type I to III) and subdivided into subtypes A, B and C (Wehbe and Schneider 1984). While the types cannot be determined in isolated skeletal material, the subtypes refer to fractures involving (A) less than one-third of the articular surface, (B) one-third to two-thirds of the articular surface and (C) over two thirds of the articular surface (Figure 10-18).

A second form of avulsion fractures of the distal phalanx involves the flexor digitorum profundus tendon (Green and Rowland 1984). Forced hyperextension may result in detachment of a portion of bone near the volar base of the phalanx. It often involves the fourth digit.

Unfortunately, for the anthropologist, the phalanges are often lost prior to or during recovery due to their small size and vulnerability to taphonomic change, particularly scavenging. Postmortem erosion also becomes a problem

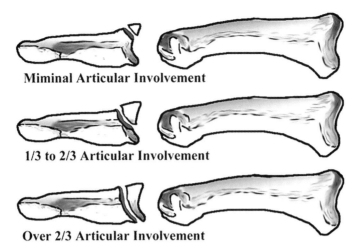

Miminal Articular Involvement

1/3 to 2/3 Articular Involvement

Over 2/3 Articular Involvement

Figure 10-18. Lateral view of mallet fracture. Mallet fractures may be confined to a mere fragment or involve separation of the entire articular surface. Attachment of the extensor tendon to the detached fragment causes the classic drop of the distal phalanx.

in interpreting any defects on these bones. Despite these concerns, detailed examination of all phalanges with documentation of location and nature of any fracture is required.

Chapter 11

THE LOWER EXTREMITY

Alison Galloway

The robust bones of the lower extremity are resistant to fracture from axial loading due to their overall and cross-sectional morphology and high bone mineral density. Even normal activities focus tremendous pressure on the feet and legs and the bone becomes highly resistant to compression. Fractures attributable to loading, which follows the normal pattern, therefore, indicate much higher energy impacts than normally occur. If, however, forces are applied in direc-tions other than those normally encountered, or there is substantial bone density loss, the bones of the lower extremity are susceptible to failure.

With each step taken, the momentum of forward movement and the weight of the upper body are met by the resistance of the substrate. The resulting strains on the body are met by the strength of the limb bones and pelvis. The pelvic girdle, which consists of the innominates and the sacrum, provides for the transmission of forces between the torso and the lower limb. In addition to its locomotor functions, the pelvis also houses the excretory and reproductive organs. The recent evolutionarily shift to bipedality and the even more recent introduction of large-brained neonates have left the pelvic girdle with narrow constraints as to the possible responses to maintain internal functions and maximize locomotor efficiency. Into this delicate, if precarious, balance we have thrown in forces far in excess of normal loading. Consequently, both the pelvis and lower limb suffer greatly with the modern application of speed, high-energy collisions, extreme sports, and interpersonal confrontations, which confer excessive force.

INNOMINATES

Pelvic fractures are associated with high mortality and, therefore, are of significance in the analysis of skeletal material for forensic purposes. Fractures are frequently complex since, although some movement is possible at the pubic symphysis and the sacroiliac joints, the pelvis is effectively a rigid ring. Fracture at any one point almost inevitably results in fracture at another location. Similarly, within the pelvis, the obturator foramina form secondary rings with the same requirement.

Mortality often depends on whether or not internal soft tissue structures have been perforated. About 4% of pelvic fractures are considered *open*, meaning there is direct communication between the broken bone and rectal, vaginal, perineal, or skin laceration (Rothernberger *et al.* 1978, Richardson *et al.* 1982). Such extreme fractures have a mortality of 50% or higher (Raffa and Christensen 1976, Rothenberger *et al.* 1978, Perry 1980, Richardson *et al.* 1982). The cause of death with open fractures is usually blood loss and hemorrhage, and survival often requires multiple blood transfusions. Subsequent infection is also a serious consideration with such pelvic injuries. Pelvic fractures are also linked to multiple major injuries elsewhere in the body (Poole *et al.* 1992).

Severe pelvic fractures usually require considerable force and are often the result of motor vehicle accidents, especially those involving pedestrians and motorcycles. Frontal crashes of 30 mph or greater or side impacts of 15 mph or greater were required to produce major pelvic fracture in one experimental study (McCoy *et al.* 1989). Although seat-restraint devices inside autos have been important in limiting some of the risks for pelvic fracture, few preventative devices can protect individuals outside the automobile in high-speed accidents. Car/pedestrian accidents are also strongly associated with pelvic fractures in both the run-under and run-over modes (Teresinski and Madro 2001). Falls from heights and sports-related accidents are also causes of pelvic injuries.

Pelvic fractures are most common in young prime-aged adult males and in older men and women (Buhr and Cooke 1959, Failinger and McGanity 1992, Ragnarsson and Jacobsson 1992). This distribution reflects two factors: propensity to engage in high-speed activities and age-related declines in bone mineral and structural integrity. While both segments of the population suffer from pelvic injuries, the severity of the high-energy impacts in the younger age group increases the likelihood of an unsatisfactory outcome. Fractures in the elderly tend to be less displaced and mortality often is attributable to secondary infections during hospitalization. Children seem less susceptible to pelvic fracture and experience a lower mortality rate (Ismail *et al.* 1996).

In one study of pelvic fractures, the pubic rami were the most common structures to be broken in either moderate or severe trauma (Ragnarsson and Jacobsson 1992). Acetabular fractures followed as a distant second, with iliac wing fractures and fractures of multiple areas forming a minor component. Other studies support the high frequency of pubic rami fractures (Lüthje *et al.* 1995).

Many different portions of the pelvic girdle can be fractured. Letournel (1980) devised a system for the identification of specific fractures in the pelvic

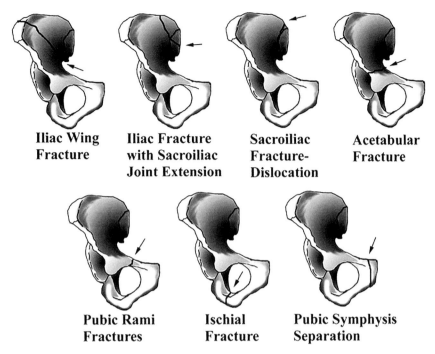

Iliac Wing Fracture · **Iliac Fracture with Sacroiliac Joint Extension** · **Sacroiliac Fracture-Dislocation** · **Acetabular Fracture**

Pubic Rami Fractures · **Ischial Fracture** · **Pubic Symphysis Separation**

Figure 11-1. Classification of pelvic fracture locations. Locations of pelvic fractures have been identified by Letournel (1980), and these identifications are useful in describing the initial location of the defect. Because of the complexity of the pelvic ring, however, multiple fractures are common. Arrows indicate the location of the fracture.

girdle without direct connection to the forces involved. This system is based on the site of injury, identifying nine locations: (1) iliac wing, (2) ilium with an extension into the sacroiliac joint, (3) trans-sacral, (4) unilateral sacral fractures, (5) sacroiliac joint fracture-dislocations, (6) acetabular fractures, (7) pubic ramus fractures, (8) ischial fractures, and (9) public symphysis separation (Figure 11-1, above).

This system is useful for defining the location of specific fractures. However, in most cases, these fractures do not occur in isolation since rupture of one part of the pelvic ring will often produce a fracture or dislocation in another portion of the ring. Consideration of the overall morphology is important for determining the forces that produced the injury.

Pelvic Ring Fractures

From the clinical perspective, the most important classification is whether the fractures are stable or unstable based on the disruption of the pelvic ring. Those interrupting the anterior, posterior or both arches of the ring are

considered unstable and involve a double fracture (Rogers 1992). Those
which do not intrude on the ring or are incomplete, and termed stable. Pelvic
ring fractures are also associated with significantly higher mortality in clinical settings (Giannoudis *et al.* 2007, Schulman *et al.* 2010).

While this is clinically important, it is of less concern forensically. Important to note, however, is that stable fractures are usually the result of falls
(Rogers 1992). Unstable fractures are usually the result of a severe trauma
such as a motor vehicle or car-pedestrian accidents. They occur more frequently in lateral impact than frontal impact crashes (Rowe *et al.* 2004). They
are extremely common in car-pedestrian accidents involving children (Paster
et al. 1974, Reed 1976). Such fractures frequently result in severe hemorrhage and soft tissue damage. When posterior portions are broken, mortality
is considerably higher (Looser and Crombie 1976). At times, pelvic ring
fractures have ben associated with ipsilateral femoral fractures to create a
"floating hip;" however, this term is not recommended clinically as it does
not generate specific complications beyond the individual fractures (Müller
et al. 1991).

The form of the disruption of the pelvic ring depends upon the direction
of the forces directed toward it. There are basically four different patterns
that will result in either ligamentous or osseous disruption (Kellam and
Browner 1992). Anteroposterior force is directed from the anterior usually
forcing one-half of the pelvic ring to be pushed outward. The second and
more common force involves lateral compression. A third force, often found
in motorcycle accidents, involves external rotation-abduction. In these
cases, the force is driven through the femoral shafts as the leg is caught and
externally rotated and abducted. The attached innominate is ripped from
the sacrum resulting in substantial fragmentation in this region. Finally,
shear forces may be involved. These often affect the bone in ways that are
unanticipated by the internal structure of the bone and so transect trabecular
patterns.

Due to the complexity of the structure, which includes not only the innominates or hip bones but also the sacrum and, to a great extent, the proximal femur, pelvic fractures have been variously classified. Bucholz (1981) and
Young and Burgess (1987) have proposed systems of classification of the location of fractures in the pelvic ring in response to the application of forces. The
latter utilizes concepts of both stability and direction of force, dividing the
fractures into those of anteroposterior compression, of lateral compression
and of combined or shear forces as described above. Many of these fracture
complexes would be included in the category of *Malgaigne* fractures, named
for the author of an extensive treatise on fractures (Malgaigne 1859). The
term *Malgaigne* fractures refers to those fractures in which there is vertical
displacement of one innominate due to either fracture in that bone or in the

associated sacroiliac joint or pubic symphysis. Unfortunately, this term does not distinguish whether the dislocation is due to vertical shearing, anteroposterior compressive, or lateral compressive forces.

Tile and Pennal (1980) have devised a classification system based on the direction of the forces and locations of the fractures. Again, the presumed principle forces of injury are anteroposterior compression, lateral compression, and vertical shear (Figure 11-2). Anterior compression involves fracture of the anterior pelvic ring, at or close to the pubic symphysis and a posterior fracture at or near the sacroiliac joint (Kellam and Browner 1992). The sacrum as well

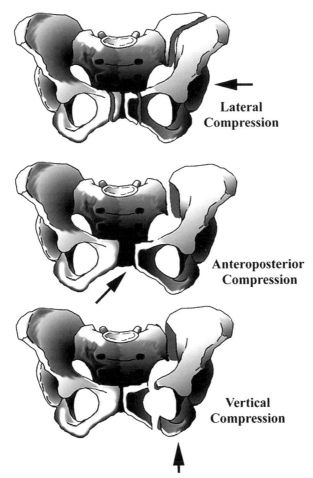

Figure 11-2. Classification of pelvic ring fractures. Classification of pelvic ring fractures by Young and Burgess (1987) and Tile (1988) is based on the direction of the force with respect to the unity of the ring. Injuries may be confined to the ligaments that bind the joints, but fractures and fracture/dislocations are also common. Arrows indicate the direction of force applied to the pelvic ring.

as one or both innominates may be involved. This produces the "open-book" or "open-clamshell" type of fracture pattern wherein one-half of the pelvic ring is externally rotated. Bilateral ramus fracturing also falls into this category. Posteriorly, sacral fracture or avulsion at the sacroiliac ligamentous attachment, which is sometimes accompanied by iliac fracture as well, is produced in sacroiliac joint dislocations (Tile 1987b). Posterior compression produces the reciprocal of the injuries produced by anterior compression with the bulk of damage occurring posteriorly (Meek 1992).

Lateral compression, the most common form of pelvic disruption, usually results in inward collapse of the innominate via fracture at the sacroiliac joint and of the rami (Tile and Pennal 1980, Meek 1992). Here the fracture pattern will reflect the location on which the force is applied (Kellam and Browner 1992). If it is placed toward the posterior part of the pelvis, fractures in the posterior ilium and sacrum will be seen. If, however, the force is applied to the anterior half of the iliac wing, the innominate will rotate inward, making the pivot point in the anterior sacroiliac joint. The anterior sacrum will be crushed. If the force continues, the innominate on the opposite side will be forced outward, usually resulting in tearing at the sacroiliac joint. Anteriorly, there may be fracturing of the pubic rami and/or disruption of the pubic symphysis. If the lateral compression is directed lower through the greater trochanters of the femora, then the fragmentation centers on the acetabulae. This action results in the contralateral or "bucket-handle"-type of fracture. On some occasions, there may be avulsion of the medial portions of the posterior iliac spine. If severe, fracture of the sacrum and bilateral fracture in the pubic arch at all four rami may be found. The rami fractures may occur on the same side or opposite the side of the point of compression (Pennal and Sutherland 1961). The innominate receiving the blow may be displaced superiorly and medially raising one crest higher than the other, the way a bucket handle is lifted above the bucket. In one variant, the contralateral pubic bone is broken outward as the innominate that received the blow is displaced to the inner portion of the pelvis. This is known as a "tilt" fracture (Meek 1992). Tile (1987b) reports that these fractures are more common in young females and the contralateral injury may extend to the anterior column of the acetabulum. Ligaments at the sacroiliac joint are usually damaged on the side of the applied force regardless of the side of fracture. Contralateral compression is less dangerous clinically because of the decreased likelihood of internal damage (Tile and Pennal 1980).

Vertical shearing is usually from forces transmitted through the femur or ischial tuberosity and is usually unilateral (Pennel and Sutherland 1961, Meek 1992). Vertical shearing fractures that involve the anterior and posterior rings may, however, extend to both sides. Posteriorly there is often iliac fracture lateral to the sacroiliac joint or sacral fracture while, in the anterior, there may be fracturing around the pubic symphysis. Anteriorly, there will be disruption of the ipsilateral or contralateral ramus unless the symphysis itself is sheared open. In violent shearing with splaying of one or both legs, the inferior hemipelvis may be torn from the upper portions with extensive soft tissue damage (Tile 1987b, Meek 1992). Avulsion of the ischial spine is also indicative of shearing action that results in gross pelvic instability (Tile and Pennal 1980). In very rare instances, shearing forces may be directed from a superior direction pushing the upper pelvis into the lower bone (Meek 1992). This is often associated with damage at the L5–S1 joint.

Biomedically, one of the most frequently cited systems is that of Tile (1988) that builds upon the previous work of Tile and Pennal (1980). It combines the concepts of stability and mechanism of injury with a determination of prognosis and treatment. Stability refers to the possibility of movement within the patient and dictates the need for fixation during surgery. Tile's (1988) Type A injuries are stable and include avulsions at the ischial tuberosity, anterior superior and/or anterior inferior spine, iliac wing fractures, isolated (4-pillar) anterior ring injuries, and transverse fractures of the sacrum and coccyx. Type B fractures are rotationally unstable but remain vertically and posteriorly stable. These include the "open-book" and "bucket-handle"-type of injuries and those due to lateral compression. This would include "tilt" fractures. Type C injuries can be unilateral or bilateral but are unstable in all directions. Typically, these include fractures through the ilium, sacrum, or at the sacroiliac joint and those associated with an acetabular fracture.

For the forensic anthropologist, pelvic fracture poses particular problems. Often the entire pelvic ring is not available for study and the direction of displacement must be reconstructed from damage to isolated elements. Taphonomic effects in the pelvic girdle, especially the consequences of scavenging, may make any attempts at deciphering injuries very difficult. Inclusion of stability factors and ligamentous damage may be problematic, since these may be difficult to diagnose from isolated bones or are seen, in some cases, as minor avulsion. Given the level of anatomical complexity and overlapping systems of classification, which rely heavily on disruption of ligamentous attachments, identification of specific areas of fracture along the lines of the Letournel (1980) system, should be the first step. The pattern of these specific defects can then be used to reconstruct the probable direction of force, keeping in mind that in some accidents the victim will have suffered a series of injuries that may have affected the pelvic ring. The use of detailed illustrations to chart the pattern of injuries, utilizing different vantage points, is helpful and photographs are critical. Use of a pelvic model in which the bones can be separated and moved may be appropriate in courtroom presentation to acquaint the jury with the three-dimensional nature of the injury complex.

Isolated Iliac and Ramus Fractures

In addition to the number of classificatory systems for describing pelvic ring fractures, isolated fractures are commonly found, some of which are given separate designations. For example, fracture of the iliac wing is known as *Duverney's* fracture (Figure 11-3). These are due to lateral compressive forces, which do not disrupt the pelvic ring.

Isolated iliac wing fractures are, in and of themselves, not usually associated with high mortality. In most cases, however, they are accompanied by extensive soft and hard tissue damage that is often life threatening (Abrassart *et al.* 2009).

Isolated fractures of a single ramus may occur (Kane 1984). This type of fracture usually affects the ischial ramus and is more common in the elderly. The most commonly cited cause is a fall from standing height and reflects the poor structural qualities of the bone. The body of the ischium may also be fractured due to falls into the sitting position, but these are reported only rarely. They are often associated with posterior dislocation/fractures, although these may not be initially clinically evident (Cosker *et al.* 2005).

Fractures of both the iliopubic and ischiopubic rami on one innominate are among the most common pelvic fractures (Kane 1984). This type of fracture can be produced by direct blows or by the indirect forces applied on the pelvic ring. More rare is an isolated fracture of the pubic body adjacent to the pubic symphysis. Berg (1979) reports that this form of injury is seen in cowboys thrown against the saddle horn.

Saddle or *straddle* fractures involve all four pubic rami without posterior arch fractures (Judet *et al.* 1964, Meek 1992, Rogers 1992) (Figure 11-3). These have often been attributable to an object striking the body in the crotch, which produces compression of the pelvic girdle, such as could occur when a motorcyclist is thrown forward onto the gas tank. They have been

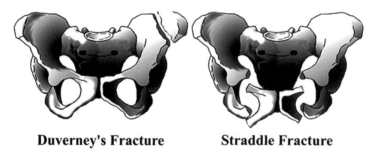

Duverney's Fracture   **Straddle Fracture**

Figure 11-3. Duverney's and Saddle fractures. Fractures of the iliac wing are often termed Duverney's fractures (*left*) and are due to lateral compression that does not disrupt the entire pelvic ring. Saddle or straddle fractures (*right*) are bilateral fractures of the ischio- and iliopubic rami due to frontal impact.

found to also result from a direct blow to the ventral surface. A similar fracture of the pubic rami can also be caused by lateral compression, but this type is accompanied by a fracture of the posterior ring. The superior rami are more often fractured than the inferior rami. In at least one reported case, the fracture was stress induced in a marathon runner (Eren and Holtby 1998).

Isolated fractures in the area of the sacroiliac joint are not common and usually result from direct trauma to the area (Kane 1984). Since the innominate in this area is relatively thick, any fractures here are usually accompanied by anterior fractures in the pubic rami or associated anterior ligamentous damage where the pelvic ring is relatively weak.

Acetabular Fractures

About one-fifth of all pelvic fractures also involve the acetabulum (Rankin 1937, McElhaney *et al.* 1976, Lansinger 1977). These injuries are mostly from motor vehicle accidents, particularly those involving a pedestrian. They are also found in industrial accidents and, in the elderly, frequently resulting from simple falls (Spencer 1989). In most cases, the femoral head transmitting forces from the foot, knee, or greater trochanter produces acetabular fractures (Judet *et al.* 1964, Tile 1987a). A blow to the knee when the hip is flexed will displace the femoral head posteriorly into the acetabular rim (Rogers 1992). Such injuries commonly occur in motor vehicle accidents when the passenger's knee strikes the dashboard. A common location in such cases is the posterior acetabular rim. Other common causes are blows to the greater trochanter, which drive the femoral head directly into the acetabulum.

Age affects the appearance of acetabular fractures. In older victims, where the forces leading to fracture are of less magnitude; acetabular fracture often appears as cracks in osteoporotic bone (Rothenberger *et al.* 1978). Epileptic seizures also have been reported to produce bilateral acetabular fractures (Granhed and Karladani 1997).

In addition to rim fractures, which can occur anteriorly, posteriorly, or superiorly, acetabular fractures include those of the supporting structures of columns as well as the roof of the acetabulum itself (Judet *et al.* 1964, Letournel 1980, Matta 1992) (Figure 11-4). The anterior column consists of the anterior border of the iliac wing, the pelvic brim, the anterior wall of the acetabulum, and the superior pubic ramus. The posterior column includes the ischial portion of the bone, the sciatic notches, the posterior acetabular wall and the ischial tuberosity.

Judet and colleagues (1964) proposed a classificatory system for acetabular fractures. They identified four simple fractures: (1) posterior lip fracture, (2) posterior or ilioischial column fracture, (3) transverse fracture, and (4) anterior or iliopubic column fracture. These simple fractures are the most common

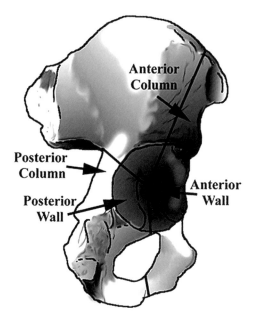

Figure 11-4. Designation of walls and columns in the acetabulum. Designation of acetabular fractures is best understood within the context of the morphology of support and articulation for the hip joint (Judet *et al.* 1964).

forms. Letournel (1980) and Templeman (1992a) modified the Judet (1964) system to include five simple and five associated fractures. The simple fractures are as follows: (1) posterior wall fractures, (2) posterior column fractures, (3) anterior wall fractures, (4) anterior column fractures, and (5) transverse fractures (Figure 11-5). Posterior wall fractures usually separate one or several fragments from the column but may result in only marginal impaction of the column itself. Posterior hip dislocations in which there is direct trauma on the flexed knee while the hip is in a right-angle flexion with little abduction produces these fractures. Blows to the sacrum in which the femoral head acts as the anvil upon which the acetabulum is driven also produce these fractures. The fragment of the posterior articular surface can be quite large although it does not infringe on the integrity of the underlying column. When the posterior column is fractured, the separated fragment is larger, usually beginning near the angle of the sciatic notch and extending to the cotyloid fossa. The mechanism of injury is postulated to be blows to the knee while the thigh is abducted and the hip flexed. Anterior wall fractures remove the anterior wall along with a segment of the iliopectinal line and may include a portion of the anterior column. Anterior column fractures separate a larger segment, passing from the superior edge of the iliopubic region through the acetabulum and into the obturator foramen. They may begin at the iliac crest and end at the pubic ramus or begin at the notch between the anterior iliac spines and extend into the pubic angle. In some cases, the fracture begins in the iliopsoas groove and extends into the midpoint of the inferior ramus. Anterior column fractures are often accompanied by a pubic fracture and are caused by blows to the leg while the hip is flexed and markedly abducted. Transverse fractures bisect the acetabulum from the medial border to the sciatic notch, usually passing through the junction of the roof and the cotyloid fossa, dividing both anterior and posterior columns. They are often accompanied by a T-shaped fracture into the obturator foramen to form an associated fracture (Gonza 1982). Such transverse fractures are induced by a blow to the greater trochanter or to the back of the pelvis while the thigh is abducted.

The associated fractures (Letournel 1980, Templeman 1992a) are (1) T fractures, (2) posterior column and posterior wall fractures, (3) transverse and posterior wall fractures, (4) anterior column and posterior hemitransverse fractures, and (5) bicolumn fractures (Figure 11-5). A vertical split passing into the obturator foramen combined with a transverse fracture produces T fractures. The ischiopubic ramus is also usually fractured. The bicolumn fractures produce a "floating" acetabulum. The name combinations describe the remaining fractures.

Often included in the acetabular fractures is a fracture complex known as *Walther's* fracture. In these, there is a transverse fracture of the acetabulum along with a fracture of the ischial ramus. The acetabular region is normally medially displaced and may be embedded in the remaining pelvic ring.

Avulsion Fractures

Avulsive fractures of the ischium may occur due to contraction of the *semi-tendinousus, semimembranosus, biceps femoris* and *quadratus femoris* muscles (Figure 11-6). These fractures are more common in adolescents and are produced by activities requiring massive muscle effort such as jumping, kicking or sudden running (Blount 1955, Sundra and Carty 1994). Avulsive fractures occur on the anterior superior iliac spine that is the attachment site for the *sartorius* muscle and inguinal ligament and on the anterior inferior iliac spine, the attachment site for one head of the *rectus femoris* muscle and the iliofemoral ligament (Kane 1984). Anterior inferior iliac spine avulsion occurs just above the margin of the acetabulum (Watson-Jones 1941). Avulsion fractures are usually seen prior to the fusion of these regions to the ilium (Blount 1955) and generally involve running and kicking activities (Sundar and Carty 1994). In more rare instances, the iliac crest may be incompletely avulsed due to contraction of the abdominal muscles (Kane 1984). In general, avulsion fractures do not affect the stability of the pelvic structure and so are less likely to be linked to a fatality. An exception may be avulsion of the ischial spines that result from violent shearing actions as described above (Tile and Pennel 1980). While rare, such injuries may speak to victim behavior prior to death and as such are of forensic interest.

Broken Bones

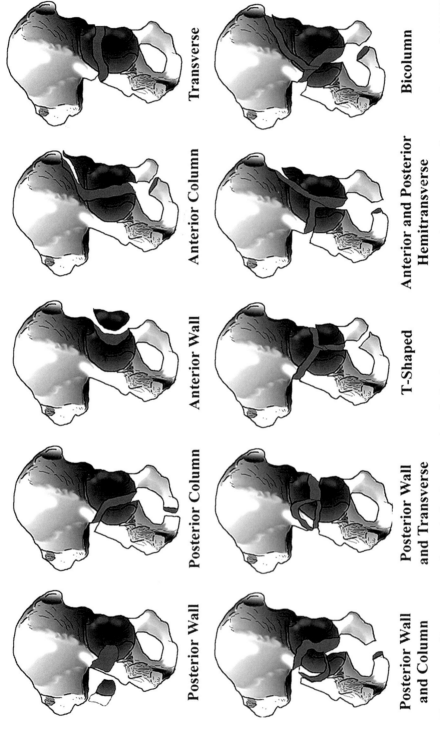

Figure 11-5. Classification of acetabular fractures. Acetabular fractures may occur in isolation or in combination. Letournel (1980) described a series of single fractures (*top row*) and added a set of fractures that are frequently found in combination (*bottom row*).

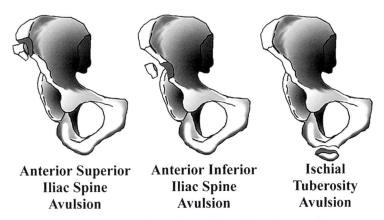

Anterior Superior   **Anterior Inferior**   **Ischial**
Iliac Spine   **Iliac Spine**   **Tuberosity**
Avulsion   **Avulsion**   **Avulsion**

Figure 11-6. Avulsion fractures of the pelvis. Within the pelvic girdle, certain areas are susceptible to avulsion fractures, particularly in subadult individuals.

FEMUR

The density of the femoral shaft protects it from many insults, but the angulation at the proximal end where it articulates with the acetabulum at the hip joint diverts the direct transmission of forces medially and jeopardizes the strength of the bone. This proximal region is also lower in bone density, subject to significant age-related losses of bone mineral, the insertion point for major hip muscles, and has a strong attachment to the acetabular bone, leaving adjacent areas of the femoral neck and subtrochanteric region vulnerable. Direct blows and wedging forces of the tibia can injure the distal femur. In this section, the focus is on traumatic injury rather than on fractures due to osteoporosis. Age-related, postmenopausal, inactivity-related or iatrogenic bone loss will, however, predispose individuals to traumatic fractures at lower energy levels than are required in younger or healthier adults. Such femoral fractures are often associated with an increase in fatigue microfractures, which can be seen histologically before any gross fracture has occurred (Freeman *et al.* 1974).

Femoral Head Fractures

Fractures of the hip and femoral shaft are uncommon in young adults (Buhr and Cooke 1959, Rogers 1992) but increase rapidly in the elderly, especially older women. In the young, such fractures are usually due to falls from great heights or to motor vehicle accidents, but, in the elderly, they may occur with only moderate or mild trauma such as falling from a standing height.

Hip dislocations are often associated with damage to the femoral head, and the innominate and femur are often combined in classificatory systems (Pipkin 1957, Brumback *et al.* 1987). Pipkin (1957) classified posterior hip

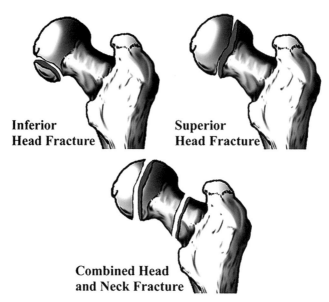

Figure 11-7. Classification of femoral head fractures. Following the guidelines of Pipkin (1957) for hip dislocations, femoral head fractures can be distinguished based on the location of the fracture line and whether it occurs in combination with femoral neck fractures.

dislocations into four types of which three involve femoral head fractures while the remaining category involves a neck fracture (Figure 11-7, above). Type I injury includes fractures inferior to the *fovea centralis* while Type II includes those fractures superior to the *fovea*. Type III combines femoral neck and head fractures. Type IV links any femoral head fracture with an acetabular fracture and may not be a distinction that can be made by the anthropologist examining isolated material.

Injuries to the femoral head may be observed relatively early since this bone forms its secondary center of ossification during the first year of life. Traumatic separation of the proximal epiphyses may occur during the birth process (Salter and Harris 1963). These separations are more common in difficult births, such as those in the breech position. Clinically, femoral head separation is of concern due to ensuing necrosis, which may debilitate the joint.

Femoral Neck Fractures

The proximal femur, which is a relatively complex structure, has many specific zones in which fractures can occur. The neck is the region between the femoral head itself and the trochanters and is marked by the intertrochanteric line and crest. Forces applied through the relatively large acetabulum, congregate and are transmitted through the femoral neck to the femoral diaphysis. Since the actual loading transmission does not lie in a direct line from the body to the knee, compressive and tensile stresses occur in this region. Juszczyk and associates (2011) showed that, in cadaver studies, fractures of the neck begin along the lateral margin from the tensile forces. Shearing forces tend to push the femoral head at right angles to the compressive forces resulting in bone failure. An analysis of trauma victims showed that, when neck fractures are found in association with ipsilateral shaft fractures, the hip must have been flexed and abducted on impact such that the femoral head was well planted in the acetabulum (Barei *et al.* 2003)

Fractures of the femoral neck are more common than intertrochanteric ones by about a 2:1 ratio (Alffram 1964), and this is especially true for women (Banks 1962, Brown and Abram 1964, Bentley 1968, Barnes *et al.* 1976). In a survey of cases, Bauer (1960) found that women outnumbered male patients by almost four to one in the patient population with this fracture. Furthermore, neck fractures in women were six times more often the result of only moderate rather than severe trauma while, in men, both levels of trauma were equally represented.

The mechanisms of injury for the femoral neck have been attributed to both direct blows to the greater trochanter and to lateral rotation (Kocher 1896). There is support for the concept of torsion initiating injury to the anterior aspect and subsequently extending through to the posterior portion. This process would account for the greater comminution typically seen on the posterior portion, which would be under increasing compression as the fracture occurs (Kyle 1992). A third possible mechanism is cyclical loading producing a stress fracture that is caused by minor torsional injury preceding a fall. These last fractures tend to be found in older osteoporotic individuals (DeLee 1984). In young adults, femoral neck injuries are typically produced by falls from a height or motor vehicle accidents (Kyle 1992). These fractures are often associated in femoral shaft fractures occurring in the same leg.

Fracture of the femoral neck can be classified as subcapital, trans- or mid-cervical, and basicervical (DeLee 1984, Rogers 1992) (Figure 11-8). The sub-capital form is the most common. This term refers to fractures immediately beneath the articular surface along the line of the epiphyseal plate. The transcervical fracture passes between the femoral head and greater trochanter. The transcervical form is quite rare, occurring primarily in adults with severe osteoarthritis. They may also be impacted (Bentley 1968). Basicervical fractures are uncommon except in children or in adults in whom some condition has already weakened this area. Basicervical fractures are actually extracapsular and are excluded by some from the category of neck fractures.

Watson-Jones (1941) distinguishes between abduction and adduction fractures of the femoral neck based upon the movement of the femoral head relative to the shaft. The former are impacted on the outer side and occur at the subcapital

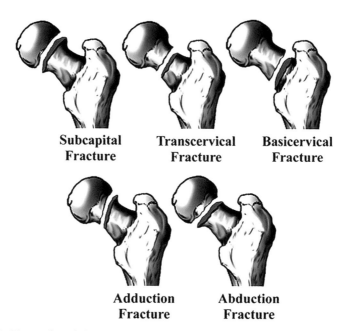

Subcapital Fracture   **Transcervical Fracture**   **Basicervical Fracture**

Adduction Fracture   **Abduction Fracture**

Figure 11-8. Femoral neck fractures. Classification of femoral neck fractures can be divided into three basic designations (top row) based on location along the femoral neck (DeLee *et al.* 1984, Rogers 1992). In addition, Pauwels (1935) distinguished adduction and abduction fractures (bottom row) based on the angulation of the fracture line.

level. The latter are subcapital, transcervical, intertrochanteric, or pertrochanteric. Skeletally, these also are distinguished by the angulation between the detached fragment and the remainder of the femur. If the angle is 45° or less, often close to horizontal, then an abduction fracture has occurred and little shearing force was involved (Pauwels 1935). Shearing forces have been active in the adduction fracture in which the fracture line is more vertical.

Intertrochanteric Fractures

The intertrochanteric region is defined as the area between the femoral neck and the lower edge of the lesser trochanter. The moment of inertia is greater in this region, despite the high trabecular component; however, this region is also subject to greater rotational forces than the neck (Harington 1982). The internal structure of this region consists of a scaffolding system of trabeculae, first described by Ward (1838), which begins in the femoral head and falls along the medial side of the femur (Levy *et al.* 1992). These trabeculae respond to the compressive forces while a second set of trabeculae from the femoral head to the lateral side are designed to resist tensile forces on the bone. Secondary arches of trabeculae cross the intertrochanteric region but tend to leave relatively barren the central region known as Ward's triangle. With age, the trabeculae in this region become thinner, which leaves this region of the bone vulnerable for collapse. Intertrochanteric fractures may be relatively simple to extensively comminuted (Harington 1982, Levy *et al.* 1992). Intertrochanteric fractures are often so extensive that they merge into the subtrochanteric region.

Intertrochanteric fractures are found in younger individuals in response to high-energy trauma, particularly motor vehicle accidents (Kyle 1992, Levy *et al.* 1992). In the later years, however, these fractures may be produced from simple falls and the indirect action of muscle contraction. While osteoporosis may be a factor, muscle atrophy and a greater propensity for falling also account for the high rates of hip fracture among the elderly. In younger individuals, the probability of additional skeletal injury is high due to the high-energy nature of the injury, but, in the older person, intertrochanteric fractures are often found in isolation. When there are other fractures in the older victim, intertrochanteric fractures are often associated with fractures of the distal radius, proximal humerus, ribs, pelvis, and spine.

The mechanism of injury includes forces applied to the greater trochanter along with torsion to the femoral shaft (DeLee 1984, Kyle 1992). Activity of the abductor muscles on the greater trochanter and the *iliopsoas* on the lesser trochanter contribute to the location of the injury. When there is less torsion and more axial loading of the femur, the fracture patterns tends to migrate distally toward the subtrochanteric region. Direct injuries, which are usually incurred in a fall, act either along the long axis of the femur or are due to forces applied to the greater trochanter.

Evans (1949, 1951) proposed a classification system for the fractures of the intertrochanteric region based on displacement and number of fragments. Jensen (1980a, 1980b, 1981) later modified Evans' system into a five-part system (Figure 11-9). In Type 1 fractures, there is an oblique two-part fracture through the greater and lesser trochanters without displacement. This fracture is expanded in Type 2 with separation of either the greater or lesser trochanter in addition to the initial break. In Type 3, a posterior fragment is detached from the greater trochanter so that there is no posterior support for the bone. Type 4 is defined by detachment of the lesser trochanter, while Type 5 combines the characteristics of Types 3 and 4. Evans (1949b) also noted reverse oblique fractures, which commonly exhibited lateral comminution. Direct blows may produce comminuted fracture of the greater trochanter that is usually confined to that portion of the trochanter, which extends above the rest of the femur (DeLee 1984).

Anthropologists working on femoral fractures should note angulation and the extent of comminution. Assessment of trabecular quality either exposed in the fractured area or radiographically may indicate any predisposing factors

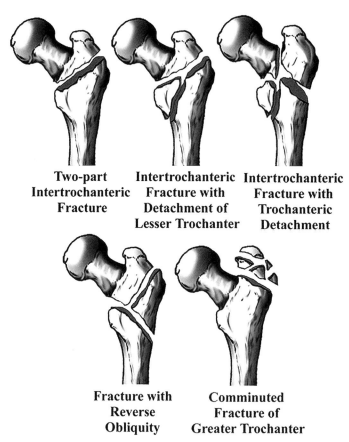

Figure 11-9. Classification of intertrochanteric fractures. Intertrochanteric fractures can be distinguished by the number of fragments, the extent of trochanteric involvement, and the direction of angulation (Evans 1949b, 1951; Jensen 1980a, 1980b, 1981).

to consider. Often fragmentation in this area is so extensive that reconstruction is difficult due to poor bone quality.

Trochanteric Fractures

Avulsive fractures of the lesser trochanter may occur in children with contraction of the *iliopsoas* muscle (Watson-Jones 1941, Salter and Harris 1963). This results from sudden abduction and extension of the hip often as the person tries to resist a force driving them toward the injured side. These injuries are most prevalent in individuals between 12 and 16 years of age (Poston 1921–1922). Fractures may also occur in osteoporotic individuals, although instances are rare. The greater trochanter can also be avulsed, however, this injury is usually confined to adolescence, between ages seven and 17 years (Armstrong 1907).

Similarly, avulsion fractures of the greater trochanter can be produced by contraction of the hip abductors and external rotators (Burroughs and Walker 2012). This action can occur in restricted hip flexion. It is more common in younger individuals prior to fusion of these epiphyses. In older individuals, poor bone quality may make older individuals more susceptible to avulsion fractures of the trochanters.

Subtrochanteric Fractures

Subtrochanteric fractures occur in the proximal portion of the shaft, between the lesser trochanter and the isthmus of the diaphysis (Schatzker 1987c; Russell and Taylor 1992). These fractures, as in the intertrochanteric fractures, may be due to the loading of the bone, which produces compression medially and tension laterally. Cochran and associates (1980) note that, in a normally loaded femur, these forces peak subtrochanterically. Failure usually begins along the tension side. Another mechanism of injury, besides axial loading, is direct lateral force applied to the upper thigh.

A bimodal age distribution is seen in these fractures with most occurring in older patients, usually after age 70 years (Arneson *et al.* 1988, Russell and Taylor 1992). The younger period of increased incidence is usually associated with high-energy trauma such as falls from a height or motor vehicle accidents. In the younger age group, these injuries are predominantly simple fractures without significant comminution (Waddell 1979). Associated trauma is also more common with high-energy trauma, especially to the long bones, pelvis, spine (Bergman *et al.* 1987), patella and tibia (Russell and Taylor 1992). Among older victims, standing falls may be the mode of injury (Russell and Taylor 1992). The degree of comminution usually relates to the level of energy. Low-energy trauma is associated with minimal fragmentation and simple fractures (transverse, oblique, or spiral), whereas in high-energy trauma, not only is fragmentation extensive but the damage encompasses larger portions of the femur. The greater fragility of the bone in older individuals, however, is translated to greater comminution in lower-energy injuries. Increased comminution is common in older patients who have experienced blows directly to the trochanteric or subtrochanteric region as well as those whose injuries are due to axial loading (Waddell 1979). Risk factors for subtrochanteric fractures in the elderly include obesity and dementia (Maravic *et al.* 2012).

A three-part classification of subtrochanteric fractures has been proposed. Fielding and Magliato (1966) divided these into Type I–at the level of the lesser trochanter, Type II–within one inch below the lesser trochanter, and Type III–one to two inches below the lesser trochanter. Waddell (1979) bases a classificatory system on pattern and stability. Type I includes transverse and short oblique fractures with little comminution. Type II consists of long oblique or spiral fractures, again with only minimal fragmentation. Type III includes all comminuted fractures. The *Arbeitsgemeinschaft für Osteosynthesefragen* (AO) classification (Müller *et al.* 1991), in contrast, divides them into simple trans-verse and oblique fractures, fractures with three major parts and a butterfly fragment, and fractures with marked comminution. Seinsheimer (1978) presented a five-type classification, which examines both fracture morphology and extent of bony damage (Figure 11-10). Type I fractures are non-displaced, Type II are two-part transverse or spiral non-comminuted fractures. Type III are three-part oblique fractures with butterfly comminution. Type IV includes fractures with bicortical comminution into four or more segments, and Type V consists of bicortical fractures with extensive comminution and extension into the trochanteric mass.

Russell and Taylor (1992) suggest an additional system that seems most useful for orthopaedic surgeons. Group I fractures do not extend into the *piriformis* fossa and include IA fractures with fractures from below the lesser trochanter to the femoral isthmus and IB fractures, which may also involve the lesser trochanter. Group II fractures extend into the greater trochanter and involve the *piriformis* fossa. Within this group, IIA fractures extend from the lesser trochanter to the isthmus and into the *piriformis* fossa but which lack significant comminution, and IIB fractures include those with significant comminution.

For the anthropologist, the Seinsheimer (1978) classification system may be more directly applicable and relevant, yet still be readily translatable into terms for the pathologist or consulting physician (Figure 11-10). Specific notation of the fracture pattern and severity and location of comminution are important. Photos and illustrations are essential for recording. Information may be difficult to obtain from weathered bone, especially bone from older individuals because the bone fragments may be quite small and difficult to recover. Scavenging activity, of course, also makes analysis of these fractures more difficult for the anthropologist.

Femoral Shaft Fractures

The femoral shafts are among the most heavily mineralized areas in the body (Galloway *et al.* 1997). Because of this, fractures of this region are rare except for those situations involving considerable force. In infants and toddlers, these fractures result from car-pedestrian accidents, falls, or being dropped (Taylor *et al.* 1994). In older children, pedestrian and bicycle accidents are the more likely circumstances. Femoral shaft fractures are at a higher level of incidence among younger adults, particularly younger males with an average age of 25–30 years. This increase most likely reflects their participation in

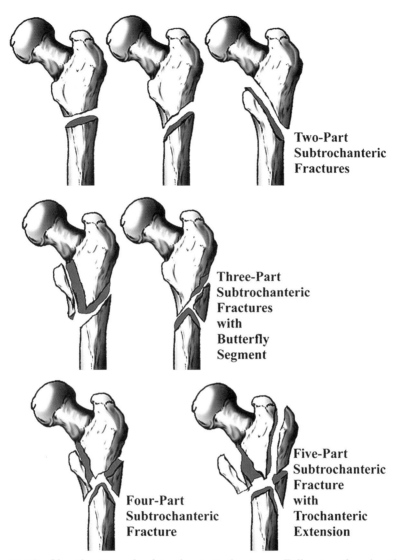

Two-Part Subtrochanteric Fractures

Three-Part Subtrochanteric Fractures with Butterfly Segment

Four-Part Subtrochanteric Fracture

Five-Part Subtrochanteric Fracture with Trochanteric Extension

Figure 11-10. Classification of subtrochanteric fractures. Following the classification system of Seinsheimer (1978), subtrochanteric fractures can be classified by the number of fragments produced and the direction of angulation. Two-part fractures can occur transversely or obliquely (*top row*). Butterfly fragments may be produced on either the medial or lateral sides (*middle row*). Four- and five-part fractures produce separation of all major segments of the subtrochanteric region.

activities in which high-energy injuries are most likely. Indeed, in adults, femoral fractures are found most often in situations such as motor vehicle accidents, car-pedestrian collisions, plane crashes, or falls from a great height (Mooney and Claudi 1984, Winquist *et al.* 1984, Arneson *et al.* 1988, Johnson

1992, Taylor *et al.* 1994, Tencer *et al.* 2002). Like fractures of the proximal femur, femoral shaft fractures also occur frequently among the elderly. Among this group, the fractures seem to be linked not only to high-energy insults but also to those of low to moderate energy. The elderly are more likely to exhibit the simpler forms of shaft fracture (Johnson 1992).

Just as the incidence of femoral fractures change with age, so does the location where these fractures are found. In children, femoral shaft fractures occurs primarily (about 70%) in the middle third of the shaft, rather than either proximally or distally. These may include birth fractures, which are often transverse fractures of the midshaft. A study in adults also showed that most fractures of the femoral shaft occur in the middle third (62.5%), followed by the distal third (21.2%) and then the proximal third (16.3%) (Winquist *et al.* 1984). Approximately half of these fractures were comminuted, with the remainder composed of transverse, short oblique, and spiral/long oblique fractures.

Shaft fractures are usually severe and are often associated with serious blood loss (Mooney and Claudi 1984). Injuries to the proximal femur, including the femoral neck, and intertrochanteric fractures may also be found together (Johnson 1992). Along with supracondylar fractures, they may be associated with fractures of the tibial shaft to create a "floating" knee. Victims of such a fracture complex have a more extensive suite of affiliated injuries.

Depending on the pattern of loading, femoral fractures follow the patterns of classic fractures of the long bones. Winquist and Hansen (1980) and (Winquist *et al.* 1984) have grouped these injuries into five categories: (0) simple without comminution, (I) small butterfly, (II) large butterfly, (III) large butterfly extending beyond 50% of the circumference of the shaft, and (IV) segmental comminution. Mooney and Claudi (1984) suggested a system based on patterns of fracture. Their system begins with division between simple, butterfly fragment, and comminuted/segmental fractures. Simple fractures are then subdivided into spiral, oblique, and transverse, butterfly fractures into those with a single fragment, those with two fragments and those with three or more fragments. The comminuted group is subdivided into those with a single intermediate fragment, those with short comminution, and those with substantial comminution. Both Müller and associates (1991) and the Orthopaedic Trauma Association (OTA) (Gustilo 1990) have expanded these classifications. The former focuses on the fracture form: Type A–simple fractures of (1) spiral, (2) oblique, or (3) transverse pattern; Type B–wedge fractures of (1) spiral, (2) bending, or (3) fragmented form; and Type C–complex fractures of (1) spiral, (2) segmental, or (3) irregular form. The OTA classification has seven categories: (I) transverse, (II) oblique, (III) spiral, (IV) spiral with a butterfly fragment, (V) comminuted, (VI) segmental, or (VII) fractures with bone loss. For both, location should be specified as to proximal, middle, or distal third of the bone.

With any of these three classificatory systems, the anthropologist should be as specific as possible. A basic description of the nature of the fracture and location are more critical than determining an exact category (Figure 11-11). Notation of comminution, bone loss, or production of distinct bone segments should be made. Bone reconstruction is often needed to determine the number and location of impacts and whether substantial bone loss has occurred. The mechanism of injury may be determined from the normal processes underlying long bone fractures (see Chapter 2).

Supracondylar, Condylar, and Distal Epiphyseal Fractures

The knee joint in humans is relatively stable in normal movement but does not cope well with severe varus, valgus, or rotational forces, especially when these are combined with axial loading, as is often the case. Loading stabilizes one portion of the joint while the other is shifted dramatically. In the femur, such injuries can affect the supracondylar and condylar regions in adults and may also affect the distal epiphysis in younger individuals. The supracondylar region extends from the top margin of the condyles superiorly to junction of the metaphysis with the femoral shaft. Condylar fractures usually involve significant damage to the articular surface as well as to the areas of attachment for the ligaments and muscles.

Distal femoral fractures are relatively common, forming about a third of femoral fractures, if those of the hip are excluded (Arneson *et al.* 1988). As with the shaft fractures, these also have a bimodal pattern of increased prevalence. The first increase is found among young adult males and these fractures are primarily due to high-energy trauma. Such fractures show greater chance of intra-articular disruption and proximal comminution (Schatzker and Tile 1987). The second rise is among the elderly, especially females, and often involves only low-energy injuries (Seinsheimer 1980, Arneson *et al.* 1988). These may occur in such relatively mild incidents such as falls onto the flexed knee (Helfet 1992). The degree of comminution is similar in both groups despite the discrepancy in energy levels. In addition, stress fractures due to skeletal insufficiency or fatigue are also found in the distal femur (Muralikuttan and Sankarart-Kutty 1999), the latter occurring especially at the initiation of intensive physical activity.

Supracondylar fractures are usually transverse or slightly oblique (Figure 11-12). Comminution of supracondylar fractures is frequently seen in association with osteoporosis (Schatzker 1987g). Seinsheimer (1980) classified these supracondylar fractures among his other distal femoral fractures and subdivided them into two-part and comminuted fractures. In general, he noted that two-part fractures occur in osteoporotic individuals while other supracondylar fractures result in significant fragmentation. These fractures can also be classified into Type A, which exclude the articular surfaces; Type B, which include one

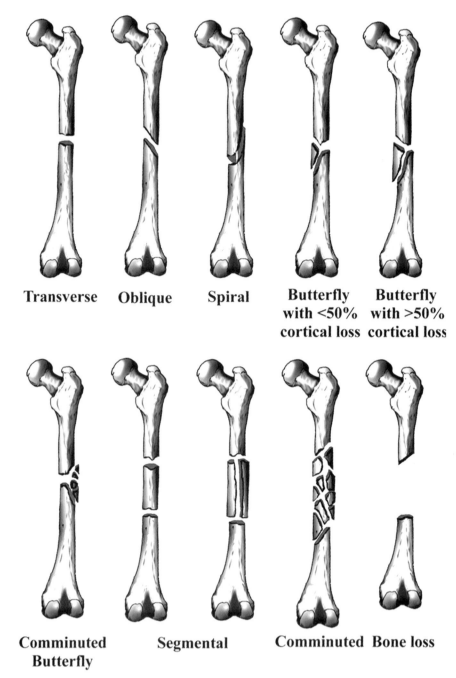

**Transverse   Oblique   Spiral   Butterfly   Butterfly
                                     with <50%   with >50%
                                   cortical loss cortical loss**

**Comminuted   Segmental   Comminuted Bone loss
Butterfly**

Figure 11-11. Fractures of the femoral shaft. Femoral shaft fractures may be simple linear fractures or with a butterfly or wedge with a varying extent of cortical involvement (*top row*). More extensive fractures include comminuted and segmental fractures or those in which there is loss of bone (*bottom row*).

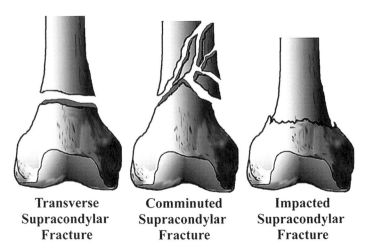

Transverse Supracondylar Fracture   **Comminuted Supracondylar Fracture**   **Impacted Supracondylar Fracture**

Figure 11-12. Supracondylar fractures of the distal femur. Classification of the supra-condylar distal femur (*right shown*) is based on location and nature of the fracture. Displacement is not considered since it is not often evident in skeletal material.

condyle; or Type C, which include both intra-articular and supracondylar fracturing (Schatzker 1987g). Impacted supracondylar fractures have also been noted (Hohl *et al.* 1984).

Fractures of the actual condyles are relatively rare except for motor vehicle accidents. Where the bent knee strikes the dashboard, the patella may be driven into the femur producing fractures (Spitz and Fisher 1980, Spitz 2005). Experimental studies suggest that the knee is more vulnerable to fracture when loading occurs with the flexion angle at less than 90 degrees (Atkinson and Haut 2001). In children, forced hyperextension of the knee may result in epiphyseal separation of the distal femur (Blount 1955). Condylar fractures are also reportedly produced by hyperadduction or hyperabduction combined with axial loading (Hohl *et al.* 1984).

Unicondylar fractures are characterized by separation of the medial or lateral condyle from the metaphysis (Templeman 1992b). Both have been variously classified, each system having features of use to the anthropologist (Figure 11-13). Seinsheimer (1980) has classified these fractures among his four basic types of distal femoral fractures in which displacement plays a role along with the actual fracture pattern. While Types 1 and 2 involve non-displaced and supra-condylar fractures respectively, Type 3 can be divided into (A) separation of medial condyle, (B) separation of lateral condyle, or (C) separation of both condyles from each other and from the diaphysis. Type 4 fractures include fractures through the articular surfaces of the (A) medial condyle or (B) lateral condyle, or (C) complete and comminuted fractures incorporating one condyle and the intercondylar notch, both condyles or the condyles and

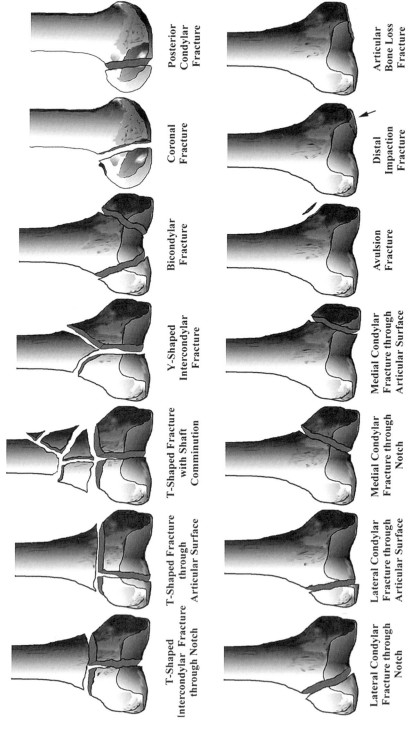

Figure 11-13. Intercondylar and condylar fractures of the distal femur. Intercondylar and condylar fractures of the distal femur (right shown) are classified by morphology, plane of the fracture and the condyle involved.

notch. Type 3 injuries typically result from simple falls in the elderly but high-energy trauma in younger patients. Type 4 fractures afflict a younger age group and are due to severe trauma. Gustilo (1990) divided these fractures into a series of forms including (1) linear through the notch, (2) linear through the articular surface, (3) avulsion, (4) posterior condyle, (5) T-shaped through the notch, (6) T-shaped through the articular surface, (7) Y-shaped through the notch, (8) T-shaped with comminution, (9) impacted, and (10) with articular bone loss. The AO classification system (Müller *et al.* 1991) also may be useful in that it addresses both condylar involvement and fracture form.

Anthropologists need to note not only the condyle involved but also the nature of the fracture, the involvement of articular surface, degree of comminution, and fracture location with respect to muscular and ligamentous attachments. This task can be accomplished with detailed photographs and charts accompanied by detailed written descriptions. A combination of the various classification systems is proposed here, which focuses on skeletal material without regard to displacement (Figures 11-12 and 11-13).

Epiphyseal fractures of the distal femur may occur at birth. This is the only epiphysis with an established center of ossification at this stage of development (Salter and Harris 1963). These will be virtually impossible to identify from skeletal material alone but may be seen radiographically on intact remains.

Osteochondral fractures of the distal articular surface can be produced by direct shearing force, rotary compression, or the action of the patella during dislocation (Kennedy *et al.* 1966). The shearing and rotational injuries may occur on either condyle while the patella injury is found on the anterior surface of the lateral condyle. Of these, fractures due to patellar dislocation are the most frequent and there may be associated damage to the medial articular surface of the patella (Hohl et al. 1984). The paucity of calcified cartilage and greater elasticity in the ligaments in subadults increases their propensity to sustain osteochondral fractures in the knee.

PATELLA

The patella is essentially a large sesamoid bone, reducing the friction and consequent wear on the *quadriceps* muscle as it passes to its ultimate insertion on the anterior tibia. Located on the point of the knee, it also bears the brunt of direct blows to this area of the body.

Fractures of the patella account for about 1% of all fractures (Boström 1972). These injuries are more common in men, but there is no greater susceptibility by side. Only on rare occasions are both patellae injured at the same time. Patellar fractures were approximately evenly divided into comminuted, transverse, and chip fractures and a cluster of other assorted forms. About 40%

resulted from falls on or blows to the knee with the rest due to motorcycle and car accidents as well as sports injuries.

Patellar fractures occur due to either direct blows or through the tension generated by the *quadriceps* muscle (Hohl *et al.* 1984, Rogers 1992, Sanders 1992, Templeman 1992c, Manaster and Andrews 1994). Direct blows can cause simple or comminuted fractures of the patella. Stellate and vertical fractures are also found (Figure 11-14). The former results from direct compressive blows, which force the bone against the femoral condyles (Schatzker 1987c, Sanders 1992). The latter, also known as marginal or longitudinal fractures, form over a fifth of all patellar fractures. Direct blows may produce chip fractures, which involve separation of a small fragment. These injuries are usually extra-articular, but the articular surface may also be involved because the articular surface strikes the femoral condyles (Watson-Jones 1941). These types of fractures are more likely to occur in older individuals whose impaired bone quality makes them prone to compression fracturing and who may stumble more easily.

The most common fracture, however, is the transverse or just slightly oblique form of fractures, usually through the midline of the patella. These may also be shifted proximally or distally and are known as *basal* or *apical* polar fractures respectively. These generally are produced by tensile stress applied to the bone during extension of the knee while the *quadriceps* muscle undergoes violent contraction. For example, these fractures may occur when a person stumbles and attempts to prevent the impact.

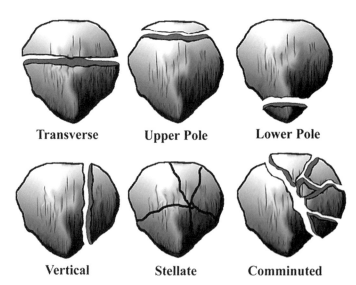

Figure 11-14. Patellar fractures. Patellar fractures are classified by the direction of fracture as well as the location of the principal fracture line.

Because the soft tissues of children are more resilient, these fractures are less common in children except by direct blows (Blount 1955, Makhdoomi *et al.* 1993). In a study of children and adolescents, patellar fractures were five times more common in boys than girls (Maguire and Canale 1993).

The forensic anthropologist must exclude the possibility of a bipartite patella prior to noting the location of the fracture and distinguishing whether it is consistent with tension or impact fracturing. These benign anomalies occur in about 20% of cases and are due to multiple centers of ossification (Sponseller *et al.* 2001).

TIBIA

The tibia has the unfortunate position of being a weight-bearing bone attached to two vulnerable joints. This bone also forms a prominent ridge along the front of the shin, well placed for blows from a number of different sources. While extremely dense in the diaphysis, the proximal end is largely cancellous bone. Distally, it sits atop a sliding joint and forms only half the brace around the ankle, the remainder being formed by the fibula. It is little wonder then that, combined with the human propensity to engage in sports and high-speed activities, the tibia is a frequent site of fractures.

Fractures Within the Knee Capsule

A number of avulsion fractures occur on the tibial portion of the knee and are here treated separately from the larger fractures of the tibial plateau (Figure 11-15). Fractures within the knee joint capsule are infrequent in younger adults except due to high-speed forces such as motor vehicle accidents or during sport-related accidents (Leffers 1992, Hess *et al.* 1994). Fractures at the tibial eminence, which are more common in children, are classified according to displacement (Meyers and McKeever 1959, Manaster and Andrews 1994). The numerous ligaments, which stabilize the knee joint, may rupture, often producing avulsion fractures at their origin or insertion points (Manaster and Andrews 1994). This is particularly true of the anterior tibial eminence, the site of attachment of the anterior cruciate ligament. These fractures are relatively unusual although possible. Minor fractures at this point may also be due to other mechanisms of injury.

Tearing of the anterior cruciate ligament (ACL) also is frequently accompanied by fractures on the posterior portion of the lateral plateau. This may result from anterolateral rotation during subluxation combined with valgus and axial forces. This induces strain on the lateral capsular ligament or lateral meniscotibial ligament (Hess *et al.* 1994). It is now often seen as a sports injury. Less common are associated avulsion fractures of the femoral attachment of

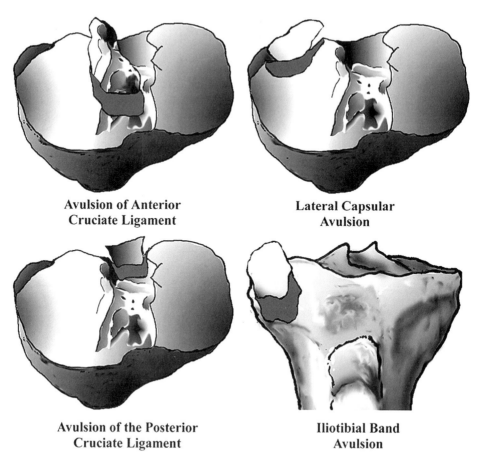

**Avulsion of Anterior
Cruciate Ligament**

**Lateral Capsular
Avulsion**

**Avulsion of the Posterior
Cruciate Ligament**

**Iliotibial Band
Avulsion**

Figure 11-15. Fractures within the knee capsule. Fractures within the knee capsule primarily affect the attachment sites of the cruciate ligaments, capsular ligaments, and iliotibial band.

the ACL following the tibial avulsion fracture (Tohyama *et al.* 2002). Usually these fractures occur between the ages of 10 and 20 years whereas, at older ages, the ligament itself is ruptured (Watson-Jones 1941).

Avulsion of the insertion of the posterior cruciate ligament (PCL) may be characterized by damage along the posterior aspect of the tibia, usually just below the joint line (Manaster and Andrews 1994). These are less frequent than avulsions of the anterior cruciate ligament (ACL) but may be produced when the knee is hyperextended (Hohl *et al.* 1984). The medial collateral ligament usually tears without disrupting the adherent bone while the lateral collateral ligament inserts on the proximal fibula and is rarely avulsed. Rupture of the iliotibial band, which inserts on Gerdy's tubercle on the tibia, may also produce avulsion fractures.

Rim avulsion fractures and rim compression fractures (Hohl *et al.* 1992) are also possible. The former are produced by tension on the capsular or ligamentous tissue of the joint with severe valgus or varus stress. These are most frequent on the lateral side of the knee and associated with avulsion fractures on the fibular head or Gerdy's tubercle. Rim compression forms, which are usually secondary to rupture of one of the collateral ligaments, increase the compression on the contralateral side. These forms are seen as localized compression of the margin or small depressed marginal split fractures.

Tibial Plateau Fractures

The tibial plateau includes the proximal portions of the tibia, which widens to support the medial and lateral menisci. This encompasses the longer medial condyle and the rounder lateral condyle, which allows for the "screw-home" mechanism that locks the knee joint. Forces inflicted either medially or laterally, axial compressive loading or a combination of these forces cause tibial plateau fractures. The fractures display a range of appearances including depression or crushing of the surface, separation of a segment or wedge of bone, and splitting.

In adults, most tibial plateau fractures are caused by abduction of the tibia while it is still under compression from the femur (Kennedy and Baily 1968, Rogers 1992). These fractures are confined to the proximal end, most often transecting the articular surface. Since the femoral condyle is more resistant to fracture, the tibia is more likely to suffer the break. Fractures of the lateral portion greatly surpass the number of fractures of the medial portion. This is due to the greater incidence of valgus forces involved in these injuries (Manaster and Andrews 1994). Pure vertical compression typically produces a T-shaped or Y-shaped fracture. Experiments by Kennedy and Bailey (1968) showed that abducting the leg with compression, when the knee is under axial loading, produces split and linear fractures. Compression fractures alone can be formed under extremes of loading (3000–4000 lbs; 1300–1800 kg) with the location determined by the flexion or extension of the knee. When the compression is increased even more, the bone is more severely comminuted. Such extremes of loading are usually produced by auto accidents and falls from heights. This injury is linked to the fender or bumper impacts attributable to car-pedestrian collisions. Only about 25–52% of these fractures result from this cause (Reibel and Wade 1962, Dovey and Heerfordt 1971, Hohl *et al.* 1974), while others result from falls and some to blows to the lateral knee joint.

The position of the knee joint during the impact will affect the nature of the fracture as well (Hohl *et al.* 1984). When fully extended, the compression forces are felt predominantly on the anterior portions of the tibial condyles, and the intercondylar notch of the femur will impinge on the intercondylar eminence of the tibia. In some sense this limits the extent of the compression by increasing the surface area active in the joint. When the knee is flexed, however, the middle or posterior portions of the tibial plateau must do all of the weight bearing because there is no contact between the distal femur and the tibial eminence when the knee is flexed. This focuses the forces of weight bearing onto smaller areas.

Tibial plateau fractures among children are more likely to be of the split form than in older victims. The bone of the tibial condyle is better able to withstand compression from the femur in younger bone and so is less likely to simply be crushed (Schatzker 1992). Split fractures of the lateral condyle from bending combined with axial loading are, therefore, more common among younger individuals. As humans age, the underlying trabecular bone is weakened and compression leads to depressed or combination split depression fractures, usually beginning in the fourth to fifth decade of life.

The tibial plateau fractures can be classified into three general types: (1) depressed fractures of either condyle with intact marginal surfaces; (2) split or displaced fractures often with some degree of depression; and (3) bicondylar fractures, which are often comminuted (Reibel and Wade 1962, Schatzker 1992). These fractures have been further classified into six types based on morphology and location (Schatzker 1987e, 1992; Hohl *et al.* 1992) or eight forms (Manaster and Andrews 1994) (Figure 11-16). Wedge or split fractures of the lateral plateau result from bending and axial forces. Some slight depression of the condylar surface may be involved. Such fractures may occur on either the medial or lateral plateau, but those of the medial plateau often involve avulsion of the tibial eminence as well. These fractures may occur in the coronal plane, usually medially and posteriorly. Split depression fractures combine significant depression of the lateral or medial plateau with an associated wedge fracture. Pure depression fractures consist of compression of the articular surface without an associated wedge fracture and often these reflect the shape of the femoral condyle that produced it. In general, split depression fractures affect younger individuals than do pure depression fractures.

In older individuals, the effects of osteoporosis produce a situation where a greater proportion of the plateau cannot withstand compression and will collapse with mild to moderate force. High-energy forces or relatively minor varus forces can produce these fractures when associated with osteoporosis. While more severe trauma will produce a split or wedge in the young, in the elderly, the bone often crumbles.

Bicondylar fractures are split fractures of both sides of the plateau, which are produced by pure axial loading to the extended knee. Finally, there is the possibility of a metaphyseal fracture that completely separates the plateau from the shaft. These fractures are also always produced by severe high-energy trauma, often with angular or rotary stress.

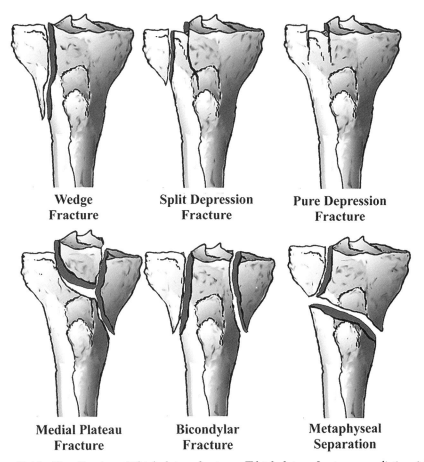

Figure 11-16. Classification of tibial plateau fractures. Tibial plateau fractures are distinguished by the location of the fracture and whether it includes depression of the articular surface.

Gustilo (1990) and Gustilo and colleagues (1992) provided yet another classification in which five categories are identified. In this system, there are distinctions as to the form of the fracture with the first type consisting of a linear fracture, which may be verical, oblique, or spiral in form, and is similar to the split fracture discussed above. Gustilo (1990) and Gustilo and colleagues (1992) also distinguish compression fractures, including both local and total defects, comminuted fractures on either or both sides of the tibial plateau, and fractures that involve some bone loss. The final group includes fractures that combine features of the other types.

A final concern in the tibial plateau is the damage done to the entire epiphysis in younger individuals. The proximal tibial growth plate is largely resistant to fracturing although anterior, anterolateral, and anteromedial displacement has been reported (Shelton and Canale 1979). In such injuries the fracture usually begins beneath the tibial tuberosity, so that the epiphysis and tuberosity are displaced as a unit. Posterior movement of the epiphysis is usually effectively blocked by the tuberosity.

Forensic anthropologists need to focus on the nature of the fracture (depression, wedge, and split) along with location (Figure 11-16). We must remember, however, relatively similar forces produce these fractures with the effects being determined by the structural integrity of the bone rather than any extraneous factor. Photographs and illustrations should accompany the description.

Tibial Tuberosity Fractures

Avulsion fractures of the tibial tuberosity may be confined to the tuberosity or extend to the proximal articular surfaces. This confinement is due to the dense attachment of the patellar ligament to the distal portion of the tuberosity (Ogden *et al.* 1980). Contraction of the *quadriceps femoris* muscles of the thigh will result in drawing the patellar ligament superiorly. These fractures of the tuberosity are more common in children and adolescents (Salter and Harris 1963) but less likely to occur in adults where there is solid fusion of the tubercle to the tibia (Watson-Jones 1941, Rogers 1992). Usually these fractures result from hyperextension of the knee with rotation of the tibia while the *quadriceps femoris* contracts and pulls on the patellar ligament. In children, this fracture frequently occurs in spills from a bicycle. Children may also experience a condition known as *Osgood's* or *Schlatter's* sprain where there is avulsion of part of the epiphysis from the tibia. This may become a chronic condition.

Fractures of the tibial tuberosity are particularly common in adolescents and are often the result of jumping activities (Hand *et al.* 1971, Ogden *et al.* 1980, Nance and Kaye 1982, Schwobel 1987). Anterior portions of the proximal tibial epiphysis may become detached as a result of these fractures in childhood although not in adolescence (Blount 1955). The anterior projection or even a larger portion of bone may be avulsed.

Tibial Shaft Fractures

Tibial shaft fractures are the most common of the diaphyseal fractures (Trafton 1992). About 30% of these will occur in victims with multiple injuries (Trafton 1992). Age distributions exhibit two peaks with the first consisting of younger adults with fractures often produced by sports-related injuries and the second peak involving adults 45–65 years old (Johner and Wruhs 1983). Fractures of the tibial shaft are common in youngsters and young adults until about 30 years of age (Buhr and Cooke 1959). The rates are approximately twice as high in men as in women throughout life until past the age of 70 years when the rates in women increase dramatically.

Fractures of the tibial shaft have many causes and are more common in the middle and distal portions. Direct blows to the bone can produce pure bending injuries, but, because this bone often bears the weight of the body at the time of impact, axial loading is also a factor altering the nature of the fracture. Because the legs are the primary means of either fleeing an impending accident or bracing for the impact, the tibia is also under compression at the time of impact. The upper body may also be turning at impact or be turned by the blow while the foot is relatively fixed on the ground, adding a rotational component.

Traffic accidents are a major cause of bending injuries to the tibial shaft although sports injuries are, too. Direct forces, such as the bending *boot-top* injuries of skiers, will be more transverse or butterflied. There may also be severe crushing of the shaft and involvement of the fibula as well as the tibia. Indirect forces, such as those produced in skiers due to twisting during spills, can result in spiral or oblique fractures (Johner and Wruhs 1983, Leach 1984, Rogers 1992). These spiral fractures may also be linked to malleolar fractures of either or both the tibia and fibula. Often automobile accidents, including car-pedestrian accidents, will produce more massive injury, with bending, compressive, and rotational components producing massive fragmentation. The role of the tibia in bracing the body often exaggerates normal compression. For example, the middle and distal shaft segments are affected in a relatively distinct pattern of segmental comminuted fracture of the tibia found in pilots from bracing against the foot pedals (Dummit and Reid 1969, Byard and Tsokos 2006). Boots often affect the location of fractures in the leg, frequently with fractures in both bones occurring just proximal to the termination of the supporting boot.

The more comminuted tibial shaft fractures produced in motor vehicle accidents and other high-energy trauma are more likely to be accompanied by other serious injuries (Johner and Wruhs 1983, Leach 1984). Comminuted fractures are usually associated with fibular fractures as force shatters both bones. Associated injuries also may be found in simpler tibial fractures. In spiral fractures, the associated fibular fracture may be placed more proximally than the tibial one, essentially forming a continuation of the spiral.

Clinical classification of the wide range of tibial fractures has been difficult and generally focuses on the extent of soft tissue damage. Johner and Wruhs (1983), however, use fracture morphology and mechanism of injury along with soft tissue damage and displacement. They grade increasing comminution A through C from simple fractures to those with a single butterfly fragment to those with several fragments. Each of these categories is then divided by the type of forces that produced them as translated into the fracture morphology. Indirect forces produce Group 1 fractures, and these range from simple spiral fractures to spiral fractures with several butterfly segments. Group 2 includes uneven or low-speed bending or bending due to four-point impact such as car bumpers. Group 3 consists of fractures produced by pure bending, high-speed impact, or crushing. Fractures are located within one of three unequal segments with the larger middle region consisting of the area where the medullary cavity is relatively narrow. While torsion is involved in the indirect fractures of all three categories, the longitudinal components of the resulting spiral fractures increase with the severity of the force. Simple spiral fractures will have one longitudinal fracture (Group A) linking the proximal and distal ends of the spiral, while Groups B and C are identified by two or more longitudinal fractures respectively. Group C spiral fractures can make multiple revolutions around the tibial shaft. Spiral length generally reflects the degree of force involved, with simple falls producing short spirals while skiing injuries produce longer spiral patterns. In fractures involving some component of bending, spiral fractures are replaced by transverse fracture patterns. Oblique fractures tend to occur when the leg is not in a weight-bearing position, probably reflecting a fixed position of one portion of the leg while the other end is moving. True oblique fractures of the tibia are reported to be rare, most containing at least some transverse component. These fractures tend to form when bending combines with compression. Simple transverse fractures tend not to occur in pedestrians hit by vehicles although they do occur as sports injuries. Car-pedestrian accidents tend to produce more fragmentation along with a significant butterfly component.

A simpler classification system by Gustilo (1992) is based upon that of Winquist and colleagues (1984) for the femora. It provides for four groups: (1) linear fractures, (2) comminuted fractures, (3) segmental fractures, and (4) those involving bone loss across the diameter. Since this system is not based on mechanism of injury but on the ease of surgical repair, its applicability to forensic analysis is limited.

The forensic anthropologist will be focusing on the location and magnitude of the fracture in order to determine the nature and direction of the force (Figure 11-17). The extent of comminution, the size and location of the butterfly segment, and the location of the transverse portions of bending fractures become critical to the interpretation of these injuries. While bending produces transverse fractures, these are quickly converted into oblique or butterfly fractures in the normally weight-bearing bones. Rotation of the body and thigh combined with fixation of the foot or the reverse can produce an element of spiraling. For this reason, reconstruction of the fragmented shaft and documentation of the injuries from multiple angles are essential.

Distal Tibial Fractures

The distal portion of the tibia is characterized by a transition to more cancellous bone from the highly dense bone in the mid-distal third. The distal

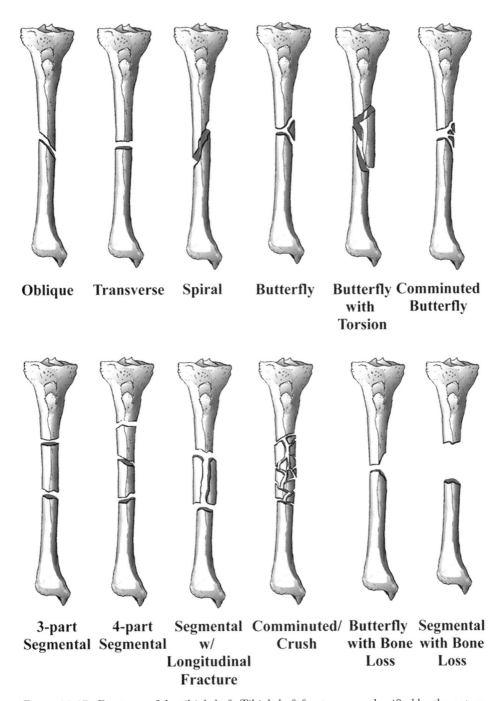

Figure 11-17. Fractures of the tibial shaft. Tibial shaft fractures are classified by the nature of the fracture line, the severity of the damage, and the number of major fragments resulting from the injury.

tibia is also the location of the complex of ligaments that support and bind the ankle joint. Tightly bound to the distal fibula, the tibia forms the medial portion of the mortise around the talus. The tibia also has a small protrusion of bone, which is often called a third malleolus, on the posterior rim. A mesh of ligaments limits movement at the ankle to maximize the efficiency of the stride. The complexity of this arrangement makes the ankle joint and the adjacent bony supports vulnerable for fracture when the movement exceeds either its normal range or magnitude.

Distal tibial fractures include those of the region of the bone above the malleolus known as *pilon* fractures and injuries of the ankle complex of which the distal tibia forms one component. These injuries may involve direct blows but often are indirectly produced by forces generated or applied to other parts of the body.

Pilon fractures are primarily located in the supramalleolar region, although there is usually accompanying fracture of the medial malleolus and posterior marginal lip (Trafton *et al.* 1992) (Figure 11-18). These fractures should be seen as distinct from fractures of the malleolus itself and typically involve greater segmentation of the distal tibia than seen in malleolar fractures. These injuries typically are produced by falls from heights or motor vehicle accidents that can produce the shearing and compressive forces, which can result in these fractures.

Rüedi and Allgower (1969) classify *Pilon* fractures into three types depending on the severity of the injury and involvement of the articular surface. These are often highly comminuted, and displacement of the resultant fragments raises clinical concerns. Forensically, the magnitude of fragmentation and angle of failure should be noted.

As the focus of injury moves more distally, the mechanism of injury may be more variable as the flexibility and complexity of the ankle joint produces a wide range of fracture patterns. Some fracture patterns are due to isolated excesses in movement, but most result from combinations of both foot and leg movement with alterations in loading as both bony and ligamentous integrity is lost. Movement of the foot and the relationship between the leg and the foot are critical for determining the injury pattern.

Most injuries to the distal tibia occur when the foot is in contact with the ground and is held down by the weight of the body. The injury itself may be induced by the rotation of the body while the foot is essentially fixated. Since the tibia and fibula form a lock around the talus, the extensions of bone around the talus are subject to fracture when the body is jarred violently. Because the leg meets the ankle joint at an angled, one side of the leg and ankle are under compression stresses while the other is under tension. These pressures affect both the bony structures and the ligaments and can result in collapse, bending fractures, avulsion fractures, and ligamentous rupture. In most cases,

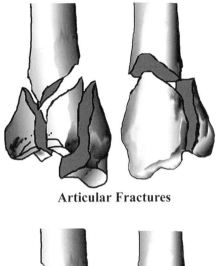

Articular Fractures

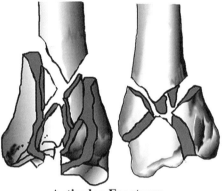

**Articular Fractures
with Compression**

Figure 11-18. Pilon fractures. Fractures of the distal tibia (*right shown*), known as *pilon* fractures, segment the articular surface as well as fragment the metaphyseal region. Dorsiflexion during compression will primarily remove an anterior segment, while plantar flexion will affect the posterior segment. When the foot is in a neutral position, articular fracture with compression produces a comminuted fracture.

one of the bones of the leg will also undergo a rotational force resulting in a spiral fracture (Rogers 1992). Initially, the side under compression is able to resist the loading, but the other side will be placed under tension resulting in ligamentous damage, an avulsion fracture or a transverse fracture. As the strength and support of the side under tension is lost, the tension and a greatly exaggerated axial load is transferred to the remaining intact portions of the ankle, often leading to collapse of this area as well.

The characteristics of the fracture hold important clues as to the events, which produced them. Transverse fractures result not only from the tensile forces but also from avulsion. Avulsion fractures are common in the ankle joint, occurring at the sites of ligamentous attachment. Oblique fractures may also be found and usually involve some movement of the talus against the malleolus or excessive loading, possibly in combination with tension. Such injuries often exhibit comminution on the side of the bone under the most compression (Wilson 1984).

Foot position in relation to the ankle and leg will also dictate the suite of injuries produced. Even pure vertical compression can produce tibial fractures with the location depending upon the position of the foot (Hamilton 1984, Wilson 1984, deSouza 1992a). Inversion or eversion of the foot directs the tensile forces along one aspect of the ankle and leg, stretching the ligaments that support the joint along that side (Tile 1987c). Dorsiflexion of the foot may result in fractures on the anterior margin of the distal articular surface (Rogers 1992), which vary from crushing of the anterior margin with mild to moderate trauma to the production of large fragments in falls or with much greater loading. When the foot is plantar flexed, posterior marginal fractures result, usually involving a large portion of the articular surface. When the foot is in a neutral position, both anterior and posterior fractures may be formed. Often these fractures are so extensive that they merge with *pilon* fractures. Fractures involving the articular surface stand in contrast with avulsion fractures, which usually incorporate only very small portions of the articular surface.

The location of fractures, as seen skeletally on the distal tibia, is important for understanding the movement involved. Most obvious are the malleolar fractures often produced by combinations of inversion and eversion of the foot, as well as abduction and adduction. Fractures of the margins of the articular surface are another common consequence of ankle injury. Anterior marginal fractures are caused by anterior capsular avulsion, which is produced by plantar flexion combined with internal rotation and adduction. Fractures may occur along the posterior edge of the fibula, which is variously identified as the posterior tibial lip, posterior tibial tubercle, posterior tibial margin, or posterior malleolus. Isolated fractures of the anterior and posterior tibial margins are relatively rare (Hamilton 1984). Dorsolateral fractures may be due to avulsion via the posterior inferior tibiofibular ligament or pressure from the talus or lateral malleolus. Dorsomedial avulsion fractures may be due to the effects of the tibial periosteum.

The complexity of ankle fractures makes classification difficult. Ashhurst and Bromer (1922) analyzed 300 fractures, devising a system that attributed these fractures to purported mechanisms (adduction, abduction, external rotation, and an assortment of other lesser causes). Unfortunately, this system did not include the marginal fractures of the tibia. The classification system of Lauge-Hansen (1948, 1950; Hamilton 1984; Wilson 1984; deSouza 1992a; Trafton *et al.* 1992) also focuses on the position of the foot and mechanism of fracture and is most appropriate for the anthropologist. In this system, the first term refers to the foot placement at the time of injury while the second term refers to the direction of talar movement relative to the leg. This system consists of four major injury suites: (1) supination-adduction, (2) supination-external rotation, (3) pronation-abduction, and (4) pronation-external rotation (Figure 11-19).

Supination-adduction fractures are a common mechanism of ankle injury. They are caused by inversion of the foot and adduction of the talus. Beginning with a fracture of the lateral malleolus or tearing of the lateral collateral ligament, this injury progresses to a shearing action on the medial malleolus as it is displaced medially by the talus. The result is a transverse horizontal fracture through the middle of the lateral malleolus and a vertical fracture of the medial malleolus originating at about the level of the distal articular surface of

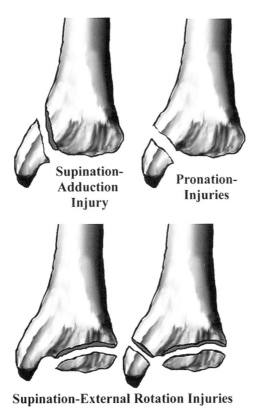

Supination-External Rotation Injuries

Figure 11-19. Malleolar fractures and mechanisms of production. Malleolar injuries of the distal tibia (*right shown*) are linked to the mechanisms of production according to the Lauge-Hansen classification system (1942, 1950). Direction of fracture distinguishes the supination-adduction from pronation injuries with the former being more vertical. Supination-external rotation injuries may progress to involve the medial malleolus but usually begin with a posterior malleolar fracture.

the tibia. There may be some impaction of the medial plafond due to this movement, which is visible as posteromedial tibial fracture just posterior to the medial malleolus. Berndt and Harty (1959) also attribute dome fractures of the talus to this mechanism.

The remainder of the Lauge-Hansen classificatory system examines injuries due to abduction (Lauge-Hansen 1948, 1950; Hamilton 1984; Wilson 1984; deSouza 1992a; Trafton *et al.* 1992). *Supination-external rotation* fractures, which account for 40–75% of malleolar fractures, are characterized in the tibia by transverse avulsion fractures of the medial malleolus. Avulsion fractures may also be present where there has been disruption of the ligaments that binds the tibia and fibula. Rotational shearing as the body falls to the side contralateral to the injury produces these avulsion fractures. Fibular failure precedes tibial avulsion in this pattern of injury, and the fibula is typically broken in a spiral oblique manner that extends proximally. If the rotation is extreme, avulsion of a fragment of the posterior tibial lip may occur. This fragment is usually triangular, conical, and about 2.5 cm long. It includes a portion of the distal articular surface. This fracture is produced by pressure from the talus against the posterolateral margin of the distal tibia. Since the locking mechanism of the ankle is destroyed, the leg often collapses. If the leg moves forward and laterally, a further fracture of the medial malleolus may occur between the articular surface of the medial malleolus and the distal tibia.

Pronation-abduction fractures are similar to the *supination-external rotation* fractures, except reversed so that the tibial failure precedes that of the fibula (Lauge-Hansen 1948, 1950; Hamilton 1984; Wilson 1984; deSouza 1992a; Trafton *et al.* 1992). This pattern is skeletally distinguished less by the tibia than by the fibula, which exhibits transverse lines of cleavage rather than a more vertical extension. Tibial involvement may include avulsion fractures of the medial malleolus or of the attachments of the syndesmotic ligaments (Tile 1987b). *Pronation-abduction* fractures often include horizontal fractures through the base of the medial malleolus (Lauge-Hansen 1950). These also are associated with avulsion fractures of the anterolateral tibial margin (Lauge-Hansen 1950), impaction fractures of the lateral distal tibial articular surface (Lauge-Hansen 1950; Trafton *et al.* 1992) and talar dome (Tile 1987d).

Pronation-external rotation fractures begin with medial failure through avulsion of the medial malleolus at the attachment of the anterior lateral malleolar ligament and the interosseous membrane (Lauge-Hansen 1948, 1950; Hamilton 1984; Wilson 1984; deSouza 1992a; Trafton *et al.* 1992). The resulting bone flake can be 2–3 cm in length. Loss of ligamentous integrity in this fracture pattern allows the talus to produce torsion between the two bones of the leg. Fractures of the posterior tubercle of the tibia at Volkmann's triangle may also occur (Tile 1987b). Spiral fibular fractures occur at or above the syndesmosis.

Fractures of the posterior margin may occur in collaboration with fractures of both malleoli due to external rotation and posterior movement of the foot (Rogers 1992). Posterior margin fractures may also be found with fractures of the proximal fibula, a combination known as a *Maisonneuve* fracture. When both malleoli are broken along with the posterior margin, this may be termed a *trimalleolar* fracture (Trafton *et al.* 1992), sometimes inappropriately called *Cotton's* fracture (Wilson 1984).

In children, distal tibial shaft fractures do not follow the adult patterns (Blount 1955). Infants exposed to direct trauma tend to produce greenstick fractures. This pattern may also be reflected in the fibula. After about age three years and into adolescence, there is usually epiphyseal damage. These have been grouped into avulsions of the lateral epiphysis, known as the *juvenile Tillaux* fracture (Bonnin 1970) and the *triplane* fracture (Spiegel *et al.* 1984) (Figure 11-20). In the former injury, the fracture line extends from the articular surface proximally across the epiphysis and then laterally along the physis. This is an avulsion fracture produced by tension on the anterior tibiofibular ligament when the foot is externally rotated. A triplane fracture involves two to four fragments of the distal metaphysis and is most common in late adolescence as fusion is occurring at this location. At first, this fracture replicates the *Tillaux* fracture, separating the anterior lateral portion of the bone that is still unfused. Then, a large posterior fragment of the epiphysis along with a portion of the metaphysis may also be broken off the diaphysis and divided, leaving the medial malleolus intact (Wheeless 1998).

For the anthropologist, ankle injuries can present difficult situations since interpretation is often dependent upon ligamentous injury and soft tissue has

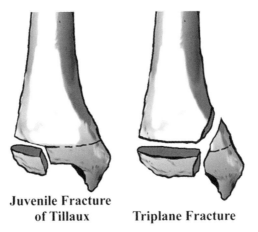

**Juvenile Fracture
of Tillaux**   **Triplane Fracture**

Figure 11-20. Ankle injuries in children and adolescents. Tillaux and triplane fractures occur along the fusing growth plate of the distal tibia (*right shown*). As the more central and medial segments are the first to fuse, fractures may deviate once these regions are reached.

often long since disappeared. Similarly, the tibia may be found in isolation or with extensive postmortem damage, which precludes reconstruction of the movements leading to fracture. Still along with documentation of the injury, the anthropologist should attempt to assess visible defects within the context of the ankle complex.

FIBULA

Lying lateral to the tibia, the long thin fibula plays an important role in the ankle joint but virtually none in the knee, except for being a ligamentous attachment site. Its primary role is to provide the lateral support at the ankle joint and the bone is ill-equiped for weight bearing. Its anatomical position leaves it vulnerable to direct blows, although it enjoys considerable protection from surrounding muscles. It is prone to fracture in older individuals due to osteoporotic changes (Hasselman *et al.* 2003, Kelsey *et al.* 2006), but its primary failure occurs in athletes (Slauterbeck et *al.* 1995, Fields 2011).

Fractures of the Fibular Head and Neck

The fibula rarely fractures in isolation but is usually linked to damage of either the knee or the ankle. The head and/or neck of the fibula may be fractured in conjunction with fractures of the tibial plateau induced by valgus (outward) forces (Rogers 1992) where it is usually associated with lateral tibial condyle fractures (Hohl *et al.* 1992). Varus or inward forces can result in avulsion fractures of the styloid process (Rogers 1992). Avulsion fractures may occur anterior to the fibular styloid where the lateral collateral ligament inserts (Manaster and Andrews 1994). The styloid itself may become avulsed due to forces produced by the *biceps femoris*, the tendon of which inserts on the styloid. Isolated simple or comminuted fractures of the fibular head tend to result from direct blows. Indirect forces, however, may also be responsible for isolated proximal fibular fractures as bilateral injuries are linked to epileptic seizures (Rawes *et al.* 1995) and parachute jumping (Hohl *et al.* 1992).

Fibular Shaft Fractures

Fibular shaft fractures can be caused by direct blows or indirectly by rotation of the foot (Trafton 1992). Usually these latter breaks are located slightly above the distal tibiofibular joint. Sometimes this fracture may occur more proximally, although these are relatively rare events (Slauterbeck *et al.* 1995). High fibular fractures in connection with ankle injuries may occur. *Maisonneuve* fractures are usually located in the proximal one-third of the shaft of the fibula but are linked to extensive soft tissue damage including ligamentous tearing in the ankle (Maisonneuve 1840, Merrill 1993). This fracture occurs when the bone is rotated externally, but the extent of rotation is limited by the strong ligamentous binding at the proximal joint. These fractures are associated with pronounced external rotation injuries at the ankle. The height of the fracture may be determined by the order of the ligamen¬tous failure with higher fractures linked to early failure of the interosseous ligament rather than the anterior tibiofibular ligament.

Pilon fractures of the tibia are frequently accompanied by fractures of the fibula (Trafton *et al.* 1992). These may be equivalent in height to those of the tibia or placed more proximally and are usually transverse or oblique in form. These fractures often indicate that some shear forces were involved as, under pure compression at the ankle, the tibia bears the brunt of the loading, often leaving the fibula undamaged (Tile 1987b). When this occurs, the ankle joint is often forced into inversion of the foot, causing excessive compressive pressure to the medial tibia.

In fibular shaft fractures, the plane of the oblique fracture gives clues as to the loading or bending direction. When the fibula is abducted, tension increases medially and fracturing begins inferiorly on the medial side, rising superiorly as it moves laterally across the bone (Wilson 1984). Comminution is common along the lateral margin. With rotation, the loading is usually posteriorly located, placing the anterior fibula under tension. Fractures then move anteroinferior to posterosuperior with comminution posteriorly.

Distal Fibular Fractures

The lateral malleolus may transmit a portion of the body weight during normal strides (Bolin 1961). Because this loading can increase dramatically with falls or other decelerating actions on the body, this portion of the fibula is prone to breakage. Malleolar fractures are linked across the joint, and a review of the tibial malleolar fracture patterns should be made in assessing those of the fibula. Tearing of the ligaments binding the two bones often results in smaller avulsion fractures at the points of attachment.

Using the classificatory system of Lauge-Hansen, discussed previously with the tibia, fibular fractures associated with *supination-adduction* of the ankle joint are characteristically transverse and at about the level of the superior surface of the talus (Lange-Hansen 1942, 1950; Tile 1987b; Trafton *et al.* 1992) (Figure 11-21). In contrast, *supination-external* rotation fractures are significantly more extensive, typically spiral or oblique fractures beginning posterior distally at the level of the distal tibial articular surface and extending anteriorly and proximally through the fibula. On the fibula, the fracture lines begin anteriorly at the talocrural joint (Lauge-Hansen 1950). The fracture initially runs dorsally and then moves obliquely and backwards. This fracture divides the fibular into two portions with the proximal portion held in place by the tibiofibular ligaments while the distal portion consists of the lateral malleolus. The fracture line is produced between the area of ligamentous attachment where the bone is less resistant to rotational forces. The spiral is "left-handed" on the right fibula and the reverse on the left leg. The tip of the distal fragment is usually 6–7 cm above the malleolar tip. *Bosworth fractures* are a variant of the supination-external rotation form in that there is posterior dislocation of the proximal fibula behind the tibia (Bosworth 1947, Hamilton 1984, Mourad 1996). These fractures may be more oblique in appearance, beginning more distally on the posterior surface. Fibular fractures in *pronation-abduction* fractures are usually transverse or oblique and laterally comminuted, being formed by bending outward of the leg. These fractures occur about ½ to 1 cm (¼ to ½ inches) above the distal articular surface and are seen moving from the distal point medially upward on the lateral side. *Pronation-external rotation* forms fractures, which are spiral or oblique and begin proximally along the anterior portion and run distally to the posterior margin. These are characteristically found well above the tibiotalar joint, at or above the syndesmosis usually 8–9 cm (20–23 cm) above the distal end of the bone. These fractures typically occur between the "surgical neck" and the fibular shaft. The actual fracture site appears to be determined by the extent of interosseous membrane rupture. Avulsion fractures also occur at the collateral ligament attachment.

The AO classification of ankle fractures emphasizes the fibular involvement and may be useful to anthropologists (Müller 1970, 1991). Three forms are recognized. Type A is produced by internal rotation and adduction, producing transverse avulsion fractures of the fibula at or below the joint line. These may be associated with medial or posterior malleolar fractures. Type B is produced by external rotation with the fracture rising obliquely from the joint line. These are often spiral in form. Type C includes simple oblique fractures moving from medial to lateral through the fibular neck due to abduction (C1), more proximally placed fractures with lateral comminution due to abduction and external rotation (C2), and fractures of the proximal fibula (C3). For types A and B, combinations of fibula fractures with medial malleolar fractures define subtype 2 from subtype 1, while the addition of a posterior malleolar fracture defines subtype 3. In general, type A is the equivalent of *Lauge-Hansen supination-adduction* fracture, type B corresponds to the *supination-external rotation* fractures with some *pronation-adduction* fractures and type C includes the *pronation-abduction* and *pronation-external rotation* fractures.

Avulsion fractures of the anterior fibula, known as *Wagstaffe's* fracture, may also occur usually in connection with *supination-external rotation* injuries. Pankovich (1979) further described these fractures, which had been reported by Le Fort (1886). Pankovich (1979) divided them into three forms. Type I

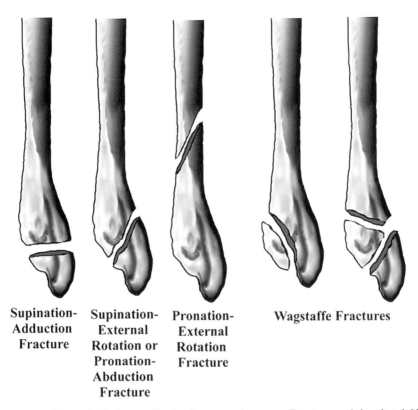

Supination-Adduction Fracture **Supination-External Rotation or Pronation-Abduction Fracture** **Pronation-External Rotation Fracture** **Wagstaffe Fractures**

Figure 11-21. Typical fibular malleolar fractures by type. Fractures of the distal fibula (*right shown*) are often an integral part of ankle injuries. The Lauge-Hansen classification system (1942, 1950) distinguished three patterns, which affect the fibula, varying by plane and location of the fracture. Wagstaffe fractures may occur with supination-external rotation.

consists of the avulsion fracture; Type II is a combination of an oblique fracture of the fibula through the distal articular surface extending superiorly and laterally and a transverse fracture above the syndesmosis; type III combines type II with an avulsion fracture of the anterior tibial tubercle.

Sometimes, distal fibular fractures are referred to as *Pott's* fractures and this term has been expanded to include fractures of both malleoli. This fracture may also be called the *Dupruytren* or *Pott-Dupruytren* fracture after another investigator whose definitions overlapped those of Pott. Serious questions as to the definition and plausibility of the original description have been raised and the term is less frequently used (Hamilton 1984).

Plastic bowing of the fibula is also reported in children, associated with midshaft fractures of the tibia (Cook and Bjelland 1978, Martin and Riddervold 1979, Trafton 1992). In these bones, natural curvature does not appear to play as great a role as it may in forearm or clavicular bowing deformation.

Anthropologists may use either the Lauge-Hansen or the AO system, but, as with the distal tibia, it is essential to view distal fibular fractures within the context of the ankle. Unfortunately, this is not always possible due to problems of recovery or taphonomic alteration of the bones. Information on the location of the fibular fracture and the nature of the break will aid in reconstructing the mechanism of injury.

TALUS

The talus forms the transition point for transmission of forces between the lower leg and foot. In addition, it must maintain a wide array of movement capabilities making it vulnerable to damage from a number of avenues. Over 60% of the surface of this bone is articular (Hansen 1992). It is essential for flexion and extension of the ankle, inversion and eversion of the foot and is active in the push-off movement during walking and running.

The talus is the second most frequently injured bone in the foot, usually due either to an avulsion fracture or a vertical or oblique fracture of the body or neck (Rogers 1992). High-energy injuries will occur in the body and neck of the talus (Hansen 1992). Fractures of the head, midbody, and posterior body are less common than those of the neck and anterior body but will be found in injuries due to extraordinary axial loading.

The clinical typology of talar fractures is dependent upon displacement of fragments, subluxation of the joint, and integrity of the blood supply to the fragments (Coltart 1952, Hawkins 1970) and thus is of less usefulness to the anthropologist. Notation should focus on location and fracture direction with solid documentation. Careful examination of the bones for shearing and avulsion fractures is also necessary.

Talar Neck Fractures

The talar neck fractures are the most common failure in this bone, accounting for about half of all talar fractures (Hawkins 1970). They occur most frequently in men in their thirties (Penny and Davis 1980). Neck fractures are usually found in situations where the foot has been under compression when there has been an impact from the substrate–such as the feet on the brake pedal of an automobile or on the floor of an airplane in a crash (Tile 1987e, Hansen 1992). Impact may produce a vertical fracture at the neck (Rogers 1992). At such times there is excessive dorsiflexion combined with the axial loading resulting in rupture of the neck. The neck is forced against the anterior margin of the tibia (Tile 1987e). Fracturing extends dorsally in the talar sulcus and ends inferiorly between the middle and posterior subtalar facet along the insertion of the talocalcaneal ligament (deSouza 1992a). This mechanism seems difficult to produce experimentally, and Peterson and associates (1976) concluded that the actual mechanism included force directed through the heel region of the foot while the ankle was braced. Rotation of the foot may also be involved as the talar body is locked between the malleoli while the foot is displaced medially. Often the medial malleolus will also fail in oblique or vertical fracture. A third mechanism of injury is a direct blow to the dorsum of the foot (Daniels and Smith 1993). Avulsion fractures are often associated with neck fractures as the ligaments become strained with the failure of the anterior bone.

Hawkins (1970) and Canale and Kelly (1976) have provided classifications of the talar neck fractures (Figure 11-22). Displacement of the head and reten¬tion of the blood supply are the prime determinants in these systems and not applicable to skeletonized material.

Talar Body and Dome Fractures

Vertical compression fractures are seen in the talar body and are placed anteriorly, posteriorly, or in the mid-body region (Rogers 1992). Such vertical fractures along with shearing fractures have been reported in falls from moderate heights (Abrahams *et al.* 1994), but these non-avulsive injuries are rare. Sneppin and associates (1977) classifies talar body fractures into (1) compressive, (2) shearing in either the coronal or sagittal plane, (3) posterior tubercle, (4) lateral tubercle, or (5) crush fractures. Shear fractures can occur in the coronal, sagittal or horizontal plane (deSouza 1992b).

Fractures of the talar dome, known as transchondral or osteochondral fractures, are probably produced by inversion forces while the foot is plantar flexed producing posterior lesions or dorsiflexed producing anterior lesions (Berndt and Harty 1959; Rogers 1992). The lateral edge can be pried off as it scrapes against the lateral malleolus. Forces generated along the talotibial or talofibular joints shear off the medial surface (Ly and Fallat 1993). Canale and Belding (1980) report that lesions located laterally tend to be shallow and wafer-shaped, while the medial lesions are deeper and cup-shaped. The latter may not be trauma related. Deep cup-shaped fractures have, however, been reported on the lateral aspect of the talar dome (Ly and Fallat 1993), probably due to forced inversion while the foot was in or close to its neutral position. The posterior margin of the dome may be chipped when the bone is wedged between the tibia and the calcaneus in extreme plantar flexion.

Berndt and Harty (1959) defined a series of stages in which these talar dome fractures may progress. Stage I represents a small area of compression. Stage II involves a partially detached fragment while Stage III and IV involve completely detached portions that, in the latter case, are dislodged from the bone. The anthropologist should note the location, nature, and extent of the damage.

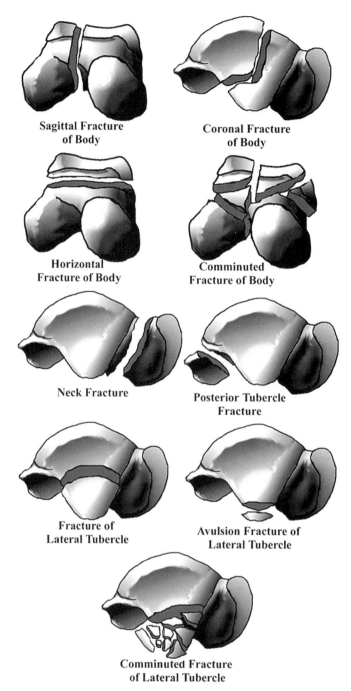

Figure 11-22. Talar fractures. Fractures of the talus (*right shown*) can affect the body, neck, or tubercles (Sneppin *et al.* 1977). The plane of fracture is used to identify body fractures, while lateral tubercle fractures are primarily identified by the extent of the fracture.

Talar Head Fractures

While fractures of the talar head are uncommon, this area may be injured during extreme plantar flexion where the force is transmitted along the axis of the foot, driving the navicular into the talar head (Coltart 1952, deSouza 1992b). Such forces may result in fragmentation of the talar head. Fractures of the talar head also tend to be associated with more complex fractures within the foot and ankle.

Avulsion Fractures of the Talus

Avulsion fractures occur at the superior surface of the neck and head, the lateral, medial, and posterior aspects of the body. In all cases, the investigator should be aware of the possibility of non-fusion of portions of the talus.

Lateral and Posterior Process Fractures

Fractures of the lateral process have gained prominence as a sports injury, becoming known as *snowboarder's ankle* (Nicholas *et al.* 1994, McCrory and Bladin 1996, Chan and Yoshida 2003). The mechanism appears to involve landing on the forced dorsiflexed and inverted foot. These can be divided into three types (Hawkins 1965, McCrory and Bladin 1996). Type 1 is a chip fracture of the inferior portion and is primarily an avulsion fracture of the anterior talofibular ligament without impacting the talofibular articulation. A large fragment, extending from the talofibular articular surface to the posterior talocalcaneal articular surface characterizes Type 2 fractures. Type 3 is a comminuted fracture often involving the entire lateral process.

The posterior process, which includes two tubercles surrounding the groove for the flexor hallucis longus tendon, is also prone to fracturing. Fractures appear to be caused by forced plantar flexion entrapping the bone between the calcaneus and the posterior margin of the tibia (deSouza 1992a, Hernandez 1994). Fractures of the entire posterior process are extremely rare (Heckman 1984). Fractures of this process may be confused with the presence of an *os trigonum*, an anomalous condition in which the lateral tubercle forms as a separate bone. The medial tubercle can be fractured when the foot is pronated and dorsiflexed, causing avulsion by the posterior talotibial ligament (Cedell 1974). Such fractures have been linked to sporting injuries involving dorsiflexion-pronation (Kim *et al.* 2003). However, others report that this can also be produced by direct trauma (Wolf and Heckman 1998). Fracture of the lateral tubercle of the posterior process has also been known as *Shepherd's* fracture (Shepherd 1882, deSouza 1992a). Stress fractures can also occur at the same region.

CALCANEUS

The calcaneus forms the heel and serves the dual function of being both a weight-bearing bone, transmitting loads from the body through to the substrate, and the attachment site for the major tendons of the calf muscles. The strong thick cortical strut within the crucial angle of the calcaneus supports the weight transferred by the talus. Internally, the calcaneus is largely cancelous bone with trabecular lines corresponding to the load-bearing stresses. Even under normal barefoot walking, the calcaneus is exposed to higher strains than the other bones of the leg and thigh (Al-Nazer *et al.* 2012). Despite the underlying fat pad, which cushions normal impacts to this bone, it is prone to injury in any event that results in massive loading to the feet. Often these injuries are bilateral and are associated with other injuries exhibiting axial compression such as vertebral fractures (Hansen 1992). Because of its high proportion of trabecular bone, the calcaneus is prone to age-related bone loss (Hoshi *et al.* 1994) increasing its fracture vulnerability.

This is the most frequently fractured of the tarsal bones (Essex-Lopresti 1952, Cave 1963) accounting for about 60% of all major tarsal injuries (Cave 1963). The majority results from individuals falling and landing on their feet, resulting in compression of the heel. This association was so strong that calcaneal fractures were once called "lover's heels"–supposedly from those jumping from a balcony while fleeing the scene of a romantic tryst. Now, motor vehicle accidents are common causes of calcaneal fracture (Hansen 1992). They are a frequent occurrence in drivers and front-seat passengers involved in frontal crashes in which the toe pan intrudes into the occupant space (Benson *et al.* 2007). All-terrain vehicles and motorcycles also are involved in accidents that result in fractures of the calcaneus (Jarvis and Moroz 2006). In many cases these fractures are also associated with fractures in the ankle and may also be linked to spinal and basilar skull fractures. In one study reported by Cave (1963), 10% of the calcaneal fractures coincided with fractures of the spine and 26% had associated extremity injuries. Most calcaneal fractures are found in males and are usually work-related (deSouza 1992a).

Romantic trysts are an unlikely precursor for toddler's fractures of the calcaneus (Laliotis *et al.* 1993), although these also are relatively common injuries. These fractures do not appear to be linked to any specific trauma and are most likely the product of the stress derived from the newly acquired skill of bipedal locomotion. Calcaneal fractures, along with talar fractures, are not common in children even though they are known to fall from heights while in pursuit of the pleasure of climbing.

The complex configuration of the calcaneus, age-related changes in the bone structure, the transmission of forces down the leg and through to the foot and the action of adherent musculature and ligaments means that the fracture patterns observed in this bone are highly variable. The severity of the breakage depends upon the weight and distance of the fall or impact and the generation of compressive forces (Hansen 1992, Rodgers *et al.* 1995).

Classification is difficult. Zwipp and associates (1993) recognized two-through five-part fractures and divided the calcaneus into five portions: the *sustentaculum tali*, the tuberosity, the subtalar joint region, the anterior process, and the anterior subtalar joint region. This system also distinguishes fractures by their impact upon the various calcaneal joints. Alternately, calcaneal fractures can be broadly divided into intra-articular fractures including tongue and joint depression fractures as well as those too comminuted to be classified and extra-articular ones that include "beak" fractures of the tuberosity, avulsion fractures of the tuberosity, along with fractures of the anterior process, medial process, *sustantaculum tali*, and body (Heckman 1984). Usually, twisting motions induce extra-articular fractures.

Intra-articular fractures are the most common form of calcaneal fracture (Cave 1963). These are usually brought about by falls from heights in which the victim lands on his or her feet (Hansen 1992, Kalla and Kaminski 1992). The inferior surface of the talus may act as a wedge producing massive disruption of the underlying bone (Heckman 1984, deSouza 1992, Rodgers *et al.* 1995). Initially the bone will fragment into two main portions with the primary fracture occurring from the plantar surface dorsally into the posterior facet of the subtalar joint. The fracture runs from the posteromedial side to the anterolateral side of the bone with further comminution occurring under the subtalar joint. The actual fracture location depends on the position of the foot at impact (deSouza 1992b). If the foot is pronated, the fracture is usually posterolateral to the posterior facet, but if the foot is supinated, the fracture occurs more anteromedially along the calcaneal sulcus. When the foot is in a neutral position, the fracture usually passes through the posterior facet.

Posterior extra-articular fractures as proposed by Essex-Lopresti (1952) form secondary to this primary intra-articular fracture. When the body fractures, the force from the posterolateral margin of the talus is passed through either an outer route through the posterior subtaloid joint or an inner route from the *sustentaculum tali* (Figure 11-23). These defects have been termed the *tongue type* and *joint depression* types of fractures. Anterior secondary fractures, both extra- and intra-articular, are also regularly found (deSouza 1992b). These breaks may extend into the cuboid facet or may travel inferiorly ending on the plantar surface. Fractures beyond these posterior and anterior breaks indicate that comminution has occurred, although generally the term does not apply to fragmentation of the lateral wall since this is a regular occurrence with calcaneal fractures.

When the forces are high, severe comminution results. In general, a triangular-shaped sustentacular fragment is produced. The anterior portion of the posterior

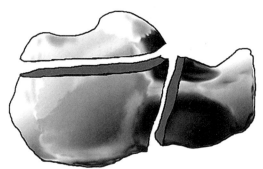

Tongue Type Fracture Pattern

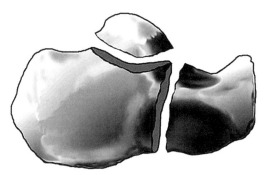

Joint Depression Type Fracture Pattern

Figure 11-23. Tongue vs. joint depression fractures of the calcaneus. Tongue fractures of the calcaneus (*right shown*) are distinguished from joint depression fractures by their location and the extent of the secondary fracture, although both share a similar primary vertical fracture (Essex-Lopresti 1952). Tongue-type fractures extend posteriorly while joint depression fractures compress or fragment the lateral articular surface.

facet may be compacted into the body of the calcaneus while the posterior portion is less severely affected. The lateral wall of the body may burst from the impact of the fibula. Fractures along the sagittal line may originate in the more vulnerable subtalar joint but continue anteriorly into the calcaneocuboid joint. Fractures of the calcaneocuboid joint often form anterior beak fractures. About 4% of calcaneal fractures are severely comminuted (Essex-Lopresti 1952).

Because of the complexity of classification and the large number of variations on the themes, many systems have been devised to identify these injuries to the calcaneus (Crosby and Fitzgibbons 1990, Sanders *et al.* 1993). DeSouza (1992b) has described a stage sequence with each of the three stages providing different options for appearance (Figure 11-24). Stage A indicates the division by the primary fracture into a tuberosity fragment and a sustantacular fragment. Within this classification, Type A1 is extra-articular with the fracture occurring

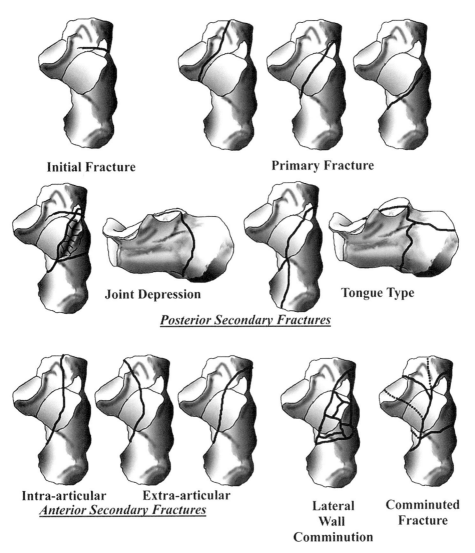

Figure 11-24. Calcaneal fracture classification according to deSouza (1992). Calcaneal fractures (*right bone shown*) usually begin with an initial failure in the coronal plane anterior to the posterior talar articular facet (deSouza 1992b). Subsequent primary facets may segment this facet or lie medial or lateral to the articular surface. Secondary fractures may occur posterior or anterior with anterior fractures distinguished by the involvement of the facet to the cuboid.

behind the posterior calcaneal facet while A2 involves a depressed posterior calcaneal facet in which the fracture is anteromedial to the posterior calcaneal facet. He notes that in some cases, the primary fracture may occur in the articular cartilage and through the facet (A3). In stage B, the tongue or joint-depression fracture type is formed and the subdivisions indicate whether one, two, or three fracture lines are formed. Stage C refers to the anterior extension of the fractures that involve the anteriolateral fragment. Here the subdivisions indicate (1) extra-articular fracturing, (2) fracture of the calcaneocuboid joint, or (3) marked comminution.

Carr (1989, 1993) approaches the classification of calcaneal fractures through the mechanisms of injury. Noting that shear and compressive forces combine to produce two separate primary fracture lines, he identified these as one dividing the bone along the coronal plane and the other running along the sagittal plane. The sagittal fracture tends to occur as the result of the eccentric loading of the bone, shearing it in two beginning at the posterior facet (Palmer 1948). This break can extend anteriorly dividing the anterior and cuboid facets. When the heel is in valgus or outward position, the fracture occurs more laterally and may avoid any articular surfaces. When the heel is in the varus or inward position, the fracture shifts more medially. When inversion of the foot is pronounced, the medial fragment may be quite small, consisting of only the *sustentaculum tali* and the middle facet (Carr 1993). Compressive forces produce the wedge-like anterolateral fragment. Laterally these fractures result in an inverted Y, pattern although the position of the posterior fracture line varies producing the tongue-type or joint depression fractures. The size and configuration of the posterior fragment determine the tongue versus joint depression distinction. The lateral wall buckles and the anterolateral fragment runs from the cuboid facet to the crucial angle of Gissane (Carr 1993).

Extra-articular fractures can be divided into two broad categories (deSouza 1992b). One group is a relatively constant pattern in which the fracture extends from the posteromedial aspect of the body to the anterolateral aspect, lying posterior to the subtalar joint. These are often produced by falls while the foot is pronated. The second group are inconstant in pattern but are also produced by falls.

Fractures that do not include the subtalar articular surface are usually of the avulsive type (deSouza 1992b, Rogers 1992). About one-quarter of all calcaneal fractures involve the anterior process (Rowe *et al.* 1963) including some that are avulsive in origin. The actual mechanism of injury to the anterior process usually appears to be forced plantar-flexion and inversion of the foot with a secondary cause being shearing or impaction from sudden dorsiflexion and eversion bringing the anterior calcaneus against the cuboid (deSouza 1992b; Roesen and Kanat 1993). This is more common when the individual is wearing high heels. Elevation of the heel causes tightening of bifurcate ligament to the point that the attachment point on the anterolateral portion of the anterior process is avulsed. Other ligaments that may be involved include the calcaneo-cuboid and anterior interosseous talocalcaneal ligaments (Jahss and Kay 1983). Norfray and colleagues (1980) argued that the origin of *extensor digitorum brevis* was responsible. Avulsive fractures are usually quite small and do not intrude into the cuboid facet joint (Heckman 1984). Clinical classification focuses primarily on the displacement as well as severity (Degan *et al.* 1982) and, therefore, is not relevant for work with skeletal material.

Non-avulsive fractures of the anterior process may also occur although these are relatively rare (Hunt 1970; deSouza 1992b). These injuries are due to forceful abduction or forced dorsiflexion of the forefoot inducing fracture of the anterior articular facet. The resulting fragment may be quite large.

Degan and associates (1982) proposed a classification of the fracture patterns in the anterior process. Their system distinguishes three types based on displacement as well as severity. Type I involves only the tip of the process, Type II does not infringe upon the articular facet, and Type III involves the calcaneocuboid joint.

Fractures of the medial calcaneal tuberosity are a rare occurrence (Heckman 1984, deSouza 1992b). This may be due to avulsion from the *abductor hallucis* and *flexor hallucis brevis* origins and attachment of the plantar fascia. The mechanism of injury also has been attributed to shearing forces during falls while the foot is in the valgus position (Watson-Jones 1941). Glancing blows to the foot while it is everted have also been cited as a causative agent (Lance *et al.* 1964).

The lateral process is also somewhat vulnerable to fracture (deSouza 1992b). This process is the origin of the *abductor digiti minimi muscle* and avulsion may occur due to glancing blows to the foot while the heel is inverted.

Fractures also may be confined to the posterior portions of the calcaneus although these are also relatively rare (Heckman 1984, deSouza 1992b, Cole *et al.* 1995). Traditionally, these have been divided into two broad categories. The superior part of the tuberosity can be broken in what is known as a *beak* fracture. These fractures are above the area usually considered to be an insertion for the Achilles tendon and probably result from direct trauma. The other form includes the avulsive fractures of the more posterior portion at the Achilles attachment site, which occur with sudden contraction of the calf muscles (Cave 1963). While this region is the attachment site of the Achilles tendon, it is generally located more inferiorly so the fractures of the superior margin have often been attributed to direct blows to this region. However, in some individuals, the Achilles tendon attachment is more superiorly placed and its rupture may be the mechanism of injury (Lowy 1969). Such avulsive fractures, which are more common in elderly women, appear to be compounded by osteoporosis.

Severe inversion of the foot leads to fracture of the *sustentaculum tali* (Heckman 1984). A secondary cause has been listed as landing on the heel. Others cite a combination of falling onto a markedly inverted foot (deSouza 1992b) or forces applied to the medial side of the foot with the heel in the valgus position (Gage and Premer 1971) as the cause. These are extremely rare (Essex-Lopresti 1952).

OTHER TARSALS

The arch of the midfoot, formed by the remaining tarsal bones, is subject to a range of injuries involving both fracture and subluxation. In general, these injuries can be divided into four groups based on location and mechanism (Main and Jowett 1975) (Figure 11-25). The first group is medial injuries produced by inversion or adduction of the forefoot. These breaks include flake fractures of the dorsal margin of the talus and navicular on the medial aspect of the foot and of the lateral calcaneus and cuboid on the lateral aspect. Longitudinal injuries, the second group, are those that occur when the ankle is plantar-flexed at impact so that the force compresses the navicular, producing shear fractures along the line of the inter-cuneiform joints. Crush fractures may also be found within this group. The third group, lateral injuries, is caused by eversion or abduction of the forefoot and includes avulsion of the navicular tuberosity and impaction fracture of the calcaneus and comminution of the calcaneocuboid joint. Plantar injuries form the fourth group. Some of

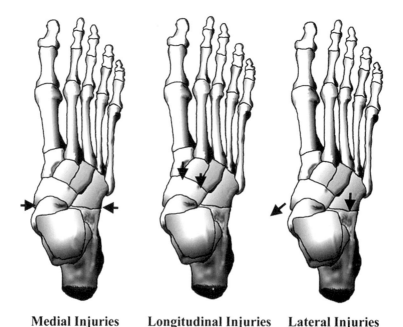

Medial Injuries   Longitudinal Injuries   Lateral Injuries

Figure 11-25. Pattern of tarsal fractures. Tarsal injuries are grouped by the mechanism of production and location of the injuries into medial, longitudinal, and lateral (Main and Jowett 1975).

these injuries are caused by the foot being twisted under the body in high-energy accidents producing avulsion fractures of the dorsum of the navicular and anterior process of the calcaneus. Others combine these injuries with impaction fractures at the calcaneocuboid joint. Finally, crush fractures may be treated separately. These fractures usually occur from weights landing on the foot and follow no distinct pattern of fracture.

Navicular Fractures

The navicular links the talocalcaneal complex to the foot and is the foundation for the medial arch of the foot. It has minimal involvement in muscle attachments and is generally well protected by the plantar surface of the foot and arch-like structure of the skeletal elements. This bone is prone to fractures from high-energy injuries and from avulsion fractures. The acute fractures to the navicular body due to direct trauma are usually associated with motor vehicle accidents or a fall from a height (Sangeorzan *et al.* 1989).

Stress fractures of the navicular are relatively common, especially among athletes (Hunter 1981, Torg *et al.* 1982). These are due to the repetitive stresses applied in running or marching, which the bone can no longer withstand, and insufficient time is allowed for healing. They are often sagitally oriented and may be incomplete (Heckman 1984). Among osteoporotics, forceful abduction of the forefoot may produce avulsion fractures of the navicular (deSouza 1992b).

Navicular fractures can be classified into four forms including fractures of (1) the tuberosity, (2) cortical avulsion of the dorsal lip, (3) the body, and (4) stress fractures (Eichenholtz and Levine 1964). Those of the body are the more serious of the injuries as it disrupts the articular surfaces. These intra-articular body fractures have been further subdivided into (1) type 1–produced by centrally directed axial force along the foot result in a transverse fracture line in the coronal plane, (2) type 2–produced by axial compression from the first metatarsal, which yields an oblique fracture line from the dorsolateral to plantar-medial surfaces, and (3) type 3–produced by a combination of axial and lateral force which produce a fracture disrupting the naviculo-cuneiform joint and the navicular becoming seriously fragmented (Sangeorzan *et al.* 1989). The second of these forms is the most common while the last of these forms is usually associated with other foot fractures.

Compression of the navicular between the adjacent bones of the foot produced by excessive flexion or eversion of the foot may pry loose a dorsal flake (Hansen 1992). Cortical avulsion fractures occur with twisting forces, usually eversion of the foot (Heckman 1984) or acute plantar-flexion with inversion of the foot (deSouza 1992b). They are most common in women. Avulsion comes from stresses placed on the talonavicular capsule and avulsion fractures through the body may occur (Rogers 1992).

Navicular tuberosity fractures can result from eversion injuries (Waugh 1958, deSouza 1992b, Rogers 1992). Such motions cause increase tension in the *posterior tibialis* tendon and anterior fibers of the deltoid ligament. In some cases, the anterior portion of the *posterior tibialis* muscle may, upon sudden contraction, produce an avulsion fracture at its insertion point on the tuberosity. This injury is often an incomplete fracture due to the complexity of the tendinous insertion on the foot (Watson-Jones 1941). This fracture must also be distinguished from the presence of an *os tibiale externum*, a congenital deformation.

Cuboid and Cuneiform Fractures

The remaining tarsal bones tend to be relatively more immune to fracturing except in high-energy situations such as motor vehicle accidents. Fractures of the cuboid and cuneiforms may occur in association with fractures in other portions of the foot and rarely in isolation except in direct impact. Classification of these fractures is extremely difficult since the bones become highly fragmented (Hansen 1992). Chip fractures of the cuboid and cuneiforms may occur from direct trauma, usually on the lateral surface of the foot (Rogers 1992).

The most frequent cuboid injury is due to abduction of the forefoot and lateral subluxation of the midtarsal joint (Heckman 1984, deSouza 1992b). This movement results in the cuboid being compacted between the lateral metatarsals and the calcaneus and produces a *nutcracker* fracture (Hermel and Gershon-Cohen 1953, deSouza 1992b). Sometimes such a motion produces only a longitudinal split through the cuboid body at the level of the intermetatarsal joint. Avulsion fractures may also occur usually involving the lateral aspect (deSouza 1992b).

Cuneiform fractures may occur secondary to tarsometatarsal dislocation (Heckman 1984). Sangeorzan (1991) found that the most common break was an oblique fracture.

One complex of fractures is the *Lisfranc* fracture of the foot, which involves major dislocations and fracturing of the cuboid and metatarsals and, sometimes, the navicular and cuneiforms (Rogers 1992, Vuori and Aro 1993). This complex of fractures appears to be increasing in incidence and is attributable to high-energy trauma (Heckman 1984, deSouza 1992b) although low-energy causes have also been reported (Vuori and Aro 1993). These fractures are attributable to both direct and indirect trauma. Heavy objects falling onto the dorsum of the foot may produce this pattern while falls produce longitudinal compression of the foot and indirect injury. In the latter instances, the foot is plantar-flexed and in an extreme equinus at the ankle. In many cases, additional rotation is involved as well, complicating the fracture and dislocation pattern. Classification of these *Lisfranc* injuries depends upon the pattern and degree of dislocation, factors usually not evident in skeletonized material (Hardcastle *et al.* 1982).

METATARSALS

The metatarsals are active in the push-off phase of walking and running and designed to resist stresses due to these activities. Their involvement in this process varies across the foot so that the first metatarsal is wider and shorter than the others reflecting its role in striding. These differences in position within the foot and structural integrity of the bone affect the frequency of injury. Two sesamoids are situated on the plantar surface of the first metatarsal, which serve to distribute the body's weight during locomotion as well as allow for the movement of the *adductor hallicis* tendon laterally and the *abductor hallicus* medially. These, too, may be injured.

The most frequently injured bone is the fifth metatarsal, followed by the third, second, first, and fourth (DeLee 1986). In part, the variation in the fracture patterns can be explained by the cross-sectional geometry of the metatarsals. Griffin and Richmond (2005) show that the middle metatarsals are the weakest in their morphology, but the second metatarsal and, to a lesser extent, the third exhibit high peak pressures during the push-off phase of walking. This phenomenon helps explain the higher incidence of stress fractures in the second metatarsal (Donahue *et al.* 2000).

Traumatic metatarsal fractures are most often associated with falls from height and motor vehicle accidents, although a wide range of causes may be involved. Blows to the top of the foot often result in a series of fractures across multiple metatarsals (Heckman 1984, deSouza 1992b). Given the staggered arrangement of the metatarsals, a fracture on the distal shaft of a medial metatarsal is usually located at the metatarsal head of a more lateral bone, therefore, multiple fractures will appear at "different" levels of each bone. Fractures of the metatarsal bases are uncommon as are fractures of the metatarsal heads. More common are metatarsal neck fractures, which often appear as multiple injuries. Indirect forces, such as when the forefoot is fixed while the hindfoot continues to twist, produce shaft fractures

As discussed previously, the metatarsals may be fractured in a *Lisfranc* injury (deSouza 1992b). While these have a number of causal mechanisms, the result is catastrophic displacement of one or more metatarsals. This results in fracture close to the base with dislocation of the adjacent metatarsals (Figure 11-26). The actual movement involved may be abrupt lateral shifting of the medial metatarsal which shears off the shaft of the adjacent lateral metatarsal, lateral movement of a group of metatarsals resulting in fracture of the more medial in the group, or splaying of the metatarsals with fracture of those at the center of the splay.

Fractures of the first metatarsal tend to be comminuted and are usually associated with significant soft tissue damage and perforation of the skin (Hansen 1992). Fractures may also occur more frequently in the head of this metatarsal in comparison to its companions. In the middle metatarsals, similar forces will

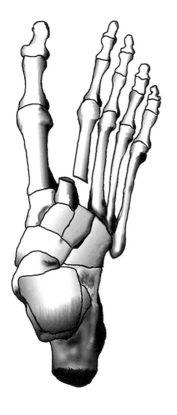

Figure 11-26. Lisfranc fracture of the foot. Lisfranc fractures may occur from a number of mechanisms, but the pattern produced involves a proximal shaft fracture of the metatarsal as well as possible injury to the cuboid and navicular.

produce fractures in the distal shaft and neck rather than the head itself. Fractures may also occur at the base of the bone. Usually these only occur with direct trauma, although indirect rotational force has been known to produce a spiral fracture of the shaft. Avulsion fractures may be found along the base of the first metatarsal where the *abductor hallucis, adductor hallucis,* and the *flexor brevis* tendons attach.

The proximal end of the fifth metatarsal is most frequently injured by an avulsion fracture. Once thought exclusively due to the action of the *peroneus brevis* muscle, these fractures are now also attributed to the lateral plantar aponeurosis being forced into acute inversion, often in plantar flexion (Richili and Rosenthal 1984). Fractures of the proximal shaft have often been grouped under the classification of *Jones* fractures, although the actual characteristics and mechanism of injury is somewhat ambiguous (Jones *et al.* 1902, deSouza 1992b, Hansen 1992). Often diaphyseal stress fractures and tuberosity and styloid fractures are incorrectly assigned to this category (Lawrence and Botte 1993). Technically, a *Jones'* fracture is a transverse fracture at the junction of the metaphysis and diaphysis without involving any of the articular surfaces outside of the inter-metatarsal joint (Stewart 1960). These are acute fractures, which often occur when the foot is adducted while the ankle is plantar-flexed

(Lawrence and Botte 1993). Diaphyseal fractures occur distal to the inter-metatarsal joint through the denser cortical bone of the proximal shaft.

Avulsion fractures of the tuberosity, known as *tennis* fracture, begin with either contraction of *peroneus brevis* or pulling on the plantar aponeurosis. These fractures may extend into the cubometatarsal joint but not into the intermetatarsal area. Avulsion fractures may also occur distal to the flare of the tuberosity. These styloid fractures appear to occur when the heel is elevated, placing the majority of the weight on the lateral aspect of the forefoot (Kavanaugh *et al.* 1978). Vertical and mediolateral forces brought to bear on the fifth metatarsal become more than the bone can withstand. About 40% of these are probably stress fractures while the remaining fractures are produced in acute traumatic events. The fifth metatarsal is also subject to *dancer's* fractures, which are spiral fractures of the cervical region (Vogler *et al.* 1995).

Metatarsal fractures are often associated with stress fractures known as "March foot" in which walking to the limit of endurance produces fatigue fractures (Jansen 1926). These occur most often in the second or third metatarsal and infrequently in the fourth and fifth, according to Jansen (1926). Meurman (1981) found that 11% occurred in the first metatarsal.

Sesamoid injuries may also occur due to direct trauma, avulsive forces, or excessive stress (Heckman 1984). Frequently these fractures are due to falls from heights or from heavy weights being dropped onto the forefoot (deSouza 1992b). Indirect fractures usually result in transverse fractures, while direct trauma causes more fragmentation. In most cases, the medial sesamoid is the most vulnerable to fracture due to the greater weight it bears (Heckman 1984, deSouza 1992b). Most of these fractures will be transverse unless associated with dislocation at the first metatarsophalangeal joint when the fracture tends to be longitudinal.

PHALANGES OF THE FOOT

The phalanges of the foot, with the exception of the big toe, are small bones ideally positioned to collide with a wide variety of objects. Generally the bones suffer poorly in such situations, although these fractures are not incapacitating.

The proximal phalanges are the most vulnerable of the toe bones due to breakage (Kelikian 1965) and of these the proximal phalanx of the fifth toe is the most commonly fractured (Chapman 1978). Fractures in the distal phalanges are similar in form to those of the fingers (Rider 1937). The middle phalanges are rarely fractured, probably due to their short, squat form. Small chips are sometimes found near the joint surface, usually produced by the "stubbed toe" phenomenon. Crushing fractures also occur as the toes are "run over" or "landed upon" by a heavy object. Fractures of the phalanges of the foot are commonly much higher in men throughout life until advanced old age.

Anthropologists usually consider themselves remarkably lucky to be able to recover any of the phalanges of the foot unless they have remained encased in a sock or shoe. The exposed foot is a primary site for scavenging activity, and the small bones are often lost in the soil or as animals transport the foot and leg. The best that can be done is to assess the type of injury and, as best as possible, the location. Healed fractures in these bones are common and may aid in the identification of the deceased.

Section III

CASE STUDIES

CASE STUDIES

Case studies are an important mechanism through which the concepts already discussed in this volume can be illustrated. A collection of nine reports is provided which illustrate several aspects of trauma analysis. These areas include (1) using the scientific method to test hypothetical mechanisms by which bones were fractured in light of the fractures evident on the bones themselves; (2) the importance of distinguishing antemortem, perimortem and postmortem injuries; (3) the often complex task of interpreting of perimortem injury; (4) what an in-depth anthropological analysis of the effects of injury involves (e.g., stereomicroscopy); (5) analysis of injury patterns across cases; and (6) anthropologists collaborating with other forensic scientists to the betterment of the case result; (7) conceding that sometimes the limited skeletal information and photos we get are insufficient, and that bringing in the forensic anthropologist early and often might produce more thorough results.

In the first case study, Crowder and Adams describe the case of a man whose remains were found at the bottom of a deep drainage ditch. Initial circumstances indicated the man either jumped from or fell a great distance. In trying to assess what forces resulted in the suite of perimortem fractures they observed, Crowder and Adams describe the perimortem trauma bone by bone then test five hypotheses regarding possible mechanisms for how the fractures were acquired. Crowder and Adams deftly use the current literature to narrow down to one plausible mechanism that best accounts for why each bone broke the way it did. In collaboration then with their medical examiner and investigators, Crowder and Adams were able to contribute evidence that resulted in the case's cause and manner of death rulings.

Zephro and Galloway use a case of an elderly woman being found dead in her bed years after her death to demonstrate how absolutely essential both gross and macroscopic examination of fracture surfaces are in determining whether the fractures occurred the ante-, peri-, or postmortem interval. This case also highlights how the age of the victim and condition of the remains at recovery can complicate the analysis requiring forensic anthropologists to truly adhere to the best practices for analyzing remains, as described in Chapter 2.

In her chapter on postcranial fractures in victims of child abuse, Jennifer Love interweaves the case of a battered child with synthesis of the literature on non-accidental injuries in children. The variably healed and healing postcranial fractures exhibited in the remains of the three-month-old infant in question were on multiple ribs, the scapulae, the sternum, several long bones, and several vertebrae. Love also provides an excellent review of how hyper-vigilant forensic anthropologists must be when examining the remains of a child and how integral to the analysis having the anthropologist present at autopsy is.

Juarez and Hughes push the boundary of how forensic anthropologists traditionally see their work: suggesting the possibility that forensic anthropologists might be able to further ongoing sociological and medical discussions by taking a reflective look at their cases once the remains have been completely analyzed and the case report submitted. Juarez and Hughes compare the kind of fractures seen on the remains of a woman killed by her husband to the kind of fractures described in the literature on Intimate Partner Violence (IPV). Juarez and Hughes do not argue that it is the job of the anthropologist to identify to law enforcement that a particular pattern of fractures will lead them to a particular perpetrator, in this case a domestic partner, rather anthropologists should be vigilant observers capable of referring law enforcement to the right literature.

The case study by Haugen demonstrates how valuable evidence can be contributed that aids both identification of the victim and determination of cause and manner of death. Haugen was able to use antemortem fractures and surgical appliances to positively identify the victim then document and describe the perimortem blunt and sharp force traumata that caused to the individual's death.

Hart provides a case study that demonstrates the positive outcome (prosecution of the perpetrator) that can be achieved when the anthropologist is involved at the death/recovery scene and the autopsy, conducts a thorough forensic anthropological examination, and provides sworn testimony about each step of the process while on the witness stand. She was able to discuss scenarios devised by both the prosecution and defense as to how the victim sustained the trauma she observed.

Nusse demonstrates how collaboration between a forensic facial reconstruction artist and the forensic anthropologist can result in life-like restorations that generate leads towards positively identifying even the oldest (37 years) of cold case victims of trauma. She provides photographs of the processes she follows and offers invaluable insight into the methods she uses when the effects of trauma and time have warped the cranial and facial skeletal elements.

Lastly, Black and colleagues describe a very violent homicide and how they collaboratively approached trying to document the multiple blows delivered to an elderly man found bludgeoned in his home. Black and her collaborators were hindered in their efforts by the fact that the case had gone cold, and all they were provided to evaluate were fragments of the cranium, scene photographs, and the autopsy records, radiographs, and photographs. Black and colleagues very effectively argue that had the forensic anthropologist been brought into the case much earlier, a more detailed understanding of the attack might have been achieved. They are even so open to peer review as to invite other experienced forensic anthropologists to propose alternate means or mechanisms to account for the extensive fracturing and fragmentation patterns they so vividly depict.

A. INTERPRETING BLUNT FORCE TRAUMA: A CASE REPORT

CHRISTIAN M. CROWDER AND BRADLEY J. ADAMS

Late one March evening in 2007, an assemblage of mostly skeletonized remains was discovered lying in a cement drainage channel. The channel was located alongside railroad tracks and below a 50-foot high stone retaining wall in the neighborhood of Harlem in Manhattan, New York City. A medico-legal investigator and a forensic anthropologist from the Office of Chief Medical Examiner (OCME) in New York City responded to recover the remains and process the scene along with the New York Police Department's (NYPD) Crime Scene Unit. The body was clothed, but was largely skeletonized with some adipocere formation and desiccated soft tissue. The adipocere was concentrated in areas that were in contact with water draining through the channel. The remains appeared to be *in situ* (in place) and were mostly articulated with minimal dispersal of skeletal elements. The body was supine, arms at the sides, with the left leg bent under the extended right leg (Figure A-1). During the recovery, the forensic anthropologist determined the remains were those of an adult male. While there did not appear to be any obvious perimortem trauma to the cranium, several perimortem fractures of the leg bones were noted during recovery. These preliminary findings at the scene presented several possible scenarios: (1) This was a homicide and body dump; (2) the decedent accidentally fell; (3) the decedent intentionally jumped; (4) the decedent was pushed or was thrown from the wall; or (5) the decedent was hit by a train which propelled his body into the nearby drainage channel. The remains were transported to the Manhattan OCME mortuary for a more thorough examination.

EXAMINATION OF THE REMAINS

The following day, the case was reviewed by one of OCME's medical examiners, and members of the agency's Forensic Anthropology Unit began a

314

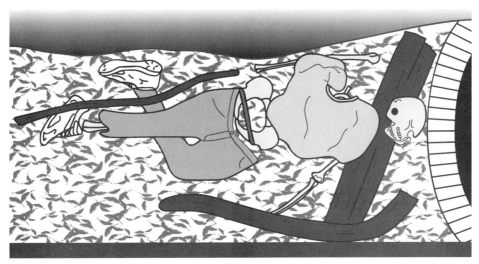

Figure A-1. Sketch map of the remains within the cement drainage channel. The channel is partially filled with wood and leaves and there is an adjoining drainage pipe near the decedent's head. Map is not to scale.

skeletal analysis to determine the biological profile (age, sex, ancestry, and stature) and interpret the skeletal trauma. The biological profile would assist in the identification process and the trauma analysis would assist in the medical examiner's determination of the cause and manner of death. Of particular concern for the medical examiner was to determine if the individual was beaten (homicide), struck by a train (accident or suicide), fell/jumped from the top of the wall (accident or suicide), or whether he could have been pushed or thrown from the wall (homicide).

While examining the remains with the medical examiner, several personal items were discovered within the pockets of the clothing; however, no identification media was located. During the maceration process, the anthropologists removed the remaining tissue from the bones and discovered a cell phone SIM card embedded within a piece of adipocere. The SIM card was turned over to NYPD detectives for their investigation.

All small bones and bone fragments were removed from the soft tissue during maceration of the remains. The resultant skeletal inventory showed that the recovery had been nearly complete, with the exception of the hyoid, sternal body, left patella, coccyx, diaphysis fragments of the right fibula, and several small hand and foot bones (Figure A-2). Several elements demonstrated evidence of rodent activity, which is possibly the reason for some of the aforementioned missing skeletal elements. In addition, there was a small amount of water running underneath the body and into a drainage pipe, which could also have resulted in the displacement and loss of some of the smaller skeletal

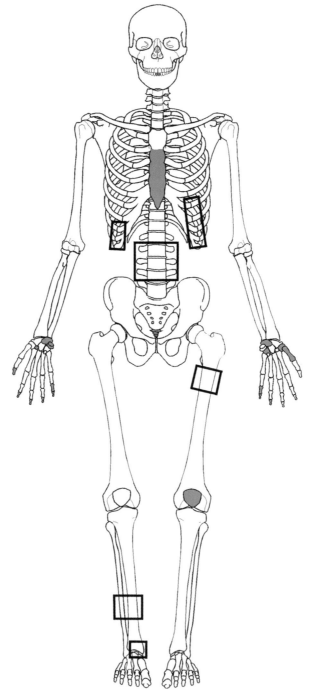

Figure A-2. Skeletal diagram indicating main areas of trauma (boxes) and missing skeletal elements (gray).

elements. The overall condition of the remains, the presence of very greasy bones, and the odor of decomposition suggested that the postmortem interval was likely less than one year prior to the date of discovery. Following maceration, a complete anthropological examination of the remains was performed to develop the biological profile and fully document the trauma.

The remains were consistent with a European (white) or Hispanic male, 25 to 35 years of age, who stood approximately 65.7 to 72 inches tall. One idiosyncratic feature present was bilateral *os acromiale* of the scapulae. No antemortem skeletal trauma was present; however, as determined during the preliminary field assessment, perimortem trauma was present on numerous postcranial elements. No perimortem trauma was noted on the cranium. The postcranial fracture characteristics were typical of blunt force trauma and the pattern suggested that they most likely occurred as the result of one traumatic event.

During the course of the anthropological evaluation, NYPD detectives were able to obtain information based on data recovered from the cell phone SIM card, which linked it to a specific individual. Further investigation showed that this person had never been reported missing, although his whereabouts were unknown. While NYPD detectives set out to gather more information based on the SIM card lead, the OCME anthropologists continued with their evaluation of the skeletal trauma.

Perimortem Trauma

Multiple areas of perimortem trauma were present on the postcranial skeleton, mostly focused on the lower part of the body (Figure A-2). The following perimortem fractures were noted:

Axial Skeleton

1. Buckle fractures (fractures resulting from compressive instability) were located near the sternal ends of right ribs 8, 9, 10, 11, and left ribs 6, 7, 8, 9, 10, 11 (Figure A-3). The transverse fracture lines are located on the pleural aspects of the ribs with the sternal end "buckling," or compressing into itself, producing internal displacement (Love and Symes 2004).
2. Lumbar vertebral bodies 2 through 4 demonstrate compression fractures, with the more extensive damage located on the 2nd lumbar vertebra (Figure A-4). The 2nd lumbar also contains a complete transverse fracture of the left lamina. Associated with the trauma to the 2nd and 3rd lumbar vertebrae is plastic deformation, which is common in blunt force injuries to bone (Galloway and Zephro 2005, Porta, 2005).

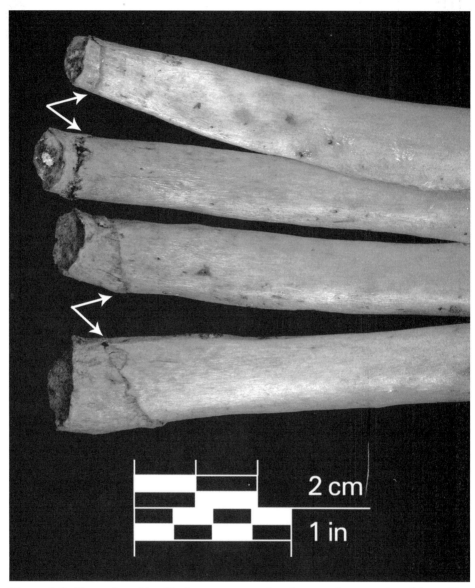

Figure A-3. Examples of buckle fractures on right ribs near the sternal end (noted by arrows). Pleural/posterior surface of the ribs pictured.

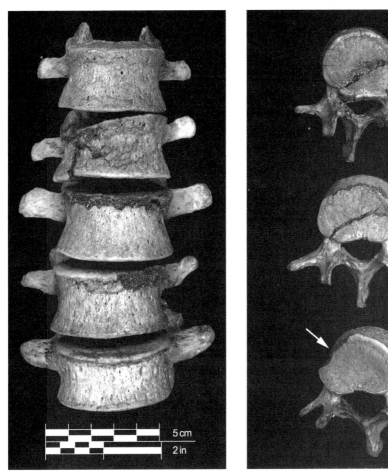

Figure A-4. Lumbar vertebral fractures. Image on left shows the anterior view with fractures to L2–L4. Image on the right shows the superior view of L2–L4 with the main fracture locations noted by arrows.

Appendicular Skeleton

1. An incomplete linear fracture is present on the base of one of the proximal hand phalanges.
2. The left proximal femur exhibits a spiral fracture below the lesser trochanter (Figure A-5). This fracture bifurcates on the posterior surface producing a comminuted fracture.
3. The right distal third of the tibia diaphysis contains a comminuted butterfly fracture with multiple radiating fractures (Figure A-6).
4. The right medial malleolus of the tibia demonstrates a complete transverse fracture with one longitudinal fracture propagating from the fracture

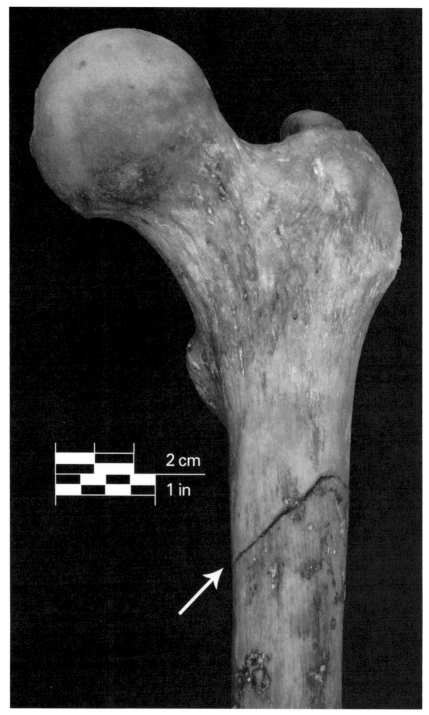

Figure A-5. Spiral fracture of the left proximal femur (noted by arrow). Scale in centimeters.

margin (Figure A-6). The fractured tip of the malleolus was not recovered from the scene.

5. The right fibula contains a comminuted fracture of the diaphysis adjacent to the fracture location on the paired tibia (Figure A-6). The superior fracture line is transverse, while the inferior fracture line is slightly oblique. The fibula demonstrates slight plastic deformation; however, a section of bone was not recovered which would have allowed further evaluation of the extent of the deformation.

6. The talus exhibits a comminuted fracture on the postero-lateral aspect of the trochlea (Figure A-7), likely due to compression contact with the tibia and fibula.

Overall, the fracture patterns suggest trauma as result of one traumatic event. The location and morphology of these types of perimortem fractures are not typical of injuries from an assault, nor would they be expected from an impact with a train. Their location and morphology are consistent with trauma seen in falls from heights (Lowenstein *et al.* 1989, Richter *et al.* 1996, Christensen 2004, Atanasijevic *et al.* 2005) with an impact on the feet. Research indicates that feet-first falls produce injuries to the lower extremities followed by compression fractures to the lumbar region, specifically at the thoracolumbar junction (Tomczak and Buikstra 1999, Christensen 2004).

The location of the rib fractures provides further information as to the amount of force and position of the body. If the transmission of force is directed up through the feet, the upper ribs (1–3) would be well protected and require extreme forces in order to fracture. The rib fractures present in this case involved ribs 6 through 11. In falls from substantial heights, unilateral and bilateral rib fractures often occur. According to Atanasijevic and colleagues (2005) the highest percent of rib fractures observed in 660 forensic cases occurred in falls from 12 to 15 meters (approximately 39 to 49 feet). In the present case, the wall measures 50 feet in the area where the body was discovered. The vertical deceleration blunt force injuries documented on the decedent are consistent with trauma as result of a fall from this height. Impact from a train would have likely resulted in more widespread fractures (e.g., upper extremities and head) and a different fracture mechanism would be apparent (e.g., horizontal deceleration vs. vertical deceleration) (Galloway and Zephro 2005). The cranium and pelvis are more frequently fractured in horizontal deceleration injuries (e.g., auto-pedestrian accidents) and it would not be typical to see compression fractures like those observed on the lumber vertebrae. The individual in this case example exhibited no cranial or pelvic trauma, which further supports a vertical deceleration fracture mechanism. According to Gupta and colleagues (1982), the frequency of cranial injuries actually decreases in falls above 40 feet. Atanasijevic and colleagues (2005) also found that only about 50% of their

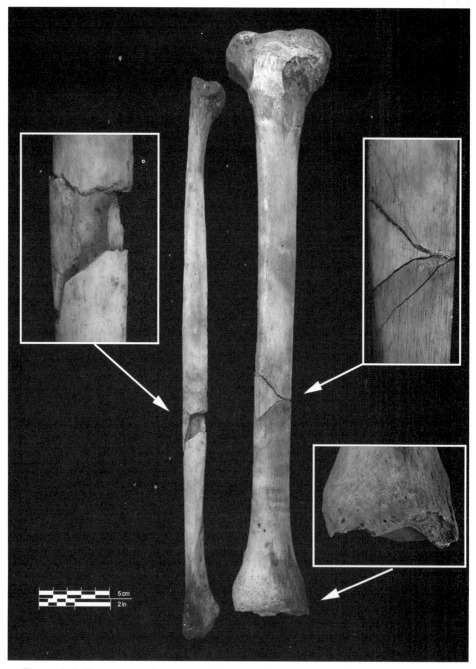

Figure A-6. Perimortem fractures of the right tibia and fibula (after reconstruction).

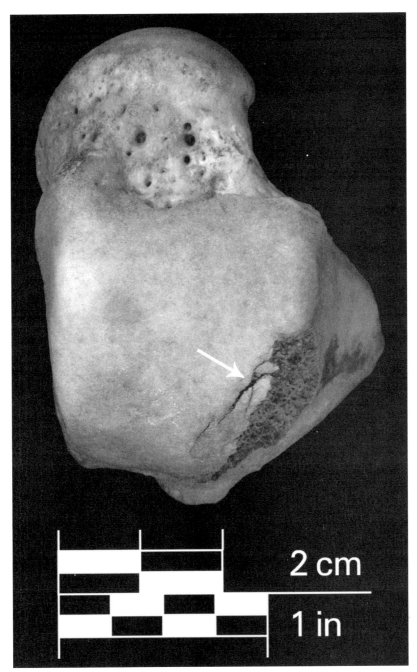

Figure A-7. Fracture of the right talus (location noted by arrow). Scale in millimeters.

cases of falls from 50 ft. had head injuries (head injuries were most frequent in falls below 7 meters and over 30 meters). This may be the result of the individual's behavioral response during the fall or simply the natural tendency for the body to change position during a free fall (Christensen 2004). The trauma observed on the lower extremities, especially the medial malleolus of the tibia and associated fracture on the talus, are typical of a feet-first vertical deceleration event (Teh *et al.* 2003). This trauma would not be expected from a horizontal deceleration event, such as an impact by a vehicle or train. While the butterfly fractures of the tibia and fibula and the subtrochanteric fracture of the femur observed in this case may be considered typical of horizontal deceleration injuries, fractures of this type from vertical deceleration events may actually result from bending loads despite their axial nature (Porta 2005). Galloway and Zephro (2005) also note that subtrochanteric femur fractures may occur in feet-first falls. Considering this, as well as the compression fractures of the vertebrae and talus, it is possible to differentiate this trauma as result of a fall from height versus impact from a train.

Based on the anthropological analysis of the fractures, it seemed compelling that the individual died as the result of a feet-first impact from a height (vertical deceleration event). Additional information, however, would be needed in order to help the medical examiner determine the manner of death (homicide, suicide, or accident).

IDENTIFICATION AND CERTIFICATION OF DEATH

In May 2007, the OCME anthropologists and the medical examiner returned to the scene in order inspect that area further (Figure A-8). With the trauma findings indicative of a fall from the top of the 50-foot wall, it became important to determine if the person could have been pushed, fallen, or intentionally jumped. Alongside the top of the wall was an 8-foot fence that ran the length of the wall, with the exception of a nearby viewing area that was protected by a decorative stone half-wall. In order for the individual to end up where he was discovered, he would need to have climbed the fence or accessed the wall's ledge from the nearby viewing area. Based on the height of the fence, it was clear that it would not be feasible for the individual to have been pushed or thrown from the top of the wall. This suggested either an accidental fall or an intentional jump.

The NYPD investigation of the cell phone SIM card traced it to a 34-year-old Hispanic male that had not been seen since May 2006. Further investigation revealed that the decedent had last been seen during the nighttime when he and another individual were pulled over by the police during a routine traffic stop. During an inspection of the vehicle, a loaded gun was discovered, and

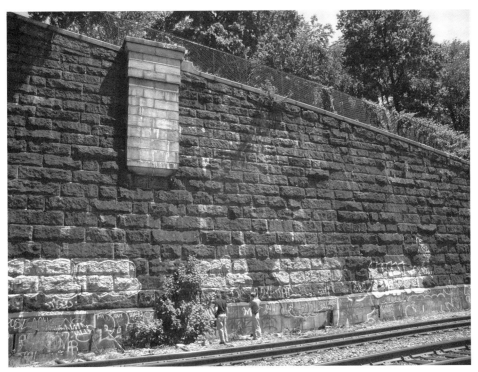

Figure A-8. View of the wall taken during daylight. Drs. Adams and Crowder are standing next to the drainage channel where the remains were recovered. The eight-foot tall fence is visible on top of the wall.

the decedent fled on foot from the police. He ran into a nearby wooded area and eluded capture from the police despite a search by additional personnel on foot and by air. The location of the traffic stop and the wooded area where the individual fled are in the same general area where the body was discovered. The biological profile constructed from the skeletal remains was consistent with the missing individual, and a comparison of antemortem and postmortem dental radiographs led to a positive identification of the remains.

The man was never officially reported missing by his family because they were under the impression that he was still in hiding from the authorities. In reality, it appears that during his nighttime flight from the police, the man scaled the fence and jumped over, not realizing that there was a 50ft. drop on the other side. It is also feasible that he accessed the top of the wall from the overlook and lost his footing as he navigated along the narrow ledge between the fence and the drop-off to the railroad tracks. Regardless of the scenario, anthropological findings coupled with the scene investigation and background information allowed the medical examiner to determine the manner of death as "accident" and the cause as "fall from height during police pursuit."

CONCLUSION

This case exemplifies how the anthropological assessment and interpretation of perimortem trauma often play an important role in assisting medical examiners with the determination of cause and manner of death. Several potential scenarios were initially possible to explain the positioning of the body at the scene and the presence of skeletal trauma. Anthropological analysis and scene investigation by the OCME, along with good detective work by NYPD personnel, allowed for the circumstances surrounding this individual's death to be fully understood.

Acknowledgements

We wish to acknowledge Dr. Roger Mitchell, who was the Medical Examiner assigned to this case, for his assistance. We would also like to thank Chris Rainwater for creating Figure A-1.

B. RIB FRACTURES IN THE ELDERLY: A CASE STUDY USING MICROSCOPIC ANALYSIS TO DETERMINE INJURY TIMING

LAUREN ZEPHRO AND ALISON GALLOWAY

The correct interpretation of fracture timing is an essential component of skeletal trauma analysis. The following case report details the discovery and skeletal-trauma analysis of an elderly female. This case illustrates the essential role of microscopy in identifying antemortem fractures even in cases where the gross fracture appears to be clearly interpretable. In addition, this case illustrates the necessity of extracting and cleaning bones prior to skeletal-trauma analysis. Imaging methods, like radiology, may miss subtle skeletal trauma especially when a body is in a non-traditional position.

DISCOVERY

In the early summer of 2001, the mummified remains of an elderly female were discovered in the home the decedent shared with her daughter. The remains were discovered during a welfare check, which was requested by a federal employee trying to contact the decedent about her retirement benefits. The decedent's pension checks, which had not been cashed, had been suspended pending confirmation of her whereabouts and welfare. Upon calling the house, the federal employee spoke with the daughter, who was uncooperative and would not divulge the current whereabouts of her mother. Alarmed, the federal employee contacted police to check the welfare of the woman.

When the officer arrived at the last known address of the mother, he approached the house, knocked on the door, and received no response. He then requested that dispatch call the residence and, again, there was no answer. The officer proceeded to contact the immediate neighbors to gain insight into the situation. Neighbors reported that the daughter of the woman seemed mentally unstable but felt confident that she could take care of her mother.

327

The neighbors also reported that they had not seen the mother in several years but that when questioned, the daughter reported that her mother was well. One neighbor reported that she heard a rumor that the mother was living with relatives on the East Coast.

Later that same day, the officer was able to make contact with the daughter. Upon hearing that the pension board was suspending her mother's checks, the daughter responded that her mother did not want anything to do with the checks or the pension board and thought it was a possible scam. When pressed as to the whereabouts of her mother, the daughter responded that the next day she would look for and give the officer the mother's phone number. After repeated requests for the information, the officer convinced the daughter to go into the house and retrieve the phone number. The daughter returned to the door approximately three times to report that she could not find the number. In the meantime, another officer arrived at the scene and began looking around the front of the residence. The second officer, looking through a window located on the front left side of the residence, saw what appeared to be the outline of a body on a bed covered in blankets. Meanwhile, dispatch received information from an out-of-state family member that the mother was supposed to be living with her daughter. Given the daughter's inability to produce the mother or the mother's current whereabouts and the scene observations made by the officers, the officers requested to enter the house. Although the daughter was initially resistant, she eventually let the officers inside. Once inside the residence, the officers confirmed that the shape under the blankets was a decaying human body. The thick layer of dust and cobwebs present in the bedroom suggested that there had been little to no activity in the room for a very long time. The decedent was lying in bed and positioned on her right side in a fetal position. The body was fully clothed and covered in bedding. The decedent's body had decomposed into the mattress and bedding and there were maggot casings in and around the body. The remains were encased in desiccated tissue and were in anatomical position. There were no obvious signs of trauma.

The daughter admitted that the corpse was that of her mother. According to the daughter, her mother had passed away six years prior, and she had not told anybody. She stated that her mother had been sick but had not sought medical attention. The daughter was afraid to tell anyone and, after the death of her mother, never let anyone inside the house again. Central to the investigation were concerns of abuse, neglect, fraud, and homicide.

INITIAL EXAMINATION

A forensic pathologist performed the initial examination of the remains. Examination revealed that the body was fully clothed in undergarments and multiple layers of outerwear, stockings, and two pairs of socks. The left sleeve of the decedent's sweatshirt was filled with used Kleenex tissue. Her underpants contained a rag-type material that was soaked with dried purge fluid. A metallic ring set with a clear stone was present on her left fourth finger. The skeleton was mostly covered in intact, mummified dermis, especially on the posterior surface of the body. The fingernails were intact and the scalp had intact matted gray hair that measured approximately 10 inches in length. The condition of the body was consistent with the decedent dying in bed and having been undisturbed for years. Full body radiographs revealed no bone fractures. Following the pathologist's examination, the remains were submitted to the Forensic Osteology Investigations Laboratory at the University of California, Santa Cruz, for forensic anthropological assessment of skeletal trauma.

ANTHROPOLOGICAL EXAMINATION

The remains were examined as they arrived (Figure B-1) and bones were extracted and cleaned with heated water and detergent. All bones were inspected grossly followed by low-powered stereomicroscopy with oblique lighting.

The remains were consistent with those of an elderly adult female, based on the presence of a ventral arch and long pubic bone, although it was noted that the subpubic angle was not very wide and the sacrum was markedly curved. Age was estimated to be elderly (60 years or older) based on the morphology of the pubic symphyseal surface and overall arthritis and loss of bone density (the skeleton was very light and friable). Ancestry was assessed as primarily "European," as indicated by a narrow nasal bridge and aperture, slanting orbits, and retreating zygomatics. Stature interval was estimated between 5'5" to 5'9½" based on long bone lengths, but significant height loss due to age must be acknowledged.

The skeletal remains contained a number of anomalies and pathological conditions although the bone was remarkably well preserved for a woman of the reported age of the decedent (94 years at the time of death). Only 11 ribs were present on the left side and the 12th rib on the right was extremely small (approximately 3.5 cm). The clavicles were of an unusual morphology although this was present bilaterally. There was eburnation of the odontoid process and dens facet of C1–2. The right articular facets of the C2–3 joint showed degradation of the joint surface. The fourth and fifth cervical vertebrae were fused along the left posterior side. The centra of the cervical vertebrae were extensively pitted on the superior and inferior surfaces, suggestive of degenerative disk disease. Arthritic changes were evident on the wrists and hand bones. The hyoid bone was bilaterally unfused and the ossified thyroid cartilage was discontinuous with a gap to the left of the midline.

Trauma

Examination of the skeleton revealed two distinct periods of antemortem trauma present on the ribs.

- There was a well-healed rib fracture on the vertebral end of left rib #10 (Figure B-2). There was excessive bony growth on the inferior margin of left rib #9 located near the angle of the rib. Left ribs 5 through 8 showed additional bony growths but to a lesser degree. This is consistent with a prior injury that had since healed but there was bony invasion of the healing region to other bones in close proximity.
- Recent antemortem skeletal trauma consisted of two broken ribs on the right side, ribs 4 and 5 (Figures B-3, B-4, B-5, B-6), and one fracture on the left rib #11 (Figures B-7, B-8a and b). The sternal ends of right ribs 4 and 5 displayed complete fractures. Left rib 11 exhibited a complete mid-shaft fracture. These breaks were not attributable to the perimortem or postmortem periods, as under magnification, bony remodeling was visible adjacent to the fracture margins. The presence of small amounts of woven bone suggests the beginning of bony callus formation and most likely indicates a time frame of 10 days to a month between the time of injury and the time of death. The fractures to right ribs 4 and 5 and left rib 11, given their anatomical placement and fracture locations, indicated at least two separate points of impact. One impact could have fractured both right ribs 4 and 5 while a second would be needed to fracture left rib 11.

No perimortem trauma or postmortem damage was noted on the bones.

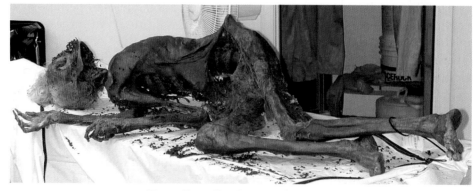

Figure B-1. Condition of the body.

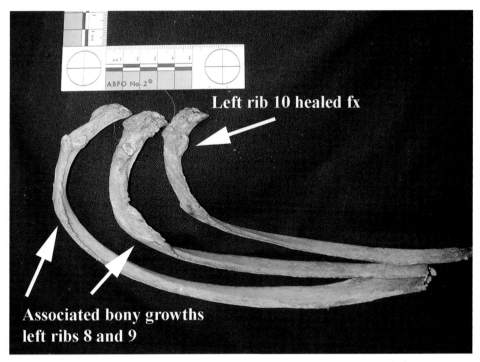

Figure B-2. Antemortem fractures to left ribs 8, 9, and 10. Bottom of scale bar is in cm.

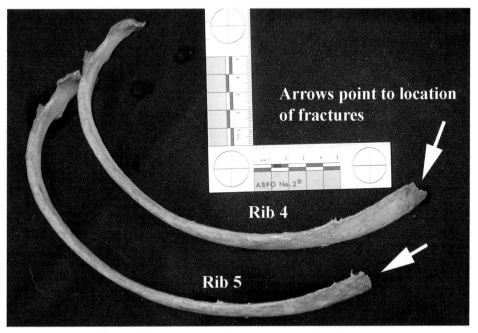

Figure B-3. Location of fractures, right ribs 4 and 5.

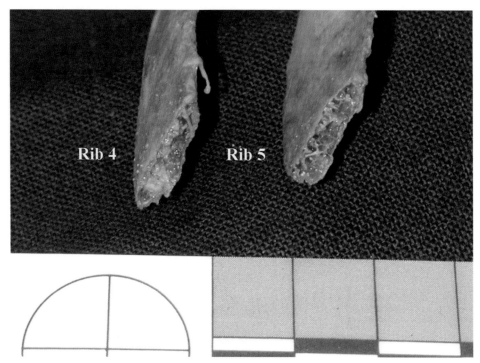

Figure B-4. Close-up of fracture margins, right ribs 4 and 5. Scale bar is in cm.

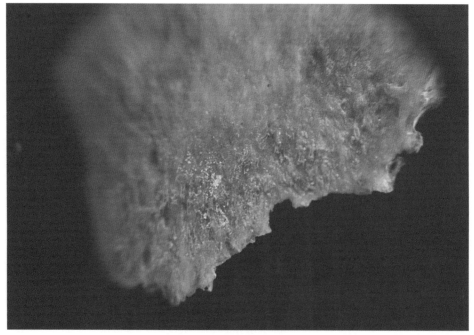

Figure B-5. Initial bone callous, right rib 4. Magnified approximately 6×, with oblique lighting.

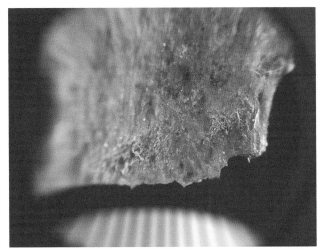

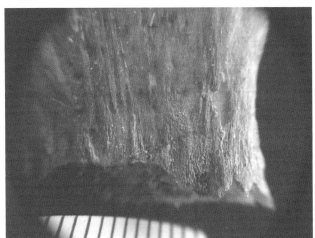

Figure B-6. Initial bone callous, right rib 5. Magnified approximately 6×, with oblique lighting. Scale bar is in mm.

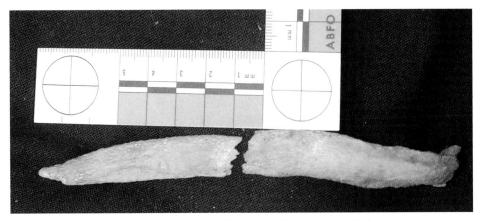

Figure B-7: Location of fracture, left rib 11. Bottom of scale bar is in cm.

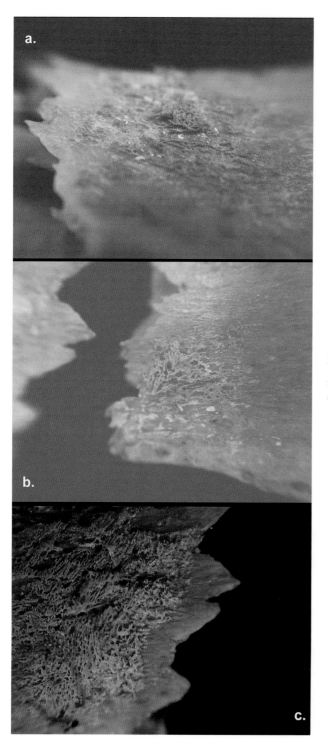

Figures B-8a, b, and c. Initial bone callus, left rib 11. Magnified approximately 6×, with oblique lighting.

DISCUSSION

Two important observations emerged from this case. First, radiology may not give full visualization of bone fractures, especially in cases where body position is flexed or the fractures are subtle. Second, remodeling on ribs may not be recognizable without the aid of a stereomicroscope. Upon initial examination, these fractures appeared to be peri- or postmortem. Given the fragility of the elderly skeleton and postmortem conditions of the body, distinguishing the difference between perimortem trauma and postmortem damage would have been difficult, if not impossible based solely on gross examination of the fractures. No tension or compression fracture characteristics were observable on the fracture margins and the bone quality, due to the very advanced age of the descendent, was very degraded and comparatively more brittle than younger bone. The poor quality of the bone likely contributed to the brittle appearance and the complete nature of the fractures. No buckling was observed. In the current case, the coroner ruled the death "undetermined" and no charges were filed against the daughter. However, the daughter did receive the attention of mental health professionals.

C. POSTCRANIAL FRACTURES IN CHILD ABUSE: ILLUSTRATED WITH A CASE STUDY

Jennifer C. Love

THE CASE

On July 2, 2006, a three-month-old female was rushed to the children's hospital after being found "gasping for breath" by the mother. Thirty minutes prior the mother had breast fed the infant and placed her supine in a bassinet. After finding the infant in distress, the mother initiated bystander CPR. The paramedics responded to the scene and found the infant asystolic and apneic. The paramedics continued CPR until they reached the emergency department. Twenty minutes after arrival, the attending physician declared the infant dead.

The infant had been born by a normal spontaneous vaginal delivery at 40 weeks gestation. Her perinatal and follow-up physical examinations were normal. The infant's last pediatric visit was at two months of age. She appeared healthy and at a normal developmental stage and received her first set of vaccinations. There was no previous history of Child Protective Services involvement with the family. The home was in disarray with clothes, dirty dishes, and stale food found throughout, but the infant's bassinet was very clean and orderly. The medicolegal investigator did note that the bassinet mattress was softer than average. In sum, there were no stark warning signs of child abuse at the scene or during the events leading to the death of the infant.

Once the autopsy began, subtle signs of maltreatment began to surface. The pathologist noted that the infant appeared well fed and measured at a normal height and weight. She was clean and her hair and nails were well maintained. Several small abrasions, ranging in size from $\frac{1}{4}$ to 1 inch were found on her neck. Several focal small subscalpular contusions, ranging in size from $\frac{1}{8}$ to 1 inch, were found on the head. A pair of small abrasions with associated subcutaneous hemorrhage was found on the superior aspect of the right shoulder. On the lower extremities, a pattern of four contusions, ranging in size from ¹⁄₁₆ to ¹⁄₄ inch and arranged in a curvilinear pattern, were located along the anterior surface of the right and left knees. Internally, all organs appeared normal and without injury.

Given the few, but unexpected contusions and the history of "found gasping for breath," the pathologist requested a full skeletal examination by the forensic anthropologist. The skeletal examination was performed following the method described by Love and Sanchez (2009). The muscles and underlying periostea were partially resected from the long bones, clavicles, and scapulae. The pleurae and intercostal muscles were removed from the internal surface of the ribs. The periosteum was removed from the ectocranium and the dura mater was removed from the endocranium. The exposed bones were examined.

Rib Fractures

Once the pleurae were stripped, posterior and lateral healing rib fractures were immediately apparent. Rib fractures, more than any other fractures in infants and children, are recognized as strong indicators of non-accidental injury (Pandya *et al.* 2009, Bulloch *et al.* 2000, Barsness *et al.* 2003, Spevak *et al.* 1994, Garcia *et al.* 1990, Feldman and Brewer 1984, Kleinman *et al.* 1996, Kleinman and Schlesinger 1997, Mandelstam *et al.* 2003, Smeets *et al.* 1990, Gunther *et al.* 2000, Maguire *et al.* 2006, Dolinak 2007). Of the various locations of rib fractures – posterior, lateral and anterior – posterior rib fractures (typically at the head and tubercle) are the most prevalent and most commonly caused by non-accidental injury (Barsness *et al.* 2003, Bulloch *et al.* 2000, Kleinman *et al.* 1996, Kleinman 1998, Kleinman and Schlesinger 1997, Bulloch *et al.* 2000, Weber *et al.* 2009, Betz and Liebhardt 1994). Posterior rib fractures are often multiple, arranged in a serial pattern, and bilateral (Kleinman 1998). Kleinman and colleagues (1996) found that of 84 rib fractures identified in 31 victims of non-accidental injury, 53 (63%) fractures were located in the posterior region of the rib. Bulloch *et al.* (2000), examining 32 cases with rib fractures, also found that posterior rib fractures were more common than anterior rib fractures, but these researchers found no significant difference in location of the fracture between non-accidental and accidental injury.

Mechanisms postulated to cause posterior rib fractures include avulsive forces applied to the rib head and posterior levering of the rib over the transverse process of the thoracic vertebra (Kleinman 1998, Bulloch *et al.* 2000, Schweich and Fleisher 1985, Weber *et al.* 2009). Kleinman and colleagues (1996) and others (Kleinman and Schlesinger 1997, Kleinman 1998, Bulloch *et al.* 2000) found that when the chest is forced posteriorly, a classic level 1 lever is formed at or near the costovertebral articulation point (the rib tubercle and vertebral transverse process). The costovertebral ligaments are stronger than the bone and excessive forces result in the failure of the rib in the region of the rib

head, neck, and tubercle. Kleinman (1998) describes, based on animal experimentation and assailant testimony, posterior rib fractures result when an
adult holds an infant by the chest while squeezing the thorax in the anteroposterior plane (possibly while shaking the infant). The infant is held facing
the adult with the adult's palms on the infant's sides, fingers on the back, and
thumbs near the midline of the chest. He also postulates that similar forces occur
when the chest is forced onto a broad surface while the back is unsupported.
Kleinman and Schlesinger (1997) report posterior rib fractures do not occur
when the anterior chest is compressed while the back is supported.

Lateral rib fractures, fractures located lateral to the tubercle and medial to
the mid clavicular line, are considered the least indicative of non-accidental
trauma. The primary reasons for the diminished specificity for non-accidental
injury are twofold: the region is more vulnerable to direct impacts (possibly as
a result of an accident); and forces associated with cardiopulmonary resuscitation (CPR) can affect the region (Bulloch *et al.* 2000, Schweich and Fleisher
1985, Weber *et al.* 2009, Betz and Liebhardt 1994, Feldman and Brewer
1984). (See Cardiopulmonary Resuscitation Fractures below.) Fractures that
are located at the most lateral point of the rib body are postulated to be the
result of anteroposterior compression that causes the bone to fail in tension
(Worn 2007). The morphologic features of an acute fracture in this region are the
best indicator as to the mechanism of force, i.e., anteroposterior compression
or direct blow (Kleinman 1998).

The anterior region of the rib, the area from the mid-clavicular line medial
through the sternal face of the rib, is vulnerable to direct blows as well as anteroposterior compression. Two fracture types are commonly found in this area:
buckle fractures of the rib body and costochondral junction (CCJ) fractures.
Kleinman *et al.* (1996) found that CCJ fractures are analogous to classic metaphyseal lesions (CML). (See Long Bones Fractures below for full description
of a CML). The fracture is a result of tractional forces applied to the chondro-
osseous joint as the chest is compressed, causing the trabeculae to fail and the
sternal face to separate from the rib as a thin disk of bone attached to the
costal cartilage. Kleinman (1998) theorizes that CCJ fractures are a result of
depression of the sternum and/or cartilages during CPR. However, several
other researchers have found that CCJs are not a result of CPR. Weber *et al.*
(2009) reviewed 546 autopsies of sudden unexpected death in infancy and
found rib fractures in 24 cases. Four CCJ fractures were identified, all were
associated with healing rib fractures and none were associated with CPR.
Smeets *et al.* (1990) reported on a single case of a nine-month-old girl with a
history of a fall two days prior to presenting at the First Aid Department of a
hospital. During a radiological examination, posterior rib fractures, cranial
fractures, and CMLs were identified. During a sonogram of the chest and
abdomen, costochondral distraction of the lower left ribs in association with

subcutaneous hematoma was identified. Based on the findings, a diagnosis of battered child syndrome was made. In addition, Ng and Hall (1998) reviewed three case studies (7-, 18-, 36-month-old children) and found a total of 10 CCJ fractures. The fractures involved ribs 6–9, were bilateral in two cases, and were not associated with CPR.

CPR fractures are rare in children, but when they do occur, they are typically buckle fractures located along the mid-clavicular line of the rib (Weber *et al.* 2009, Love and Symes 2004, Betz and Liebhardt 1994, Feldman and Brewer 1984). Buckle fractures are incomplete, linear fractures that result from a failure in compression (Love and Symes 2004). The fractures are typically serially and bilaterally distributed along the mid-range ribs (3rd–6th). *In situ*, there is often no to very little hemorrhage associated with the injury.

Fractures of the first rib have received special attention in the literature (Kleinman 1998, Strouse and Owings 1995, Vikramaditya 2001, Schweich and Fleisher 1985). The first rib is uniquely located within the chest. It is positioned under the shoulder girdle and therefore protected from direct blows. Strouse and Owings (1995) state that the first rib typically fractures through the subclavian groove, a weak point of the rib. They and others infer that the bone often fails due to muscle contractions associated with violent shaking (Strouse and Owings 1995, Vikramaditya 2001, Schweich and Fleisher 1985). Vikramaditya (2001) reported two cases of isolated 1st rib fractures identified in adolescents after vigorous activity. He attributed the fractures to be the result of stress generated from opposite forces exhibited by the scalene and serratus muscles.

THE CASE

As a result of the recognition of the rib fractures *in situ*, all 24 ribs were removed from the decedent. Left rib 7 and the anterior portion of left rib 6 were retained for histopathological examination. The remaining ribs were processed in a water-soap bath following standard macerating process (Love and Sanchez 2009). A total of 24 rib fractures were identified. The fractures were located at the CCJ of right ribs 3–8 and left ribs 1–9, neck of right ribs 5–7 and left ribs 6–8, lateral region of right rib 7 and left rib 6–8, and the anterior region of right rib 6 (Figure C-1.) Additionally, while a swell of subperiosteal new bone formation (SPNBF) was present on the internal surface of right rib 5, no fracture was associated with the SPNBF. All the fractures were healing and were found to be in one of two healing stages, organizing bone callus or open fractures with minimal SPNBF. The CCJ fractures were also healing, as evidenced by the thickened trabeculae and lacy bone of the periphery.

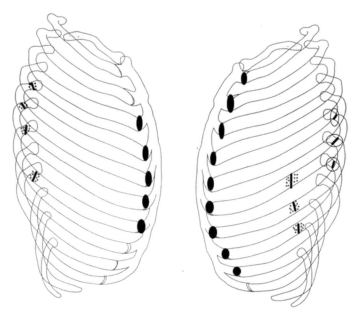

Figure C-1. Distribution of fractures observed on the ribs. Stippling surrounding fractures represent SPNBF. Encircled fractures represent large fracture calluses. The blackened costo-chondral junctions (CCJs) are fractured.

Long Bone Fractures

The skeletal examination of the long bones revealed classic metaphyseal lesions (CMLs) at numerous locations and a relatively thick layer of SPNBF along the shaft of all the long bones. A CML is considered the long bone fracture with the greatest specificity to non-accidental injury (Johnson 2009, Kleinman 1998, Kleinman and Marks 1995, Kleinman and Marks 1996). It is a trans-metaphyseal disruption of trabeculae of the primary spongiosa, and occurs when indirect torsional or tractional forces are applied to an extremity. The delicate nature of the immature trabeculae, the loose attachment of the periosteum to the diaphysis and the firm attachment of the perichrondrium to the epiphysis all contribute to the bone failing at the specific location (Kleinman 1998, Leonidas 1983; Worlock *et al.* 1986, Pierce *et al.* 2004, Johnson 2009). The loose periosteum transmits most of the dynamic force associated with the trauma to the metaphysis where the trabeculae of the primary spongiosa are weaker than the cartilage of the epiphysis (Kleinman 1998, Leonidas 1983). CML are most common during the first and second years of life (Kleinman 1998).

CMLs are considered specific for non-accidental injury primarily because the forces associated with the trauma are not typically generated during a fall

(Leonidas 1983, Klienman 1998, Johnson 2009). Kleinman *et al.* (1995) examined 31 victims of child abuse and found 64 CMLs. They reported the most common sites for a CML are the proximal and distal tibia and the distal femur. Worlock *et al.* (1986) retrospectively compared children with non-accidental injuries to children with accidental injuries. The authors found 17 CMLs, which all were observed in cases of non-accidental injury in which the child was under the age of 18 months. They concluded that CMLs are not a very common fracture, making up only 17% of the fractures recorded in the non-accidental injury cases, but that they are only seen in abuse cases. Conversely, Caffey (1957) noted that birth trauma, especially breech delivery, may result in CML.

Historically, CMLs have been called bucket handle or corner fractures. The terminology is based on the radiological appearance of the fractures. The forces cause the physeal surface of the bone to separate from the metaphysis creating a disk-shaped fragment of bone that remains adhered to the epiphysis. Typically the disk is thicker along the periphery and thinner in the middle. Radiographically, the fracture appears as a line or a translucency through the metaphysis that dips deeper into the metaphysis at the edges of the bone, hence the bucket handle or corner fracture appearance (Kleinman *et al.* 1985, Kleinman and Marks 1995, Kleinman and Marks 1996).

Shaft, metaphyseal, and epiphyseal fractures are not considered specific for non-accidental injury. The long bone fractures observed in children are similar to the long bone fractures observed in adults and the mechanism of injury is also similar. The two exceptions are CML (discussed above) and epiphyseal separations. Epiphyseal separations, in contrast to CMLs, are primarily cartilaginous injuries, although they can extend into the bone. Epiphyseal separation occurs more often with accidental injury, especially in older children. Salter and Harris (1963) studied these fractures experimentally induced in rabbits and identified five types (see Chapter 5). Types I and III involve only the cartilage. Type II and IV extend into the metaphysis in a similar pattern as a CML. Type V involves the chondro-osseous interface (see Figure 5-3). Kleinmen (1998) hypothesizes that given some of the shared features between CML and epiphyseal separation, the forces causing these injuries are similar and the level of force determines if the failure is a CML or an epiphyseal separation.

No long bone fracture type is pathognomonic for non-accidental injury. Differentiating accidental from non-accidental long bone fractures is dependent on age and developmental stage of the child and the history of the traumatic event as well as type and location of the fracture (Lonergan *et al.* 2003, Pierce 2004, Rex and Kay 2000, Skellern 2000, Thomas 1991, Taitz 2004, Kemp *et al.* 2008). Several researchers have found a significant relationship between cause of an injury, accidental or non-accidental, and age of the child (Strait 1995, Worlock *et al.* 1986, Pierce *et al.* 2004, Taitz *et al.* 2004, Johnson 2009, Pandya *et al.* 2009, Loder and Feinberg 2007, Schwend *et al.* 2000). Pandya *et al.* (2009) compared 500 child abuse victims to 985 accidental injury cases (ages birth to 48 months) and found that the odds of a tibia/fibula fracture are 12.8 times, humeral fracture 2.3 times, and femoral fracture 1.8 times more likely the result of child abuse if the child is younger than 18 months. Conversely, in children 18 months and older, the occurrence of humeral fractures and femur fractures were 3.4 and 3.3 times more likely the result of an accidental injury. Pierce *et al.* (2004), through a literature review, found that among infants 40–80% of long bone fractures are from abuse. Coffey *et al.* (2005) conducted a retrospective study of a regional pediatric trauma center and found that 67% of lower extremity fractures in patients less than 18 months were linked to child abuse, while only 1% of lower extremity fractures in patients 18 months and older were linked to child abuse.

Researchers have attempted to identify trends in the location and type of fractures resulting from non-accidental injury. Kemp *et al.* (2008) conducted a thorough literature review in an attempt to identify criteria useful in distinguishing fractures resulting from accidental and non-accidental injury. They included studies that reported skeletal trauma in children less than 18 years old and found that the probability of abuse given a humeral fracture was between 0.48 and 0.54 and a femoral fracture was 0.28 and 0.43, depending on the definition of abuse. Worlock *et al.* (1986) performed a retrospective comparison of fracture patterns observed in accidental and non-accidental injuries in children under the age of five years. They found spiral humeral fractures were significantly more common in the group of non-accidental injury ($p < 0.001$). Beals and Tufts (1983) conducted a 22-year retrospective study of femur fractures identified in children younger than three years and reported that fractures resulting from non-accidental injury tended to be buckle fractures of the distal metaphysis and proximal diaphyseal fractures. However, the most common fracture was the mid-shaft fracture, which occurred in both accidental and non-accidental injury. Additionally, Arkader *et al.* (2007) examined the occurrence of complete metaphyseal fractures of the distal femur recorded in two level-1 trauma centers over a 10-year period. They found 29 fractures of which 20 had occurred in infants. Fifteen of the 20 fractures were confirmed to be the result of child abuse or highly suspicious for abuse. The five fractures resulting from accidental injury were due to birth trauma, fall from a swing, dropped by a sibling, fall from a bed and MVA. Rewers *et al.* (2005) conducted a review of the cases entered into the Colorado Trauma Register over a four-year period. They found that among children younger than three years, falls were the most common cause of femoral fractures followed by non-accidental injury. The non-accidental femoral fractures tended to be a more distal and a combined shaft-distal pattern.

Humeral and femoral shaft fractures are documented as the most common long bone injury observed in children, both in cases of accidental and non-accidental injury. Loder and Feinberg (2007) conducted a retrospective review of child abuse cases with identified perpetrator. They sorted 1,794 abuse cases into four groups based on age: infants (birth to 1-year); toddlers (1–2 years), children (3–12 years), and adolescence (13–20 years). Forty-nine percent of all fractures occurred in the infant group, and the skull, followed by the humeral and femoral fractures were the most common. Banaszkiewicz *et al.* (2002) conducted a five-year retrospective study of medical records of infants with long bone fractures. They found 74 cases of skeletal fractures of which 46 were cranial, 14 femoral, seven humeral, and five tibial fractures. King *et al.* (1988) reviewed the chart and radiographs of 189 battered children aged one month to 13 years. A total of 429 fractures were examined. The most commonly fractured bone was the humerus, followed by the femur and tibia.

Of the long bone fractures, the humeral shaft, humeral supracondylar, and tibial shaft (Toddler) fractures are considered the most common accidental injury in infants and children (Kemp *et al.* 2008). Shaw *et al.* (1997) conducted a six-year retrospective study during which four physicians reviewed the medical charts of patients under the age of three years with humeral shaft fractures. The physicians found that 82% of the humeral shaft fractures were a result of an accidental injury. Kemp *et al.* (2008) reviewed 32 published studies of skeletal fractures in children aged less than 18 months and found supra-condylar fractures were most commonly associated with accidental injury, specifically falls. Conversely, Strait *et al.* (1995) conducted a three-year retro-spective study of children less than three years old treated for a humeral fracture. They found non-accidental injury as the cause of the humeral fracture in 36% of the patients less than 15 month of age, 20% of the fractures were supracondylar and 58% were spiral/oblique.

Accidental tibial fractures are often isolated fractures located on the mid and distal regions of the tibia. This type of fracture is classified as Childhood Accidental Spiral Tibial (CAST) fractures. Often the spiral fracture is oriented from superolateral to inferomedial. CAST fractures are most common in children aged 2–6 years. The mechanism is torque or rotational force applied to the lower extremity associated with a fall or an immobilized foot (Mellick and Ressor 1990). CAST fractures are easily recognized on radiographs. Toddler Fractures are considered a subset of CAST fractures. They are non-displaced oblique or spiral fractures of the distal tibia that are difficult to recognize on radiographs (Kleiman 1998). Mellick and Ressor (1990) conducted a prospective study of 14-months in which 10 reports of isolated spiral tibial fractures were examined and a retrospective study of five years in which social work service records of child abuse cases were reviewed. Of the 10 examined fractures, nine were due to accidental injury and were found in children ranging in age from 21 months to 44 months. The only non-accidental fracture was the result of a physical assault by a babysitter and the child was nine months old (non-ambulatory). The retrospective study identified only three CAST fractures in 33 cases of skeletal injury. Additionally, Schwend *et al.* (2000) found that spiral femoral shaft fractures were common in ambulatory children and the authors equated them with Toddler Fractures. They stated femoral shaft fractures can occur at relatively low energy levels, including low-level simple falls, and are non-specific for non-accidental injury.

THE CASE

After the skeletal examination was concluded, collimated radiographs were taken of each extremity joint. The following long bones were removed and processed: right humerus, right ulna, right and left radii, right femur, left tibia, and left fibula. CMLs were found on the distal metaphysis of the right humerus, right ulna, right and left radii, left femur, left tibia and left fibula and the proximal metaphysis of the right humerus, left femur, left tibia, and left fibula (Figure C-2). The exposed trabeculae of the CMLs were thickened and rounded indicating a period of healing. No callus formation was observed in association with any of the CMLs. Finally the shafts of all the retained long bones were encased with SPNBF.

Additionally, the higher definition radiographs showed defects consistent with CMLs on the distal left humerus, distal left ulna, right proximal, and distal tibia (none of which were retained). The defects were consistent in radiological appearance to the confirmed CMLs observed on the retained paired bones.

The distribution of the rib fractures was consistent with an anterior/posterior constriction of the chest with posterior levering of the ribs against the transverse process of the vertebral column. The long bone fractures were consistent with shear force applied to the ends of the long bones, at nearly every joint. The constellation of fractures distributed throughout the whole body was consistent with the infant being held by the thorax and shaken. The rib fractures were consistent with the squeezing and posterior levering of the chest as described by Kleinman (1998). The uniform distribution of the CML was consistent with shear forces resulting from flailing of unsupported limbs. The healing pattern was consistent with a minimum of two traumatic episodes: (1) organizing rib fracture calluses; and (2) open fractures with minimal callus formation, SPNBF covering the long bones and the thickened and rounded trabeculae of the CMLs. No perimortem trauma was observed on the retained bones.

Ultimately, the pathologist ruled the cause and manner of death as undetermined. No acute trauma, pathological condition, or toxicological findings were identified that could have caused the death. In the comment to explain

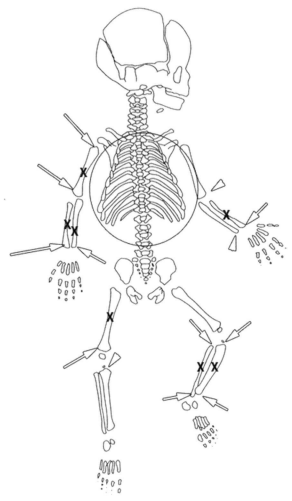

Figure C-2. Distribution of fractures throughout the decedent. Arrows mark the location of CMLs identified on processed bone. Arrowheads mark the locations of CMLs observed on the radiographs. The Xs mark the processed bones covered with SPNBF.

the classification, the pathologist acknowledged the autopsy finding indicating significant injuries at various stages of healing. She also stated an asphyxial mechanism of death could not be excluded based on the autopsy findings.

The highlighted case exemplifies a number of fracture types considered highly specific for non-accidental injury. Additionally, Kleinman (1998) identifies complex skull fractures, scapular fractures, sternal fractures, and spinal fractures as being highly specific for non-accidental injury. In contrast, he states simple skull fractures and clavicular fractures are commonly caused by accidental injury (Kleinman 1998).

Scapular Fractures

Scapular fractures in children are rare and considered highly specific for non-accidental injury (Kleinman 1998, Coote *et al.* 2000). Kleinman (1998) theorizes that scapular fractures are due to indirect forces generated by violent traction and torsion of the humerus. His theory is based on the anatomical structure of the shoulder and the concomitant pattern of fractures observed in abused children. The scapula is attached to the clavicle at the acromial and coracoid processes through the acromioclavicular and coracoclavicular ligaments. These attachments create a stable unit with the predilection for the bone to fail along the two processes. Scapular fractures are noted most often in children with typical fracture patterns involving the posterior region of the upper ribs and the shoulder girdle and are most likely the result of abnormal forces generated during shaking or abnormal rotation or traction of the upper extremity (Kleinman 1998). The most common location of a scapular fracture is the middle third of the acromion. Fractures of the corocoid and inferior glenoid margin have also been documented as a result of non-accidental injury, but are less common (Kleinman 1998).

Supporting the postulated indirect mechanism of injury, several researchers have reported avulsive fractures of the acromion resulting from muscle spasms. Kalideen and Satyapal (1994) prospectively studied 171 neonates with tetanus over a five-year period and found 10 patients with bilateral symmetrical avulsive fractures of the right and left acromial processes. Tetanus results in muscle hypertonia and spontaneous contraction of agonist/antagonist muscles. In the shoulder, the deltoid muscle abducts against the concomitant adduction forces resulting in the avulsion of the acromion. Coote *et al.* (2000) report a case of bilateral acromial fractures in a patient of malignant infantile osteopetrosis. The fractures were noted on chest films taken a day after the patient had two witnessed seizures. The authors stated that the acute deltoid muscle contraction against the weak bone resulted in the avulsive acromial fractures at the deltoid muscle attachment sites.

Sternal Fractures

Historically, sternal fractures in children have been considered highly specific for non-accidental injury. Additionally, sternal rib fractures were believed to be associated with significant blunt force injury to the thorax. Kleinman (1998) states sternal fractures are indicative of massive force, typically direct, applied to the thorax and in absence of a significant injury they should be considered suspicious for inflicted injury. However, several researchers have found sternal fractures resulting from relatively minor trauma. Hechter *et al.* (2002) conducted a retrospective review of radiographic and clinical charts of all documented sternal fractures observed over an 11-year period at a large pediatric hospital. They found 12 documented fractures; four in children under three years and eight in children over three years of age. One fracture was classified as probably and one fracture as possibly the result of non-accidental injury; the children were 1.5 and 2.5 years old, respectively. The other 10 fractures were the result of accidental injury. The most common location of the fracture was the proximal region of the *corpus sterni*, followed by the manubrium and the lower region of the *corpus sterni*. The authors concluded that the fractures of the sternum are uncommon in children but not highly specific for non-accidental injury. Ferguson *et al.* (2003) also conducted a retrospective study. They reviewed the hospital records of children who received a plain radiograph or computed tomography (CT) scan of the thorax after trauma over a 40-month period. They identified 12 cases with sternal fractures; the age range was five years to 12 years. Seven sternal fractures resulted from direct blows and five from hyperflexion. All of the fractures were isolated injuries, and none were caused by motor vehicle accidents. Eleven of the 12 fractures were non-displaced fractures of the anterior cortical of the first and second sternebrae. One direct blow resulted in a fracture at the manubriosternal joint and a posterior displacement of the *corpus sterni*. All of the accidental injuries occurred during common activity such as a fall from a trampoline or bouncy structure (4 cases), fall from bicycle (4 cases), fall from a 5–6 feet height (2 cases), and fall from a standing position (2 cases). Finally, DeFriend and Franklin (2001) reported two cases in which children sustained sternal fractures from a fall off a swing. One child, an eight-year-old, fell onto her chest and sustained a fracture of the proximal region of the *corpus sterni*. The other child, a seven-year-old, fell onto her back and her legs went up over her shoulders causing hyper-flexion of her torso. She also sustained a fracture in the proximal region of the *corpus sterni*.

In sum, authors of the current literature recognize sternal fractures as relatively rare and postulate that the flexibility associated with the costosternal, sternoclavicular, and sternomanubrium joint reduces the incidence. There is also a consensus that sternal fractures are more common in accidental injury and are the result of relatively low levels of trauma. Finally, sternal fractures are most commonly in the proximal region of the *corpus sterni*, rarely displaced and effectively treated with analgesics.

Vertebral Fractures

Vertebral fractures are rare in children and reportedly account for 1–3% of child abuse fractures (Kleinman 1998, Bode and Newton 2007, Sieradzki and Sarwark 2008, Kemp *et al.* 2010). The low incidence of spinal fractures is due to the increased elasticity of the spine as a result of the ligamentous composition

(Kemp *et al.* 2010). Kleinman *et al.* (1992) found 165 fractures in 31 child abuse victims; only one was a spinal fracture. Most often, spinal fractures involve the vertebral body. When the posterior column is involved, typically it accompanies a vertebral body fracture. Vertebral body fractures have been categorized into three patterns: (1) mild compression deformity with intact end plates; (2) fracture of the anterosuperior end plate with no loss of vertebral body height; and (3) a combination of compression deformity with anterosuperior end plate fracture (Kleinman and Marks 1992, Kleinman 1998). The fracture of the anterosuperior end plate typically results in an osseous fragment (Kleinman and Marks 1992, Kleinman 1998). The mechanism associated with spinal fractures is hyper-flexion and/or hyperextension with associated axial loading and rotation (Kleinman 1998, Ranjith *et al.* 2002).

A predilection for thoracolumbar region fractures is documented in the literature (Levin *et al.* 2003). Levin and colleagues (2003) reviewed plain films, CT, and MRI of seven thoracolumbar fractures with listhesis in child abuse victims aged six month to seven years. They noted the most common location of the fracture was at the level of L1/L2. Bode and Newton (2007) and Sieradzki and Sarwark (2008) each report a single case of child abuse with a thoracolumbar fracture-dislocation. The level of the fracture was T12/L1 in both cases.

Additionally, several case reports have documented bilateral spondylolysis of the C2 (*Hangman's* fracture) with associated spondylolisthesis (Kleinman and Shelton 1997, Kleinman 1998, Ranjith *et al.* 2002) (see Chapter 9). Spondylolysis of C2 is recognized as an injury secondary to hyperextension. In childhood the injury is most commonly associated with a fall or motor vehicle accident, but also has been documented in non-accidental injury (Kleinman and Shelton 1997, Kleinman 1998, Ranjith *et al.* 2002, Kleinman 2004).

Kemp *et al.* (2010) conducted an in-depth literature review of published studies and case reports of spinal trauma identified in child abuse victims less than 18 years old. They found reports of 25 child abuse victims with non-accidental spinal injuries: 12 individuals had cervical injuries (median age 5 months), 12 individuals had thoracolumbar injuries (median age 13.5 months), and one child had cervical, thoracolumbar, and sacral injuries (age not mentioned). The authors state that the pediatric cervical spine is particularly vulnerable to injury for four reasons: (1) the underdevelopment of intervertebral joints; (2) the horizontal orientation of the facet joints; (3) the relatively large size of an infant's head; and (4) the low tone of the neck musculature. Ten of the 12 children with cervical trauma had musculoskeletal injury. The types of musculoskeletal injuries observed in their analysis include *Hangman's* fracture at C2/C3, anterolisthesis, compression fracture of the vertebral body, and bilateral pedicle fractures. Eleven of the 12 thoracolumbar injuries had musculoskeletal injuries, which included lesions at T11–T12, fracture dislocation and compression of the vertebral body. The mechanism of injury was known in eight cases, and included: four cases of shaking (3 with cervical injuries and 1 with thoracolumbar injury); two cases of throwing (1 child landed in a jack-knife position with thoracolumbar hyper-flexion); 1 case of spanking; 1 case of "rough play"; and 1 case of forcefully slamming onto a hard surface in a seated position (injury of the cervical, thoracolumbar, and sacral vertebral regions).

SUMMARY

No fracture is pathognomonic for child abuse, but several fractures are considered highly specific for non-accidental injury. The presented case highlights many of these fractures. However, when diagnosing child abuse, the age of the child, multiple fractures at various stages of healing, and inconsistencies between the history and the fracture pattern are the best indicators of non-accidental injury.

D. INTIMATE PARTNER VIOLENCE (IPV): DEMOGRAPHICS, SKELETAL INJURY PATTERNS, AND THE LIMITATIONS

CHELSEY A. JUAREZ AND CRIS E. HUGHES

INTRODUCTION

When analyzing human skeletal remains in the forensic context, one role of the forensic anthropologist is to observe and describe skeletal trauma. Throughout this process of observation and description, specific patterns of defect location or timing of injury may be recognized as consistent with particular contexts that could create such patterns of defects. However, as discussed in Chapter 2, it is outside the scope of the forensic anthropology case report to make connections between the relationship of defects (i.e., patterns) and the identity of the perpetrator or the manner of death that could potentially generate such patterns. The circumstance(s) or context in which the skeletal defects occur cannot be determined solely on the basis of the skeletal evidence. Such interpretations are the responsibility of the case investigator, who has access to the multiple lines of information and evidence for a given case.

While the pattern of traumatic defects are not linked with context in the case report, this knowledge may be relevant in other aspects. For example, the forensic anthropologist may provide scientific research references, which might assist the death investigator in supporting or refuting his/her hypothesis for a particular context.

Although forensic anthropologists are not responsible for incorporating such interpretations in case reports, they have a duty to the sub-discipline and to anthropology in general. We are responsible for being cognizant of and contributing to the scientific research of peer-reviewed literature that demonstrates the connections between patterns of skeletal defects and events that can (or cannot) produce such patterns. If no research exists to document the presence or absence of these relationships, then there is no scientific/statistical documentation with which to provide the investigator.

Forensic anthropological analyses and research have been able to make substantive contributions in some areas of patterns of skeletal defects. Research on the relationship between child abuse and patterns of skeletal defects such as timing, location, fracture type, and mechanisms of force is available (Merten 1983; Cook *et al.* 1997; Galloway 1999; Marks 2009, Ross and Abel 2011, Love this volume). Human rights abuses have also been addressed extensively, relying on the context and known histories to support the skeletal analyses (Brogden *et al.* 2003; Kimmerle and Baraybar 2008).

However, much less attention has been paid to the study of chronic abuse in adults. Chronic abuse connotes repeated events of violence over time, which may or may not leave evidence on the skeleton. One type of chronic abuse in adults is intimate partner violence (IPV), which is synonymous with domestic abuse. IPV includes forms of physical, sexual, or psychological harm by a current or former partner or spouse (Smith and Farole 2009). In the majority of cases, IPV occurs over a long period of time resulting in a documentable history of soft tissue and/or skeletal injuries (Campbell and Glass 2009). At the extreme, IPV may result in the death of the victim, forming a case of intimate partner homicide (IPH).

The purpose of this chapter is three-fold: (1) to discuss the victim demographic and traumatic injury patterns associated with IPH, (2) to introduce the most current data on patterns of skeletal injury common in cases of IPV, (3) to illustrate a case study in which IPH is known to have occurred that demonstrates the complexity of this abuse in a forensic anthropological setting. Core to this discussion is that IPV is defined by the relationship between the victim and the perpetrator, something not determinable through skeletal analysis.

INTIMATE PARTNER HOMICIDE (IPH)

IPH is the form of IPV that results in the death of the victim and may or may not be tied to skeletal evidence of previous abuse (healed or healing bone defects). Since the remains of these individuals may be referred to the forensic anthropologist, it is important that practitioners be familiar with the available research. Here, we discuss the demographics of IPH victims and the research on patterns of IPH trauma.

When the victim/perpetrator relationship is known, females are six times more likely to be IPH victims than males (Cooper and Smith 2011). Because of this disparity, the majority of the literature focuses on data for females, and therefore females are the focus of this chapter as well. However, it must be acknowledged that IPV/IPH is not confined to female partners nor to heterosexual couples. Although overall rates of IPH have declined during the past 25 years, 63% of all female homicide victims died at the hands of an intimate partner (Violence Policy Center 2011). Recent medical studies indicate that 75% of all cases of homicide involving intimate partners show a history of IPV (Campbell and Glass 2009), thus suggesting the likelihood that evidence of chronic IPV may appear within the cases seen by forensic anthropologists. These data also show that the risk rises for women in their late teens and does not drop substantially until after the age of 60.

Ethnicity/race and incidence of intimate partner violence/homicide are correlated, but IPV/IPH is a world wide issue spanning a variety of demographics. Here, we focus on the data for the United States. In the U.S., the age and race at highest risk for IPH are African American females between the ages of 20 to 29, followed by white females aged 30 to 39 years (Violence Policy Center 2011). For ethnic groups such as Latinas, the picture of IPH becomes much more complex and is impacted by legal issues such as immigration status. The most recent comparative rates of IPV between Latinas and non-Latinas have been reported as roughly equal between groups (Denham *et al.* 2007; Catalano *et al.* 2009). Regional studies investigating IPV/IPH within Latina groups suggest that immigrant Latinas have lower rates of IPV than U.S born Latinas. However, immigrant Latinas experience higher rates of IPH than non-immigrant Latinas (Runner *et al.* 2009).

Life events and marital circumstances appear to correlate to greater risk of homicide. Studies suggest that divorced or separated women have the highest rates of IPH (Rennison and Welchans 2000, Biroscak *et al.* 2006). Ease of divorce and financial arrangements at divorce or separation also affect a female partner's ability to leave a relationship prior to homicide in the course of IPV (Gautheir and Brankston 2004). However, separation does not guarantee safety from a male abuser. Available statistics suggest that, while spouses have traditionally been the most common perpetrator, increasingly, non-marital intimate partners are responsible (Fox and Zawitz 2007). Other studies suggest that pregnancy increases the risk for violence against women. In their 2002 study of ongoing domestic abuse victims, McFarlane and colleagues found a statistically significant increase in attempted and completed homicides during pregnancy as compared to victims who were not pregnant.

Beyond basic demographic information, little research has focused on the injuries associated with IPH. The only data that touches on the actual circumstances of IPH is weapon use (Fox and Zawitz 2007, Puzzanchera *et al.* 2012). In cases of female IPH, guns remain the most commonly used weapon. However, this trend is changing: since 1980, gun use has decreased 16% and now represents around 51% of IPH cases (Cooper and Smith 2011). Blunt force trauma represents approximately 20% of cases[1], and sharp force

---

1. The actual percentage for BFT may exceed this number as 12% of cases were classified as "unknown weapon" by the FBI Supplemental Homicide Report 2012.

trauma represents 15% of cases (Puzzanchera *et al.* 2012). Beyond weapon use, the large majority of research on the actual bodily injuries caused by violence focuses on non-fatal IPV, since almost all studies collect data on IPV survivors via survey or medical records. For IPH data, medical examiner and coroner records are the appropriate sources of information regarding the formal identification of IPH; however, practitioners must await the prosecution of the crime to divulge case data.

Review of Relevant Ipv Literature

Beyond IPH, research on non-fatal IPV injuries is also relevant to the forensic anthropological context, in that the majority of IPH victims were victims of chronic IPV while alive (Campbell and Glass 2009). In the context of forensic anthropology, this relationship between IPH and chronic non-fatal IPV suggests that the skeleton of IPH victims may exhibit antemortem fractures from instances of IPV. It also highlights the importance of recording ante-mortem injuries in all remains, even when homicide may not be suspected.

With few exceptions, the demographics of sex, race, and ethnicity for IPV victims mirror that of IPH victims. IPV against women is much more common than against men, representing 22% of all violence against women, versus 5% of all violence against men (Truman 2011). African American women experience IPV in rates twice that for white females, whereas Latinas appear to have IPV rates roughly equal to white non-Latinas (Catalano *et al.* 2009). In addition, women with disabilities are twice as likely as women without disabilities to be victims of IPV (Armour *et al.* 2008).

The general topics of interest to IPV injury research have focused on the mechanisms of injury and the location and pattern of IPV injuries. Studies on IPV and non-IPV injury cases overwhelmingly demonstrate that, blunt force trauma followed by sharp force trauma are the most common types found (Le *et al.* 2001, Sheridan and Nash 2007). Data collected for research on IPV comes from either surveys or medical/emergency room records. Therefore, data collection is biased towards those injuries that require medical attention. This chapter focuses on blunt force trauma and IPV including the mechanisms, patterns, and locations of injury associated with IPV and descriptive analysis of a case study.

Mechanism of Injury

IPV is an intensely personal assault and much of the violence comes through manual contact (punches/slaps) or by being beaten with a blunt object (U.S. Bureau of Justice 2006). While impacts from the hands can result in contusions, abrasions, and lacerations, it is the fractures that are most important to the forensic anthropological analysis. Impacts from a fist have an increased force and are more likely to result in fractures (Sheridan and Nash 2007). Le *et al.* (2001) report that fists caused 67% of the injuries due to domestic violence. Other blunt objects, such as bottles, sticks, or pipes were used in the remaining study cases. Strangulation is another common occurrence in IPV and is usually done manually rather than with a ligature (Strack *et al.* 2001).

Location and Pattern of Skeletal Injury

Injuries to the head, face, and neck have been consistently documented in IPV literature (Tintinalli and Hoelzer 1985, Berrios and Grady 1991, Muelleman *et al.* 1996, Fanslow *et al.* 1998, Greenfeld *et al.* 1998, Greene *et al.* 1999, Perciaccante *et al.* 1999, Le *et al.* 2001, Petridou *et al.* 2002, Crandall *et al.* 2004, Biroscak *et al.* 2006, Arosarena *et al.* 2009). The most comprehensive approach to date is Wu *et al.*'s (2010) metadata analysis of IPV research literature. The authors analyzed the incidence of IPV injuries to four separate regions: (1) head, neck, and face; (2) trunk; (3) upper extremity; and (4) lower extremity. The head-neck-face was the only region to be a statistically significantly associated with IPV. Even more specifically, Le *et al.* (2001) identified the middle third of the face as the location of highest risk for IPV trauma.

Crandall *et al.*'s (2004) work supplements these findings by comparing the risk of facial injury from a variety of circumstances. The authors utilized a sample of women aged 16 to 69 in acute care hospitals in the U.S. from 1997 to 1998 for a total sample size of 92,480 with 705 patients identified as presenting with intentional injury. Their analysis demonstrated that blunt trauma to the face was statistically more likely to occur in intentional violence than from motor vehicular accidents or falls. In addition, as a group, the victims were younger than those in the other categories, particularly in contrast to victims of falls whose average age was considerably older.

In addition to research of trends in IPV injury location, several studies have examined whether specific fractures are statistically associated with IPV. Arosarena *et al.* (2009) sampled 326 combined medical and dental records of adult female facial trauma victims with recorded trauma causation (fall, motor vehicle accident, IPV, and non-IPV assault). The authors determined that statistically significant correlations exist between injury type (e.g., motor vehicle crash, fall, assault by unknown assailant) and injury pattern (i.e., skeletal fractures). Zygomatic complex fractures, orbital blowout, and intracranial injuries were found in higher than expected frequencies among IPV patients. In contrast, assaults by an unknown assailant correlated more significantly with mandibular fractures. Trauma from a fall was more likely to have a combination of nasal fractures and alveolar ridge fractures, and motor vehicle crash victims manifested statistically more mandibular fractures, intracranial injuries, and alveolar ridge fractures.

In comparison to cranial trauma, there are far fewer published studies documenting postcranial trauma in IPV cases. Wu and associates (2010) found no difference in thoracic, abdominal, and pelvic fractures between IPV patients and those with injuries from falls or motor vehicle accidents. Upper and lower extremity injuries were found to be less frequent than expected in IPV patients. Le and colleagues (2001) found that the vast majority (81%) of fractures/dislocations involved the face. Of the postcranial fractures/dislocations, most were found on the chest, followed by the arms and hands, and a few injuries to the legs. It is possible that the upper limb injuries are attributable to defensive moves by the victim (Galloway 1999, Sheridan and Nash 2007, see Chapter 7). Reliable statistics on correlating forearm defensive fractures to deflection of violence, however, are minimal.

In sum, the present literature emphasizes the head-neck-face region as the most frequent location and the only region of the body to be statistically associated with IPV – an association not found with other circumstances studied thus far (Crandall *et al.* 2004, Arosarena *et al.* 2009). Furthermore, orbital "blow-out" fractures, zygomatic complex fractures, and intracranial injuries are associated with IPV versus other studied circumstances (Arosarena *et al.* 2009).

It is extremely important to emphasize the distinction between statistical significance of association of these factors with IPV versus the exclusive occurrence of these factors within IPV. Head-neck-face injuries, and the specific fracture patterns associated with these injuries, are in no way unique to IPV. They certainly occur in non-IPV circumstances as well. What this research demonstrates is that the frequency in which these patterns occur in association with IPV in contrast with other circumstances of injury are great enough to reach statistical significance. IPV in its very nature is complex, and the majority of its manifestations (emotional abuse, threats, soft tissue violence) are outside the realm of the skeleton. Even when antemortem skeletal trauma is present, the current IPV literature makes clear that there are no traumatic "indicators" *unique* to IPV, and the simplest pattern for chronic abuse in the form of multiple stages of healing may or may not be present. The following case study demonstrates the complex context of IPV and IPH, and the extent to which forensic anthropological observations can contribute.

FORENSIC ANTHROPOLOGY CASE EXAMPLE OF KNOWN IPV

The case selected for this section displays an array of perimortem trauma. This case is of particular interest because it represents a case of known IPH with no skeletal evidence for previous IPV. Some injuries are consistent with IPV trauma while other patterns were not.

In the fall of 2006, the Forensic Osteological Investigations Laboratory (FOIL) at the University of California, at Santa Cruz received the partial remains of a single adult female. The remains had been recovered after the husband of a recently missing woman led deputies to the location of the body. Probable identification was based on the information from the husband. Anthropological analysis for biological profile and trauma was requested.

FOIL anthropologists estimated the skeletal remains to be a female, age 20–25 years, of possible Hispanic identity. No antemortem trauma was found on the remains. Perimortem blunt and sharp force trauma to the body was extensive (Table D-1).

TABLE D-1
BREAKDOWN OF TRAUMA BY TYPE
AND BONE/REGION

Bone / Region	Sharp Force Trauma (SFT) Description	Blunt Force Trauma (BFT) Description
SKULL		Minimum of 7 direct impacts
UPPER FACIAL	2 SFT defects on the frontal bone at midline	Blunt force impact 2mm superior to the right orbit resulting in radiating fractures and complete fracture of the frontal bone.
MIDDLE FACIAL	0	Complete obliteration of nasals. Extensive periorbital fracturing, with obliteration of the ethmoid, lacrimals, and sphenoid resulting in orbital blowout. Significant malar obliteration, zygomatic complex fracturing and a Le Forte 1 facial fracture.
LOWER FACIAL	Cuts at (a) midline, (b) inferior margin on left, (c) R body, (d) R ascending ramus,	Fracture at (a) R ascending ramus and (b) at midline
NEURO-CRANIUM	23 SFT defects around cranial vault	BFT impacts to R occipital and temporal bones and to R and L sides
VERTEBRAE		
Cervical	8 impacts on C2–7	Fracturing associated with SFT
Thoracic	18 impacts resulting in 23 defects	Fracturing associated with SFT
Lumbar	5 impacts resulting in 17 defects	Fracturing associated with SFT

(Continued)

Bone / Region	Sharp Force Trauma (SFT) Description	Blunt Force Trauma (BFT) Description
RIBS	SFT on most ribs, both sides	Fractures to left and right ribs 1–11, not focused on any aspect
STERNUM	SFT on anterior manubrium	Depressed fractures to upper sternal body
CLAVICLES	1 SFT on each clavicle	Fracturing associated with SFT and additional fracture on midshaft R clavicle
SCAPULAE	3 SFT impacts to R scapula resulting in 5 defects; 1 SFT impact to L scapula	Fracturing associated with SFT
HUMERI	4 SFT impacts to R humerus and 5 to L humerus, resulting in 27 defects	Fracturing associated with SFT.
RADII	5 SFT insults to R radius and 3 SFT insults to L radius, resulting in 11 defects	Fracturing associated with SFT
ULNAE	3 SFT insults each to R and L ulnae, resulting in 10 defects	Fracturing associated with SFT
HANDS		
Carpals and Metacarpals	2 SFT impacts to R palm/wrist; 5 SFT to L palm/wrist and dorsal	hand/wrist
Phalanges	5 SFT defects on proximal phalanges, 3 SFT to middle phalanges, resulting in 14 defects	Fracturing associated with SFT
FEMORA	3 SFT impacts to each femur at distal ends	
PATELLA	4 SFT defects on R patella	
TIBIA	1 SFT defect on L tibia	
TOTAL	177 defects	

TABLE D-1
BREAKDOWN OF TRAUMA BY TYPE
AND BONE/REGION *(Continued.)*

Perimortem trauma to the cranium (Figures D-1 and D-2) is prevalent and includes all of the documented patterns of IPV-associated fractures, specifically zygomatic complex fractures, orbital blowout fractures, and intracranial fractures (Arosarena *et al.* 2009). Trauma to the midface was the most extensive and in certain areas demonstrated complete obliteration of bony structures. Also documented was extensive mandibular fracturing, a fracture type not statistically associated with IPV in Aroserana and colleague's work (2009).

The postcranial skeleton shows extensive perimortem trauma (both blunt and sharp force). The assailant confirmed that he disarticulated the body for transport and burial. Anthropological analysis suggests that dismemberment included the following segments: head, shoulder girdle, upper arms, forearms, hands, right ribs, left ribs and spine, pelvis and thighs, right leg, and left leg. It was not possible to distinguish cuts inflicted during the fatal assault (if any) from those associated with dismemberment. In addition, much of the post-cranial fracturing is associated with sharp force trauma. The presence of trauma to the ribs and forearms are most notably common to our case and IPV data. Because of the extent of the damage, it was not possible to separate the purely blunt force-derived fractures on the radii and ulnae, relative to those associated with the sharp force trauma. The presence of trauma to the vertebral column, lower extremities, hands, and wrists was also documented.

The skeletal remains were later positively identified as the wife of the assailant, and she had a history of documented spousal abuse (IPV). Interestingly, her demographic profile contained several "flags" indicating that she was a person more likely to experience IPV: she was a young (21 year old), mentally disabled, undocumented Hispanic immigrant, and mother of three children. In other ways, this case is atypical for IPV/IPH trends. Although guns are the most commonly used weapon in IPH assaults, the weapons used in this case were limited to sharp and blunt instruments. Another important point to emphasize is that no antemortem trauma was documented, even though later investigation information confirmed a history of IPV. This proves the point that chronic abuse may not leave osteological indicators.

CONCLUSIONS AND RECOMMENDATIONS

An ongoing collection of information about the causes, characteristics, and consequences of violence is essential to building a comprehensive understanding of IPV/IPH. When compared to the available literature on IPV injuries, the case study presented here exhibited all of the fractures statistically correlated with IPV. However, it also exhibited fracture types statistically correlated with non-IPV scenarios. This reality underscores the complexity between known data, i.e., the fracture patterns correlated with IPV, and unknown potential

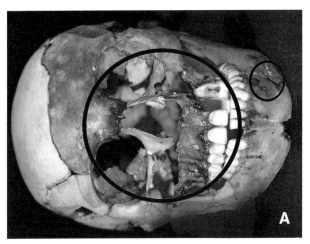

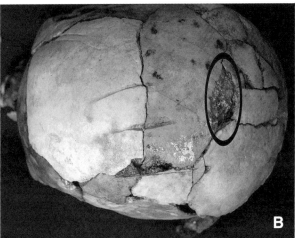

Figure D-1. Anterior (A), superior (B), and inferior (C) views of skull from known IPV case. Areas outlined in ellipses indicate areas of impact. Due to the extensive fracturing, these impact sites sometimes encompass large areas (A), as the exact impact is not discernable, but the fracturing patterns suggest that an impact to the general area occurred.

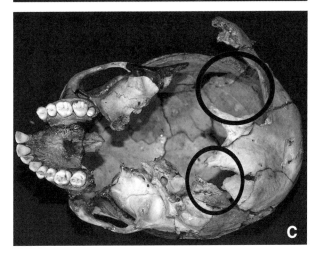

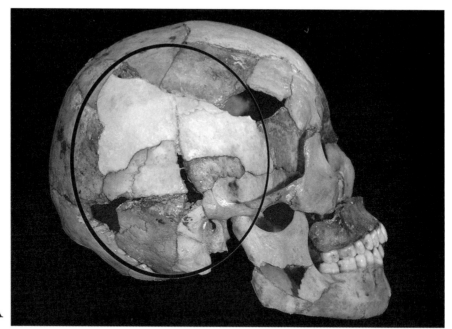

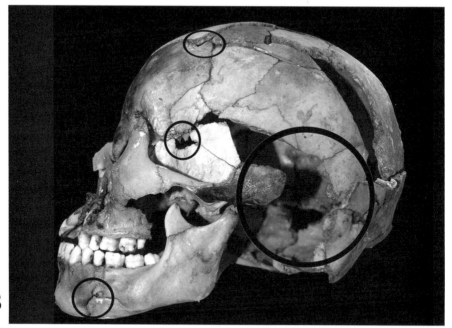

Figure D-2. Lateral views of the skull. Areas outlined in ellipses indicate areas of impact. Due to the extensive fracturing, these impact sites sometimes encompass large areas (A), as the exact impact is not discernable, but the fracturing patterns suggest that an impact to the general area occurred.

patterns of IPH. IPV and IPH are different scenarios, and while there maybe similar fracture types correlated with both, this relationship is not known and more research on IPH fracture patterns is needed. Forensic anthropologists are in a unique position to contribute data on fracture patterns of cases later determined IPHs by investigators. These data can serve as a comparison to established trends for IPV, and contribute to a more comprehensive understanding of IPV and fracture patterns potentially correlated with IPH. As documentation of IPV- and IPH-related skeletal trauma continues to grow, forensic anthropologists will have a clearer grasp of what to expect when faced with a potential case of IPV/IPH. Although no fracture or fracture pattern is diagnostic of IPV, the trends discussed below serve as reminders of the current understanding of IPV/IPH.

1. Most victims of IPV are involved in ongoing abuse, and therefore antemortem trauma may be present.
2. Although not unique to IPV, periorbital fractures, zygomatic complex fractures, and intracranial injury in women correlate statistically with IPV.
3. Fracturing to the nasals and mandible, while documented in IPV, is not statistically correlated with IPV. In contrast, these two fracture types have been statistically associated with assaults by unknown or unidentified assailants.

E. A MYRIAD OF MECHANISMS

Gina Hart

Forensic anthropologists are being called upon with higher frequency to interpret traumatic events in medical examiner cases. In these instances, anthropologists can aid pathologists by examining and determining the mechanism of trauma (ballistics, sharp force, or blunt force trauma). In some instances, the mechanism of trauma is not always clear or multiple mechanisms of trauma may be at play. The following case study describes an instance where witnesses presented the anthropologist with a myriad of possible trauma mechanisms, as well as statements that conflicted with what the man accused of the crime confessed to having done.

THE CASE

An auto body shop owner in urban New Jersey got into an altercation with one of his mechanics on a Friday in the fall of 2006. Reasons for the conflict are unknown, but one observer stated that the auto body shop owner believed that the mechanic was using drugs at work. Two witnesses stated that they saw the perpetrator hit the victim over the head with a handgun, but their accounts vary in the number of times that they saw the victim get struck. One witness stated that he saw the perpetrator hit the victim once, while the other stated that he saw the victim being beaten repeatedly. Both witnesses then stated that they heard a shot and then saw the victim fall to the ground, but neither actually saw him being shot. The witnesses then saw the perpetrator holding the smoking gun, and they believed that the victim had been shot in the head, because there was blood coming from his mouth. The perpetrator threatened the witnesses, telling them that they did not see anything happen. All of the surviving parties then left the shop.

In the days following the events that ensued at the body shop, someone came forward to tell the victim's wife what happened in the body shop. The wife then went to the police and told them the story. Police went to the body shop the week after the incident only to find a sign stating that the shop was closed. Investigators obtained a search warrant and searched the body shop, discovering blood near a vehicle bay. The perpetrator's vehicle was then searched and a substantial amount of blood was discovered in his trunk. The perpetrator had previously fled the state but was later apprehended in Washington, DC, by United States marshals. He was transported back to New Jersey, where he eventually agreed to take authorities to the body. He led police to an urban area in New Jersey, where the body was located in a vacant lot under a piece of sheet rock. It had been a month since the victim had been murdered, and the remains were almost completely skeletonized. The tasks of identifying the remains and determining the cause of death were at hand. While in custody, the perpetrator stated that he would not give a statement or sign anything.

Anthropological Examination

The autopsy took place the morning after the remains were discovered. The pathologist requested the presence of the forensic anthropologist to examine and analyze the bones for trauma and to verify the possible identification of the victim. The remains were complete, and mostly skeletonized with some desiccation of the tissues and the presence of insect pupae. Both the anthropologist and the pathologist grossly examined all remains at time of autopsy. The anthropologist removed from the body areas exhibiting trauma and elements aiding in demographic information. The skeletal elements removed included the skull, mandible, all cervical vertebrae, all of the ribs, the sternum, the left and right pelves, a portion of the left hand, and the right femur. These bones were macerated in a mixture of water, powder detergent, and hydrogen peroxide. The anthropological findings indicated that the remains belonged to a 35–55-year-old black male. The body was later positively identified via dental records as the suspected victim, a 43-year-old black male.

Antemortem Trauma

The skeleton was examined for any evidence pertaining to the timing of injuries (antemortem, perimortem, or postmortem), as well as signs of any disease processes. Only one site of antemortem trauma was present and it was on the facial skeleton: an inferior orbital rim fracture with an orbital floor fracture to the left eye. The fracture had completely remodeled after being knit back together with a metal plate that measured 2.5cm and was anchored by five screws (Figure E-1).

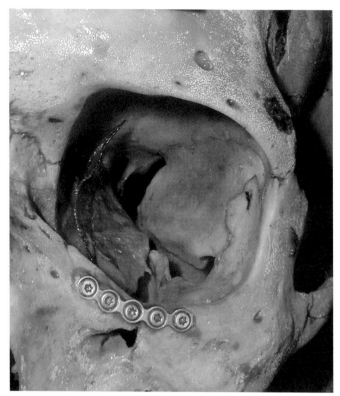

Figure E-1. Surgical hardware, which had been used to reconstruct an antemortem orbital rim fracture.

Perimortem Trauma

The Skull

The skull, mandible, and cervical vertebrae were of particular interest because of the statements given by the witnesses that the victim had suffered blunt force trauma (via pistol whipping) and ballistics trauma. These skeletal elements were closely examined for any perimortem injuries both during the autopsy and after maceration. No evidence of gunshot wounds was present on the skull. The only evidence of trauma was a single depressed fracture on the skull (Figure E-2). The fracture, which is located on the superior aspect of the left parietal, runs perpendicular to the sagittal suture. It is 1 cm in length and 2 cm from the coronal suture. The bone surrounding the fracture exhibited evidence of a hematoma. The presence of the bone contusion is gross evidence of biological reaction to trauma and indicates that this is a perimortem injury.

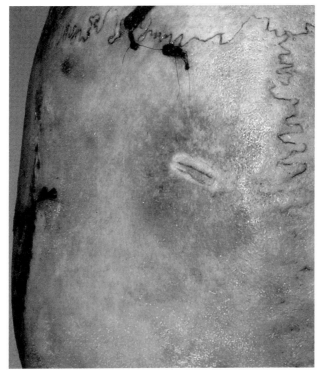

Figure E-2. Depressed fracture with bone contusion to left parietal.

Fourth and Fifth Cervical Vertebrae (C4 and C5)

Additional trauma was present to the 4th and 5th cervical vertebrae (Figure E-3). An incomplete fracture runs horizontally along the vertebral arch of C4, starting at the inferior border and traveling to the left of the spinous process, passing through the process itself, and terminated near the right superior articular facet. A small amount of deformation is present to the inferior aspect of the fracture, indicating that this is a perimortem injury.

The vertebral arch of C5 exhibited a complete fracture to running vertically and lateral to the left and right laminae. The spinous process was never recovered, possibly due to transport of the body by the perpetrator from the primary to the secondary scene. There is a dark discoloration to the fracture surfaces, which is possibly the result of powder residence or lead wipe. No evidence of this was found in the radiographs. This injury appears to also be perimortem because of the deformation present.

The mechanism of trauma for these injuries cannot be determined because of the complex appearance of the cervical vertebrae fractures and the absence of an impact site.

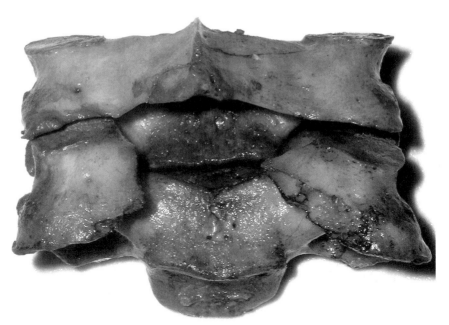

Figure E-3. Linear fracture to the vertebral arch of C4 and complete fracture to the vertebral arch of C5.

Left 2nd Metacarpal

The anthropologist performed a cursory skeletal survey at the time of autopsy and then a detailed examination of the elements removed. The only other perimortem injury noted was to the left second metacarpal (Figure E-4). The comminuted metacarpal fracture is consistent with a defense wound (Chapter 7, this volume). This fracture involves the mid-shaft and distal end of the bone. The bone has a shattered appearance and displays a significant amount of deformation. Not all of the bone fragments are present. This indicates that a high amount of energy created the injury and that the injury occurred at or around the time of death. The mechanism of trauma could not be determined but most likely was the result of a gunshot wound or blunt force trauma with a rapid loading rate and a small focal point (see Chapter 3, this volume).

After the Analysis

The healed orbital fracture was found to be consistent an old antemortem injury that the victim had. At autopsy, it was recognized as a possible aid in identification if medical records and antemortem x-rays could be found and the injury corroborated.

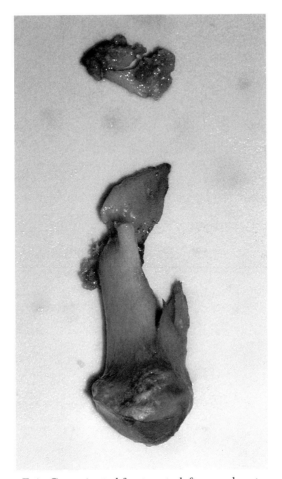

Figure E-4. Comminuted fracture to left second metacarpal.

The anthropological report aided the associated pathologist in determining the cause of death to be gunshot wound and blunt force injury and the manner of death to be homicide. The case went to trial in 2008. The pathologist had since left the state, so the chief medical examiner rendered autopsy testimony. Since the pathologist slated to testify was not available, the anthropologist's testimony was critical. She was the only expert witness who was present at the time of the examination. The testifying pathologist attested to the cause and manner of death while the anthropologist discussed the nature and location of the skeletal injuries.

The perpetrator pled not guilty and, after the trial proceedings ended, a jury found him guilty of aggravated manslaughter, aggravated assault, possession of a weapon for an unlawful purpose, and improper disposal of human remains. He is currently serving 35 years in a New Jersey prison.

CONCLUSION

This case study describes an example where witness accounts were clarified and vetted by the trauma analysis. Additionally, this case demonstrated how important trauma analysis can be to case prosecution. The case resolution achieved would not have been possible without the medical examiners and forensic anthropologist working in tandem. In this case, the traditional scope of anthropological examination was expanded to include a comparative analysis of the traumatic events and the confessions. Differentiating between the various mechanisms of trauma (ballistics, sharp force, and blunt force trauma) is an important aspect of daily casework, because the bone is typically the best witness.

F. BLUNT FORCE TRAUMA TO THE CHEST: TWO CASES OF COMPLEX RIB FRACTURES

JENNIFER C. LOVE, MERRILL O. HINES III,
AND STEPHEN K. WILSON

The primary responsibility of the medical examiner's office is to independently investigate all homicides, suicides, accidental, and unexpected deaths. The medical examiner reconstructs events surrounding a death by conducting physical examinations of the body and scene. Often to assist in reconstructing the forces that impacted the body, a forensic anthropologist is asked to examine traumatized bones.

In the following two cases, forensic pathologists found numerous fractured ribs and requested a trauma consultation from a forensic anthropologist. The anthropologist removed the fractured ribs from the decedent, processed them to remove all soft tissue, and reconstructed each fracture. The fracture types, associated biomechanical forces, and distribution pattern were interpreted to assess the minimum number and direction of impacts received by the decedent. In both cases, the decedent was in police custody at the time of death, and several witnesses in affidavits described the events surrounding the death.

CASE 1

A 51-year-old male with a history of chronic ethanolism was arrested for the assault of a police officer and resisting arrest. During the arrest, a physical altercation occurred between the arresting officers and the male. Following the arrest, the man was taken to the jail and examined by emergency medical services (EMS). The man refused medical treatment. While in custody, the male was witnessed unable to walk without assistance. Approximately 5½ hours after his arrest, the man was found unresponsive in the holding cell. EMS declared the man dead, and he was transported directly to the medical examiner's office.

The witness statement given by the first of the two arresting officers stated the event began when the officer observed the man hiding in the bed of a pick-up truck. The officers requested the man exit the pick-up truck. When the man attempted to exit, the first officer noted the man was trembling and assisted him. While the first officer was placing the male's hands on the back of his head, the man tensed, began shaking, and tried to pull his hands away. The officer swept the man's legs with his right leg. The officer and the male went to the ground, the male landed on his stomach with the officer on top of him. The officer got up into a kneeling position and placed his left knee on the man's shoulders and tried to pull the man's left arm behind his back. The male began kicking at the second officer and struck him in the legs several times. The man rolled over onto his back and grabbed the first officer's left leg with his hands. The officer gave the man a knee strike to his side. The man released the officer's leg but then grabbed the officer's shoelace and boot. The officer delivered a second knee strike to the man's side. At this point, the second arresting officer gave the man several knee strikes. The man attempted to spin around and kicked at the second officer's leg, striking him in the shin. The first officer struck the man with an elbow strike to his right forearm as the man pulled his hands under his body near his waist. Thinking the man was reaching for a weapon, the first officer stuck the man with his knee several times in the left side and leg. Finally the officers were able to subdue the man and handcuff him. While escorting the man towards the patrol car, the man tripped over a median, fell onto his stomach and struck his forehead on the concrete. The man was then placed into the back of the patrol car and taken to the jail.

The second arresting officer gave a similar account of the event. One notable difference was that the second officer reported that the officers applied knee and elbow strikes to the male's back and legs to prevent injury to the officers while subduing the violent behavior.

During the autopsy, the examining pathologist noted extensive acute blunt force injuries. On the head and neck, he noted subcutaneous contusions and abrasions with no skull fractures or intracranial hemorrhage. He observed subcutaneous contusions, abrasions and petechial hemorrhages, bilateral rib fractures, bilateral parietal pleural laceration, bilateral pulmonary contusions, and bilateral hemothoraces in the chest. He also noted bilateral antemortem rib fractures that had long since remodeled and had recognizable calluses. On the extremities, he documented subcutaneous contusions, abrasions, and petechial hemorrhages. Additionally, the man had a history of chronic heavy ethanol consumption. In evidence of this history were a fatty liver, chronic pancreatitis, and atrophic brain changes. The medical examiner classified the cause of death as blunt impact thoracic trauma with rib fractures, pleural lacerations, pulmonary contusions, and hemothoraces with the chronic ethanolism as a contributing factor, and the manner of death as homicide.

Anthropological Examination

The pathologist requested the forensic anthropologist do a trauma analysis of the ribs. The anthropologist removed the acutely fractured ribs (right ribs 8–12 and left ribs 9–11) and documented healed fractures located on the remaining ribs *in situ.* The anthropologist removed the soft tissue from the retained ribs and reconstructed them prior to analysis.

A total of 10 antemortem and 14 perimortem fractures were observed. The perimortem fractures were located primarily in the posterior region of the ribs. The fractures were complex and suggested an involvement of an axial loading force transferring through the bone in a posterior to anterior direction. The signature of the axial load was observed as longitudinal fractures extending anteriorly and posteriorly through the cortical bone from the transverse fracture and the splaying apart of the cortical bone (Figure F-1). The heads of right ribs 8–10, 12 and the left ribs 11 were incompletely fractured (Figure F-2). The fracture types and distribution pattern observed in the posterior region of

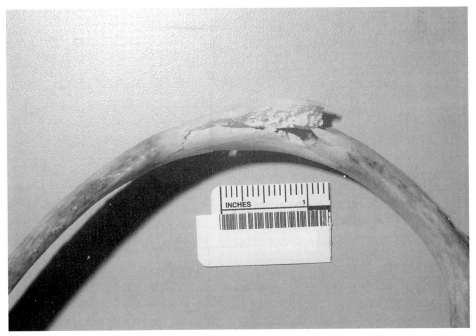

Figure F-1. Right rib 9. The reconstructed fracture is located with in the mid to posterior region of the rib body. Note the deformation consistent with an indirect blunt force impact. Scale bar in inches.

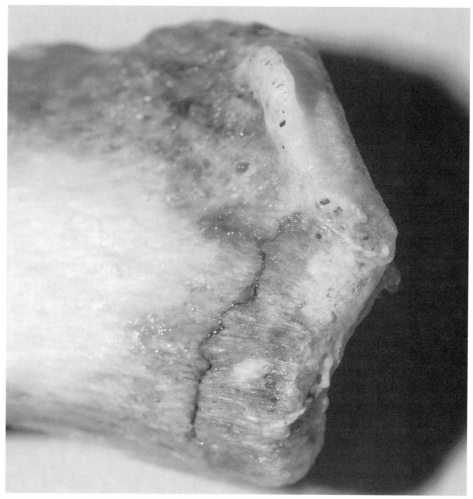

Figure F-2. Right rib 8. The incomplete transverse fracture only involved the internal surface of the rib head.

right ribs 9–12 and left ribs 9–11 (Figure F-3) were consistent with a minimum of one impact to the mid back in a posterior to anterior direction with an object of relatively broad surface area.

Serial rib fractures were also observed in the sternal end of the rib shafts of right ribs 8–11. The fractures were complete and transverse. Longitudinal fractures extended posteriorly from the transverse fracture only in right rib 8. The remaining three fractures were simple and consistently transverse. The cortical bone at the fracture sites was very thin. Signatures of failure in compression or tension were not observed. The lack of detail at the fracture margins precluded interpreting the direction of force.

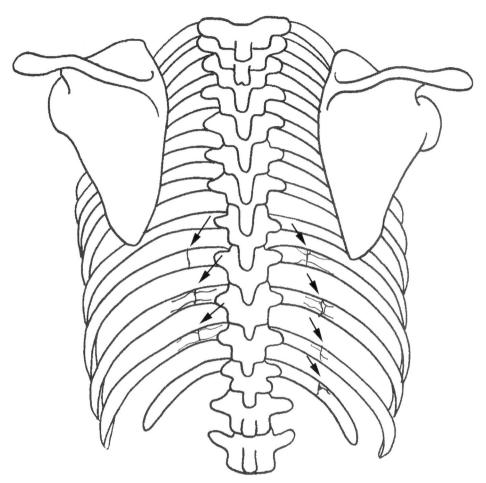

Figure F-3. Diagram with arrows illustrating the distribution of the posterior rib fractures.

The perimortem fracture pattern was consistent with a minimum of one blow to the mid back in a posterior to anterior direction with the right chest supported or braced against something or a minimum of two blows: one to the mid back in a posterior to anterior direction and one to the right anterior chest in an anterior to posterior direction. All of the antemortem fractures were completely healed, and the number of traumatic episodes, the direction of force, nor the age of injury could be estimated. Ultimately, the perimortem rib fractures and distribution pattern were consistent with fall or knee strikes to the man's back. In general, the ribs were notably light and friable. The trabecular bone density was somewhat reduced. Reduced bone density has been associated with chronic ethanolism (Chakkalaka 2005). The quality of the ribs likely made them more susceptible to fracture.

CASE 2

A 50-year-old male was arrested for outstanding warrants and taken to jail. One day after he was taken into custody, the male complained of stomach problems, was taken to the hospital and given the anti-emetic Phenergan. The hospital staff noted that the man's hands were shaking, but that the patient was alert, awake, and oriented. Radiographs and CT scans showed no skeletal injuries. The differential diagnoses included seizures and ethanol withdrawal. The following day, the man was released from the hospital and taken back to the jail.

Upon returning to the jail, the man was noted to be agitated and incoherent. The jail staff opted to move the man to the violent cell (V-cell) for his personal safety. The man resisted the transfer. One of the transferring officers swept the man's leg, bringing him to the ground. The transferring officer and a co-worker carried the man to the V-cell and left him on the floor. After exiting the cell, the officers instructed the man to remove his clothes and dress in a suicide vest, an article of clothing designed to reduce the risk of an inmate injuring him/herself. The man refused. After approximately 10 minutes of directing the man to remove his clothing, three officers entered the cell to forcefully undress the man. The first officer entered the cell and struck the man in the chest driving him to the back wall. The officer then supported the man as he dropped to the floor. The second and third officers entered the cell and held the man's arms while undressing him. The officers then exited the cell with the man's clothing. Approximately three hours after the incident, the man was found unresponsive. EMS pronounced the man dead. The medical examiner's office transported the decedent to the morgue for an autopsy.

During a follow-up interview, the officer who brought the man to the ground in the V-cell demonstrated his actions to the interviewer. The interviewer reported that the officer placed his head on the interviewer's sternum and then wrapped his arms around the interviewer's mid chest in a "bear hug." The interviewer noted that the officer performed the proper technique used by football players to drive opponents back. He further noted that although the officer was demonstrating the move more slowly and with less force then used against the man, he could feel the officer's strength. The tackling officer denied slamming the man to the ground, punching him, or witnessing others punching the deceased. When ask if he could have broken the man's ribs during the tackle, the officer stated it was possible.

During the autopsy, the examining pathologist noted that the man had blunt chest and abdominal trauma which included multiple acute rib fractures; splenic laceration; subcapsular hemorrhage of the liver; and subcutaneous contusions of the chest, back, and abdomen. He also noted subcutaneous contusions of the upper and lower extremities. The man was found to have changes in the liver (micronodular cirrhosis with steatosis) consistent with chronic ethanol use. He classified the cause of death as blunt chest and abdominal trauma with multiple rib fractures, splenic laceration, and hemoperitoneum, and the manner of death as homicide.

The pathologist requested a trauma analysis of left ribs 3–9 and anterior segments of right ribs 3–4. The anthropologist retained the ribs during the autopsy. All of the soft tissue was removed and the ribs were reconstructed prior to forensic anthropological analysis.

Anthropological Analysis

Twelve acute fractures were found on the nine ribs the medical examiner submitted to the forensic anthropologist for analysis. The fractures were distributed along the mid clavicular and lateral regions of left ribs 3–6 and along the lateral regions of left ribs 7–9. The fractures located along the lateral regions of left ribs 3–6 were relatively simple, ranging from complete oblique fractures to complete butterfly fractures (Figure F-4). All

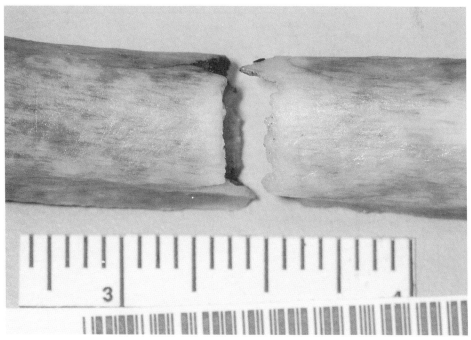

Figure F-4. Left rib 4. The complete transverse fracture representing the simple fractures observed along the lateral regions of left ribs 3–6. Scale bar in inches.

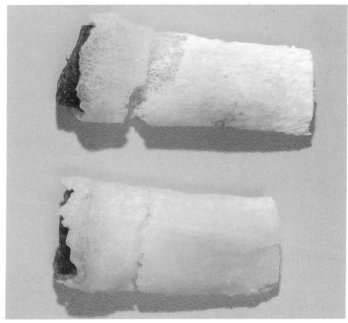

Figure F-5. Left ribs 5 (top) and 6 (bottom), external surface. The incomplete buckle fracture of rib 6 illustrates the folding of the cortical bone. The fracture type was observed in the sternal region of left ribs 3–6 and right ribs 3–4

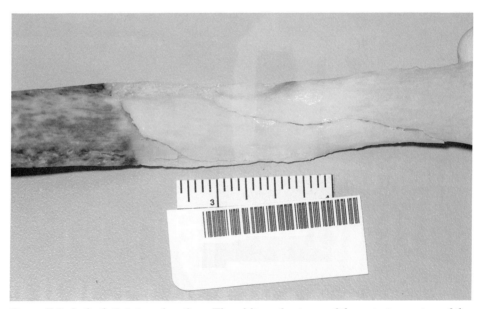

Figure F-6. Left rib 8, internal surface. The oblique fractures of the anterior region of the rib body illustrating the superior to inferior twist of the bone prior to failure. The label is under the caudal margin of the bone. Scale bar in inches.

of these fractures failed in tension along the internal surface. The anteri-orly located fractures of left ribs 3–6 and right ribs 3–4 were more complex. The compromised cortical bone had folded into itself, consistent with axial loading (Figure F-5, facing page). The fractures of left ribs 7–9 were pri-marily oblique, consistent with a downward twisting of the ribs (Figure F-6, facing page).

The fracture distribution (Figure F-7) and fracture types suggested a minimum of one left to right, superior to inferior impact to the left anterolateral chest with an object of intermediate size. There was no evidence of healing and the fracture margins were sharp. The findings corroborated the scenario described by the tackling officer; however, the location of the fractures sug-gested that the site of impact was the left lateral flank instead of the center of the chest.

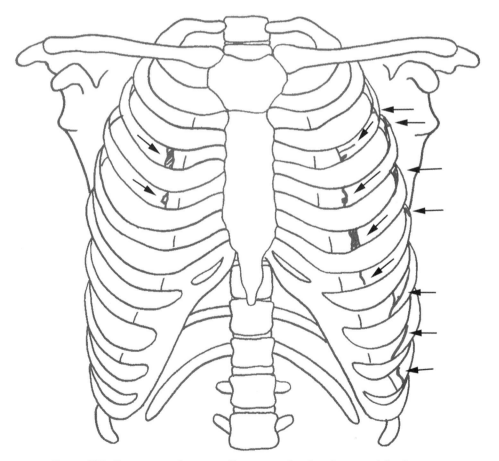

Figure F-7. Diagram with arrows illustrating the distribution of the fractures.

DISCUSSION

In these two cases, the skeletal trauma analyses performed by the forensic anthropologist resulted in detailed descriptions of the fracture types and distribution patterns. These analyses provided independent examinations and reconstructions of the forces impacting the body during the events surrounding death. Ultimately, the anthropological findings corroborated the statements offered by the officers involved in the physical altercations.

G. MANAGING TRAUMA IN FACIAL RECONSTRUCTIONS

Gloria L. Nusse

When case files go cold or human remains are too disfigured to publish photographs by which to narrow the list of possible identities, medical examiners or coroners' offices often request forensic facial reconstructions. Forensic facial reconstructions involve putting clay at pre-determined average thicknesses on different landmarks of the skull to give the bones a face. The following cases present challenges that may occur while implementing normal techniques of facial reconstruction due to fragmentation of the skull. Skulls may become fragmented during autopsy and postmortem transportation and storage, from ante- and perimortem trauma, or from damage due to decomposition or burial conditions. Perimortem blunt force trauma may result in fracture and depression of the cranial and facial bones. In addition, blunt force damage may occur from natural elements such as animal activity or from handling of the remains during investigation and autopsy. There may be tool marks, knife marks, or bullet patterns evident on the skull.

The skull consists of 23 separate bones and 6 ossicles of the inner ear. During the postmortem interval and/or due to trauma, any of the bones, particularly those of the face, which are fragile, may become damaged, disarticulated, or lost. Some damage may be of sufficient magnitude as to preclude the creation of a satisfactory reconstruction. For example, the practitioner should be cautioned that, when half of the face is missing, the artist has only half the necessary information. Experience and knowledge of facial anatomy help the practitioner to determine whether sufficient landmarks remain to safely guide reconstruction of the missing portions. The following case studies illustrate how the artist overcame the obstacles of bone trauma to complete a reconstruction that could then aid in the investigation.

In order to begin the reconstruction process, a mold of each skull is created for the reconstructions. In the case of severe trauma, the author finds it imperative that an exact replica of the skull is made either by molding and casting or sculpting in clay. Clay modifications replace the bony landmarks and the actual sculptures are fashioned upon the cast replica of the skull. This allows the artist to preserve the original skull for study and consultation during the reconstruction process. In this text, the face is not covered for reconstructing, rather, this study focuses on managing the skeletal remains in preparation for facial reconstruction.

The types of damage found on these skulls came from blunt force trauma, fire, missing dentition and dental arcades, autopsy cuts, unrecovered or unreconstructable bones, and postmortem warpage and loss of bone quality. These problems span the spectrum from antemortem, through perimortem, and postmortem causes. All presented unique problems for the artist to solve.

CASE 1

In 1979, a young woman's body was found on the beach in a northern county of California. She had been beaten, stabbed, and shot, and her body was burned. The coroner ruled that the death had occurred in the previous 24 hours. Her face was burned beyond recognition. Despite publicity and postmortem sketches created in 1979, she remained unidentified for 23 years. Her body was buried in a county cemetery and exhumed in 2002 for another attempt at identification.

During the time the body remained unidentified, the county cemetery flooded many times. When the grave was opened, it was saturated with water. The water and acidic conditions of the soil had caused the bones to become disarticulated, extremely brittle and somewhat distorted. Her skull was in several fragments. The teeth, extracted with segments of alveolar bone during the 1979 analysis, had been placed in county storage. Unfortunately this facility had moved several times during the ensuing decades and the teeth could not be found. Photographs of the teeth with a scale, morgue photos, and many other details of the case existed, but the actual teeth along with attached bone remained missing. The fragmented burned skull fragments and reports with the photos were delivered to the forensic artist for reconstruction.

By the time Case 1 arrived at the artist's studio, the victim's temporal bones, the greater wings of the sphenoid, and portions of the maxillae were crumbled and broken. The calvarium was detached and the zygomatic arches were separated and in pieces, especially along the right side. As bad as the fragmentary remains were, the greatest problems were the missing teeth and parts of the surrounding maxilla and mandible. Before making the mold of this

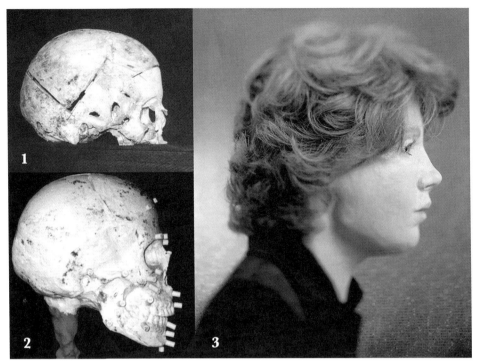

Figure G-1. Case 1, remodeled skull and lateral view of reconstruction.

skull, the artist remodeled the missing sections with clay using the opposite side as a guide for wholly missing parts (Figure G-1).

The nasal bones had curled upwards, causing them to disarticulate from the frontal process of the maxilla. This transformation may have started with very minor thermal damage when the body was burned. The consulting anthropologist examined the bone under magnification and concluded that the bone, although burnt, had sustained the majority of damage from being wet during its long burial. The splaying and separation of the nasals were likely warpage from water exposure. In any case, the original configuration of the nasal bones also had to be reconstructed by the artist.

CASE 2

In 2003, a body was found wrapped in a canvas bag and hidden in the shrubbery off the parking lot of a chain restaurant. Inside the bag was the partially decomposed body of a young female homicide victim. After several unsuccessful attempts at identification, a forensic artist was called to make a

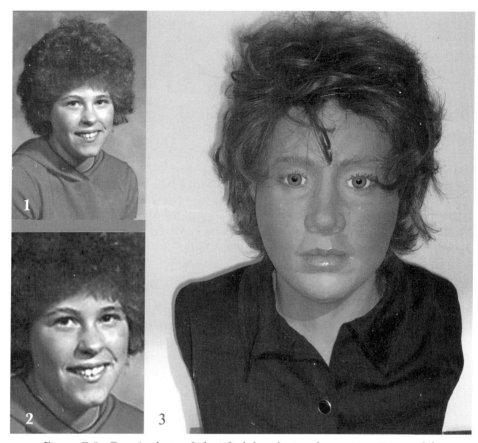

Figure G-2. Case 1, photo of identified decedent and reconstruction model.

facial reconstruction in hopes of generating additional leads. The community had adopted this young girl and buried her remains in an elaborate vault in a local cemetery. An anthropologist was asked to exhume the remains. Once exhumed, the facial skeleton was examined. The maxilla and parts of the mandible had been completely resected, severely damaging the facial skeleton. The artist, along with a forensic anthropologist and an odontologist, had access to the body for only 24 hours, beginning with the exhumation at dusk. Many details emerged in this second examination that were useful for the reconstruction, such as closer estimation of hair color, determination of ancestry, and estimation of age at death.

As with Case 1, regions of the face regions had to be reconstructed prior to molding. In addition, missing sections had to be replaced with clay. Only at this point could the artist begin the process of reconstruction of the facial features. This case resulted in the young woman's positive identification.

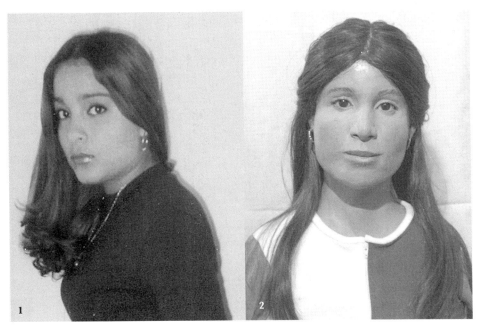

Figure G-3. Case 2, photo of identified decedent and reconstruction model.

CASE 3

A body was fished out of an irrigation canal in 1971. The female victim had been stabbed numerous times. Despite extensive media coverage, she remained unidentified, her remains were interred in a Jane Doe grave, and she went unidentified for 37 years. When her body was exhumed decades later from the county cemetery, her skull had badly decayed. Extensive water damage had produced erosion of the cortical surface and the bone had become brittle, friable, and warped. The calvarium did not fit evenly with the facial skeleton. The initial investigation's reports included many photographs. While all of the bones were present, the bone quality was so fragile that it required special treatment before the artist could begin work.

The bones were extremely fragile and friable. In particular, the bones were eroding and fragmentary along the temporal bones and zygomatic arches. There was a 4mm gap in zygo-temporal suture and an erosion of the facial surface of the maxilla on the right side. The cranial calotte, removed during autopsy, had become extremely distorted. There was also a postmortem radiating basilar fracture that had, over time, become distorted and warped. The surface of the skull was especially soft and the cortical layer crumbly. Given all these problems, it was only with great patience that the pieces were gradually coaxed together in a satisfactory matter. There was still some distortion of the

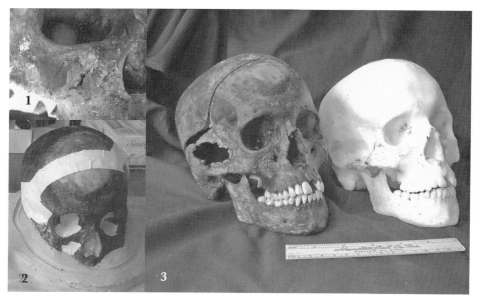

Figure G-4. Case 3, skull and mold preparation with cast of skull.

posterior cranial cap along the old autopsy cut. This was bridged with artist's tape, which is non-acidic and removable. After clearing this procedure with the investigating agency, the surfaces of the bone were treated with a mold-release

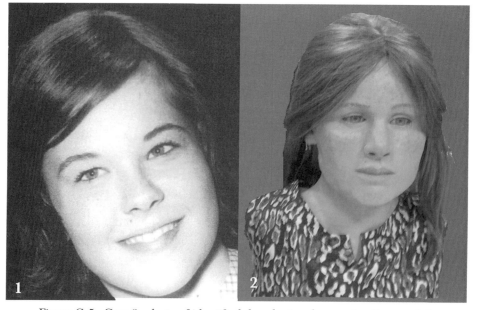

Figure G-5. Case 3, photo of identified decedent and reconstruction model.

agent. A mold was made of the skull using methods previously published by this author (Nusse 2003).

CASE 4

A young girl's body was discovered in the woods, the victim of a brutal attack. The right side and posterior aspects of the skull exhibited extreme perimortem blunt force trauma. The blows she sustained were so vicious that half of her skull was completely crushed. Impact points and tool marks could be seen on the parietal and occipital bones. All that remained relatively intact of her skull was the left half of her facial bones along with the orbital rim of the zygomatic bone on the right side. Her nasal aperture was mostly intact as was the nasal spine. However, by the time the remains were sent to the artist for reconstruction, the mandible was missing. Extensive

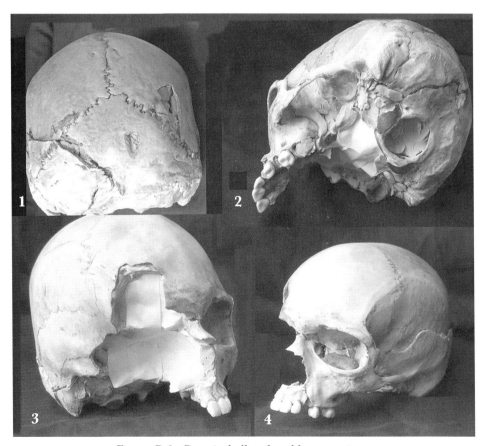

Figure G-6. Case 4, skull and mold preparations.

documentation of the initial investigation was available for the case along with hair samples.

Because evidence of the blunt force trauma was still present, the artist had to document and to protect the impact marks. The material used for mold making is specially formulated for use on injured human tissue. The mold was made of the skull as it was, and no remodeling was performed on the actual skull (Figure G-7). A mold was made of the left half of the skull, including the lateral left side and a partial medial surface of the face. A separate mold of the lateral orbital rim of the zygomatic bone on the left side was also completed. The features on the left side provided the guide for remodeling the missing parts on the right side. The cast of the orbital region of the right zygomatic bone was subsequently fit into the clay on the right side (illustration 4).

Case 4 had a missing mandible in addition to the blunt force trauma. The author used Krogman's method of calculating a visual arc representing the length and arc of the lateral mandible (Krogman 1962). The medial measurement of the mandible was calculated according to the George Mandibulofacial index for average females (George 2007). This reconstruction was calculated at 70.1mm. The replacement mandible was fashioned from an extra cast mandible, modified to meet the requirements of the calculated indices for Case 4. It was cut and fit to the mandibular fossae of the temporal bone (Figure G-8).

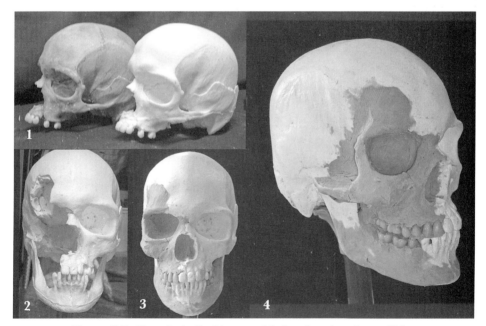

Figure G-7. Case 4, skull with remodeled and replaced mandible.

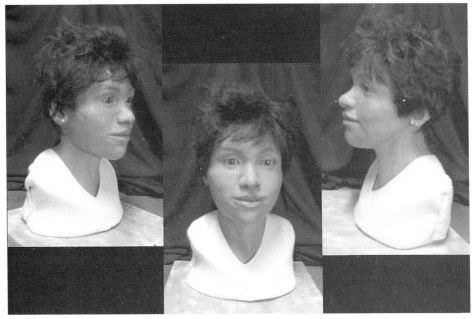

Figure G-8. Case 4, facial reconstruction, decedent unidentified as of this writing.

Fragmentation, Missing Pieces, and Reconstruction

Fragmentation of the skull can often be severe and the artist must always evaluate the feasibility of a reconstruction before commencing. In some cases, commissions must be refused if the damage is too severe. However, there are often ways to accommodate to the current state of the bones. Fragmented remains for the cases presented here were glued carefully together with glue such as model airplane cement, which is reversible with acetone, with white glue that is reversible with water, or with museum wax for temporarily holding parts together. Small rectangles of card stock and pieces of tongue depressors were affixed to the inside surface help to suspend pieces, as were pieces of re-movable artists tape. The pieces were held loosely in place at the beginning to allow the subsequent pieces to fit.

Because the skull often retains evidence of impact points and imprints of the weapon used, the artist must document and protect all such markings. Sharp instruments must never touch the bone directly and any sensitive data must be protected with thin foil or plastic. The artist always consults with the investigative agency before proceeding with any process that may affect these marks. For example, in Case 3, it was necessary that explicit permission be granted for the artist to use a mold release agent on the very fragile and eroded bones.

Removal of the brain during autopsy is done with a Stryker saw, which destroys approximately 1 to 2mm of bone. This gap can be easily filled and the calvaria glued in place using flat toothpicks to fill this space. If there is plastic distortion of this intersection, the artist can place the distortion near the posterior aspect of the skull since it may be obscured by hair. The author tries to keep the anterior, lateral, and medial facial planes as intact as possible.

When the teeth have been removed during autopsy for radiographic identification, as seen in Cases 1 and 2, these areas need to be reconstructed. The care taken at the time of the removal varies. In Case 1, a Stryker saw was used, leaving a smooth cut. Had the teeth been recovered, the gap could have been accommodated in the same manner described in the section describing removal of the calotte. In Case 2, the teeth had been removed using root clippers. As a result, the maxilla was shattered along with the temporal condyles, coronoid processes, and the condylar necks of the mandible. In this case, spacing of the frontal region of the face had to be matched and filled in to approximate the correct space as well as correct placement of the mandible since the mandibular condyle and condylar neck were missing. Even though the teeth were present, it was treated as if it were edentulous to accommodate the missing parts. This was possible because the mandibular notch was present.

By the time the skeletal remains are delivered to the artist, the mandible is usually separated from the cranium. In order to fit the mandible correctly to the cranium, it is necessary to achieve the correct angle of the mandible in alignment with the rest of the skull. This artist uses the method outlined by Gatliff in Taylor's *Forensic Art and Illustration* (2001) for fitting an edentulous skull. This fitting is accomplished by placing a standard wooden pencil so that it passes over the mandibular notch then through to the other side along the inferior aspect of the cranium behind the pterygoid plates and rests on the opposite side. A wire is then inserted into the casting between the mandible and the cranium to accommodate the occlusal fit and mandibular angle (Figure G-9). A small piece of toothpick is inserted to create a gap between the teeth to mimic the relaxed position of the occlusal bite in life.

When parts are missing altogether, they must be remodeled in clay. The author has found that it is best to mold the skull with the parts missing and then remodel the replica skull. The artist sculpts in the missing parts with oil-based clay using the surviving side as a guide and matching sides for the missing parts.

This remodeling process can be particularly critical when the dentition is involved. Often the upper teeth and surrounding alveolar process and horizontal ramus are missing due to removal for radiographic analysis. As occurred in Case 1, the artist then must use available records. In Case 1, an old photo taken of the intact maxilla and mandible with a scale bar was found in the case file. After consulting the dental report written on the case in 1979, the artist enlarged the photo of the teeth to life size. This image was then printed

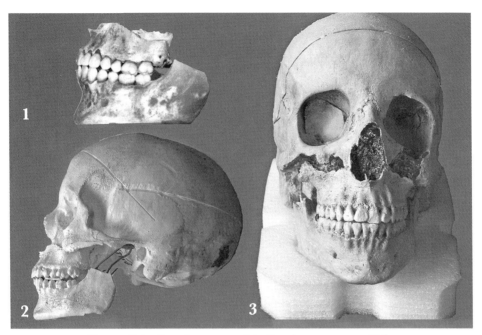

Figure G-9. Case 2, casting of skull with wire in mandible.

on a transparent piece of acetate. The acetate was then trimmed and fitted along the barrel of mouth in a contoured fashion. The transparency of the acetate allowed the underlying bone to be positioned to accommodate the cut bone. An Adobe Photoshop© image of the same was created (Figure G-10). The rolled acetate fit better with the actual skull because this allowed for distortion in the old photograph. These composite photographs were used for consultation in sculpting the missing parts in clay.

When the mandible is missing, techniques similar to what is described in Case 4 should be followed. A basic model of a mandible, matched for approximate size and sex, should be used as the foundation. The George Mandibulo-facial index may be used to fit the mandible size to that of the victim's cranium.

SUMMARY

Facial reconstructions have been widely adopted, especially to reinvigorate cases that have gone cold. Unfortunately, these remains are often badly damaged, making reconstruction of facial features more difficult. The cases described above, along with the techniques used, demonstrate there are ways the artist can handle even badly damaged bones to produce a good reproduction while ensuring the integrity of the skull for further analysis.

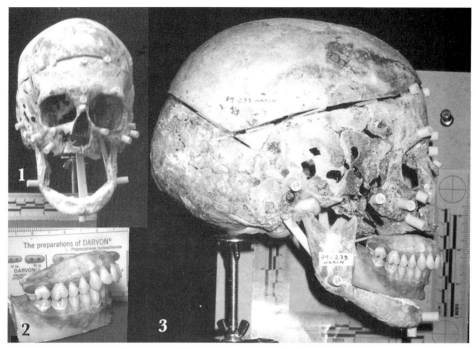

Figure G-10. Case 1, assembled skull, teeth and composite image.

H. HEALED TRAUMA AND HOMICIDAL VIOLENCE IN THE CASE OF A HOMELESS MAN

Gwendolyn Haugen

On a March day, two individuals were searching for aluminum cans along the side of a major interstate highway in rural Missouri when they noticed a tennis shoe in the brush. Upon closer examination, they observed skeletal remains protruding from the shoe extending into a pant leg that was positioned slightly upslope. The couple immediately contacted the local sheriff's department for assistance. A relatively complete set of skeletonized human remains, partially concealed by large stones from the chest to head area, was identified at the scene (Figure H-1). The remains were positioned on the ground, which sloped to the east, with the head to the south and the feet to the north. Also associated with the remains were clothing and possible bedding materials. The head was covered with what appeared to be a shirt and faced slightly west. No identification media was found with the deceased. The sheriff's department reported to the medical examiner's personnel that transients were known to live on both sides of the highway in this area because it was known as a popular spot for panhandling. Sheriff's department personnel performed a detailed recovery of the remains and all associated evidence. The human remains and associated clothing were removed *in situ* and transported to the medical examiner's office for examination.

INITIAL EXAMINATION

An inventory of the remains revealed a virtually complete human skeleton clothed in two shirts (one long sleeve and one short sleeve), black jeans, underwear, socks, and tennis shoes (Figures H-1 and H-2). The shirts had been pulled up and wrapped around the skull leaving the torso exposed. The body had been supine with the left arm raised above the head and bent at the elbow and the hand area preserved under the skull. The right arm was positioned downward along the right side of the torso, and the legs were extended and

391

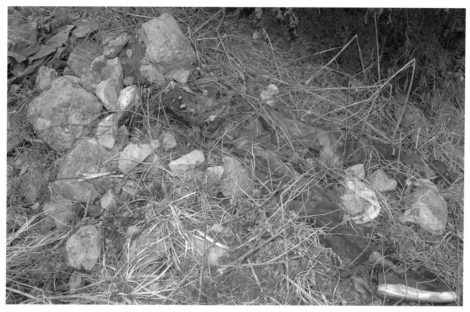

Figure H-1. Skeletal remains in the context of discovery.

parallel. The shirts were removed to reveal the skull, which was positioned on its left side. The remains were well preserved. Adherent to the remains were local plant materials and some soils that were determined to be consistent with the context of discovery. The condition of the plants indicated that the body had been in contact with the ground surface for an extended period of time. Pupal insect casings were observed, but no active maggot infestation was noted. The state of preservation of the remains was interpreted to indicate a postmortem interval of ten months or more.

Anthropological Analysis

The remains were in an excellent state of preservation and necessitated merely minimal maceration (Figure H-2). The biological profile categorized the individual as male of European ancestry who was approximately 50–59 years old at time of death. His mean living stature was 73 inches (6'1"). In addition, the dentition exhibited damage consistent with chronic use of crystal methamphetamine.

Evidence of Trauma

The skeleton exhibited evidence of both ante- and perimortem trauma. Each instance was photographed and described. The extensive antemortem

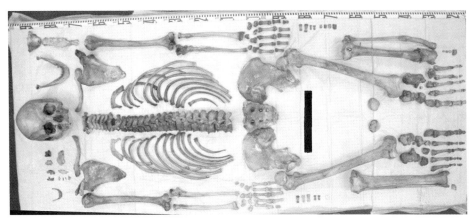

Figure H-2. Skeletal remains following maceration. Scale is in centimeters.

trauma with surgical appliances ultimately aided in positively identifying this individual. Each instance of antemortem trauma was documented.

Antemortem

It was immediately apparent that this individual had been involved in a serious antemortem traumatic incident that required surgical repair and stabilization of the skull, left arm, and left leg. Additionally healed injuries to multiple ribs and two hand phalanges were observed. The medically-treated fractures of the face (left maxilla), left arm, and left leg appeared to have been sustained at the same time based on the degree of bone remodeling observed. Because all of the evidence of fracture remodeling and callus development was similar, it was inferred that antemortem injuries were all sustained in the same traumatic incident. The injuries were as follows:

1. Skull: Fracturing of the left maxilla extending into the left zygomat had been surgically repaired with three mini plates and screws. Two orbital floor implants were also present in the left eye orbit. A healing fracture was observed to the left frontal at the superomedial aspect of the orbit (Figure H-3).
2. Ribs: Left ribs 2, 7, and 9 exhibited healed fracture areas to the medial and lateral aspects. Right ribs 2, 3, and 9 also exhibited healed fracture areas to their medial and lateral aspects.
3. Left Arm: The proximal ulnar diaphysis exhibited a fracture that had been stabilized with a plate and six screws (Figure H-4). The plate exhibited a service mark and a serial number, both of which were recorded as possible aids to the identification of this individual. The 5 proximal hand phalanx exhibited a healed fracture at the distal aspect.

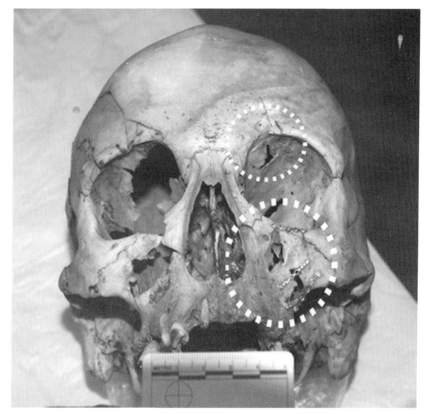

Figure H-3. Surgical mini plates and screws that were used to repair the right maxilla (bottom elipsis) and healing superomedial orbital fracture (top elipsis). Both elipses denote areas of antemortem trauma. Scale bars in millimeters.

4. Right Hand: The right first distal hand phalanx exhibited a healing sharp trauma defect to its medial aspect. A second, indeterminate distal hand phalanx exhibited a healing sharp trauma defect to its distal end.

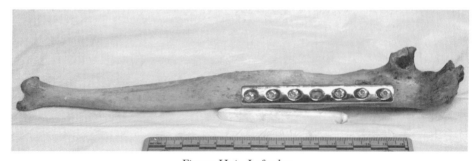

Figure H-4. Left ulna.

5. Left Leg: The tibia had been stabilized with a full-length diaphyseal rod and two screws (one proximal and one distal). It appeared that the tibia had fractured obliquely subsequent to the surgical stabilization (Figure H-5). The oblique fracture occurred just superior to the distal screw. This fracture appears to have displaced the distal screw and was never medically treated. Extensive evidence of bone remodeling was observed in the form of periosteal reaction. An oblique fracture was also observed on the distal articulating surface of the tibia. The fibula exhibited a healed oblique fracture to the distal diaphysis. This fracture appeared to have occurred at the same time as the oblique fracture of the tibia and was also not medically treated (Figures H-5–H-7). The intramedullary tibial rod was removed revealing additional service numbers and a

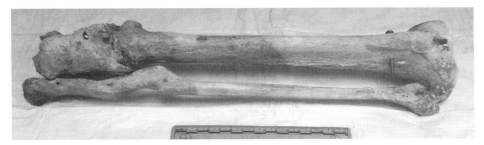

Figure H-5. Left tibia and fibula, lateral articulated view. Scale bar in millimeters.

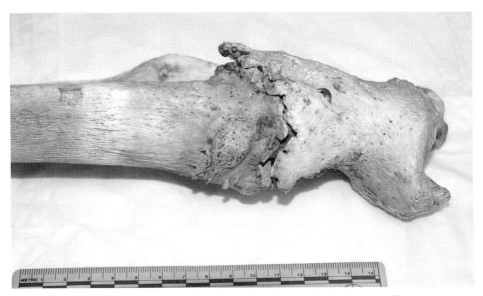

Figure H-6. Distal aspect of left tibia. Medial view. Scale bar in millimeters.

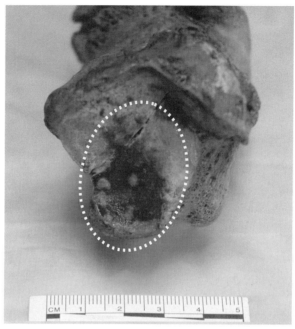

Figure H-7. Distal articulating surface of the left tibia. Ellipsis denotes area of trauma.

service mark. These were also recorded as a possible aid to the identification of this individual.

Perimortem Trauma

Considerable perimortem trauma was also observed and consisted of both blunt and sharp-force trauma. The injuries are described as follows:

1. Skull: Blunt-force trauma was observed to the right side of the skull with comminuted fracturing of the temporoparietofrontal and orbital regions (Figures H-8 and H-9). This area was partially reconstructed to facilitate analysis.
2. Sternum: A sharp trauma defect was observed on the left latero-distal aspect of the manubrium.
3. Ribs: Three left ribs and one right rib exhibited perimortem trauma. Left rib 3 exhibited sharp force trauma with the sternal end missing postmortem. Left rib 7 exhibited probable blunt force trauma to the sternal aspect. Left rib 8 had a hinged fracture present at its sternal end. Right rib 8 exhibited blunt-force trauma with the sternal end missing postmortem.
4. Cervical Vertebrae: C4 exhibited sharp force trauma bilaterally on the superior articular facets. C5 exhibited a perimortem fracture to the right superior articular facet.

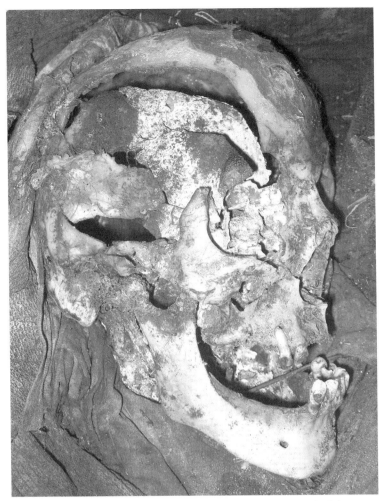

Figure H-8. Right side of skull as viewed upon removal of shirt.

5. Right Hand: The distal diaphysis of the number 1 proximal hand phalanx
   was fractured obliquely and the distal tip was missing postmortem.

SUMMARY

Personnel from the State Highway Patrol Crime Laboratory researched the
serial numbers and service marks from the intramedullary tibial rod and the
ulnar plate, and a list of hospitals receiving these appliances was generated by
the company. A hospital in Tulsa, Oklahoma, had received both the ulnar plate
and the intramedullary tibial rod. The hospital was contacted and the patient's

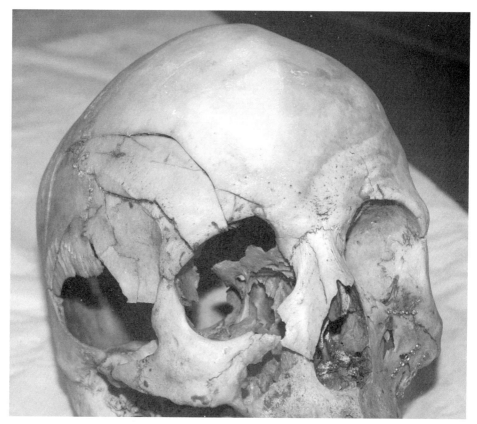

Figure H-9. Oblique view of right side of skull after maceration of tissue and partial reconstruction. Scale bar is in millimeters.

medical records were requested and received by the Medical Examiner's Office. The records revealed that five years prior to discovery of the remains, a white male, then 47 years old, had been the victim of an auto-pedestrian accident in which he was struck on his left side. The man's injuries necessitated extensive surgery and a three-month hospital stay.

The medical examiner took into consideration the findings of the forensic anthropologist and certified the cause of death as homicidal violence based on the blunt force trauma to the head and blunt and sharp force trauma to the chest and neck. This case is an excellent example of how properly classifying blunt force into the ante-, peri-, and postmortem periods can both help lead to the identification of the deceased as well as contribute to the determination of cause and manner of death. Despite the wealth of identifying information the skeleton exhibited, no leads have successfully led to the capture and prosecution of any suspects in the case. However, it remains under investigation.

I. AN ANTHROPOLOGICAL CONUNDRUM

Sue Black, J. Smyth, Alastair Bentley, Caroline Erolin,
and P. Randolph-Quinney

In the late winter of 2007, a 92-year-old man (MFB) was found dead in the rear bedroom of his bungalow. He had reportedly last been seen alive that morning. Police found no evidence of forced entry or of theft, nor any of the weapon(s) that had been used by whomever committed the crime. He was lying face down in a large pool of his own blood with a section of the left frontal lobe of his brain on the floor beside him. While the injuries to the soft tissue of his face were not insubstantial, the injuries to the bone were much more devastating than originally conceived.

A forensic anthropologist had not been involved in the original postmortem examination and the postmortem images came for anthropological assessment some seven months later when it was clear that an obvious solution to the cause of the trauma (skeletal and soft tissue) was not forthcoming. Unfortunately, the body had been released for burial, and while the calotte had been retained, cleaned, and reconstructed, the remainder of the skull had been interred with the rest of the remains. Much of the analysis, therefore, had to be undertaken based on postmortem images and discussions with the pathologist and the police. Radiographs had been taken, but they did not confer any additional information.

This case study will demonstrate that even given a limited amount of bone, a few photographs, and associated radiographs, a forensic anthropologist can describe evidence otherwise not collected. However, this case provides a prime example of the limitations imposed when the anthropologist is not involved from the very beginning: the very best one might be able to contribute is description, rather than an interpretation based on the descriptors.

FORENSIC EXAMINATION

When fresh and still fleshed, the remains were autopsied. The preliminary external examination revealed the following facts that are relevant to the analysis of the skeletal injuries presented:

- Blood seeping from left ear.
- Two faint red abrasions, each about 2mm in diameter on the left side of the forehead 8cm to the left of the anterior midline and 5cm superior to the glabella.
- A red abrasion (2.5×1.5cm) on the left side of the forehead, 6cm to the left of the anterior midline and 4cm superior to the glabella.
- A red abrasion (0.8×1cm) on the right side of the forehead, 3.5cm to the right of the anterior midline and 5.5cm superior to the glabella.
- Purple bruising to the upper left eyelid.
- Purple-blue peri-orbital haematoma around the right eye.
- An oblique cut (7.4cm in length) extending from the medial end of the left supraorbital ridge to the prominence of the left cheek (around the inner canthus of the left eye). Fishtailing was present at the upper end of the cut with seven stellate punctuate abrasions forming two interrupted curves.
- Comminuted fracture of the left nasal bone.

The autopsy of the musculoskeletal system and internal organs revealed the following (other non-related features were recorded but are not relayed in this communication):

- Tearing of the rhomboid major and minor muscles on the right side.
- Extensive bruising across the occipital, frontal, and superior aspects of the inner surface of the scalp.
- Extensive comminuted fracturing of the calvarium, most obvious in the parieto-occipital region, but extending to both lateral aspects of the skull.
- Gaping fracture extending from the inferior border of the left zygomatic bone extending vertically between the nose and orbit and then vertically through the frontal bone, just left of the midline, into the area of comminution in the parieto-occipital region. Comminuted fracturing of the right supra-orbital ridge and adjacent area of the frontal bone.
- Ragged deep sagittal fracture of the base of the skull to the left of the midline passing to the left of the hypophyseal fossa and extending to the junction with the petrous part of the left temporal bone.
- Comminuted (ring) fracturing around the foramen magnum.
- Extrusion of the left frontal lobe of the brain.
- Bilateral comminuted fracturing of the maxilla and comminuted fracturing of the left nasal bone and medial part of the left orbital margin.
- Transverse fracture through the upper part of the body of the sternum at the level of the second intercostal space.
- Anterolateral fractures of the fourth to eighth ribs on the right side, with no obvious associated bruising.

The neuropathologist's report revealed:

* Detached region of left frontal lobe measured 6×5cm.
* Posterior section of this detached portion showed a fairly clean cleavage plane.
* Little underlying neurodegenerative disease.
* No well defined haemorrhagic tract.
* No evidence of an acute stroke.

In summary, the pathologist's findings were as follows:

* Toxicological analysis was negative for alcohol and common drugs.
* Death due to severe head injury had resulted in extensive fracturing of almost all major bones of the skull.
* There was a "tear" in the skin overlying a gaping fracture to the left side of the nose through which a sizeable portion of the left frontal lobe of the brain had been expelled.
* The extent of the fracturing of the skull and facial bones strongly suggested more than one forceful impact; however, there was a small number of relatively minor injuries to the scalp, which was surprising. These gave no clear indication as to how the extensive fracturing was sustained.
* The distribution of blood at the locus indicated that the head injury must have occurred within the room in which the deceased was found. There was nothing at the death scene to offer a plausible explanation as to how such a severe head injury could have been sustained as a consequence of an accident, and the medical examiner concluded that MFB was the victim of a fatal assault via a weapon or weapons unknown.
* The nature and pattern of the injuries suggested multiple impacts, one of which was likely to have been a blow delivered by a weapon/implement to the left side of the face between the eye and nose. The other injuries were likely due to blunt force trauma but there were no appreciable marks on the skin to help to ascertain how they had been sustained.

ANTHROPOLOGICAL ASSESSMENT

The calvarial portion of the skull (Figure I-1) and an area associated with the left orbit, maxilla, and nasal region (Figure I-2) were the only skeletal material retained and transferred to the anthropologist for examination, although supplemental information was available from the postmortem photographs and radiographs. Figures I-1 and I-2 show the reconstruction of the skull with anatomical realignment of the skull fragments. These cannot be directly compared with the appearance of the skull at the time of the post-mortem when the fragments were in a slightly different alignment. Due to

Broken Bones

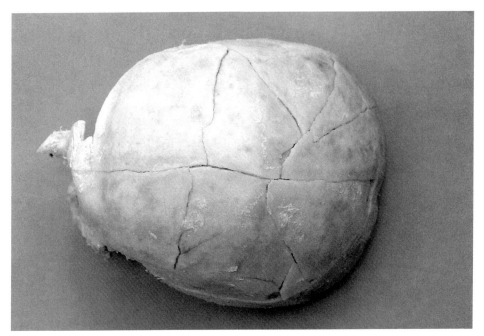

Figure I-1. Retained, cleaned, and reconstructed calotte.

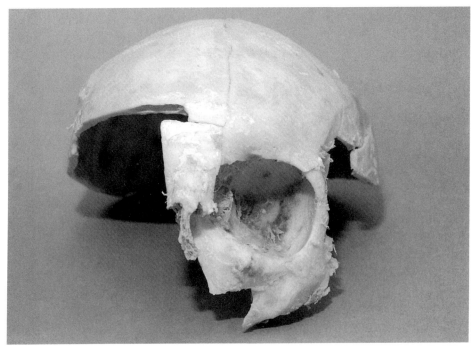

Figure I-2. Retained, cleaned, and reconstructed facial elements.

the sensitivity of this case, we cannot show the original postmortem images, but the subsequent illustrations (Figures I-3–I-8) are representations from the postmortem images and therefore show the more realistic alignment of the fragments.

The images make clear that several episodes of trauma had occurred to the skull, and one of the first processes to be carried out was a sequential analysis of individual injuries in an attempt to predict the number of events and the order of their occurrence. The extensive fragmentation of the skull further complicated the interpretation of the injury patterns as a shattered skull behaves differently from one that is intact. Each sequential impact must be analyzed with the pre-existing level of fragmentation borne in mind.

At least five identifiable impacts or traumatic events were proposed, and a tentative sequential progression was suggested. The external soft tissue trauma was of limited assistance in the interpretation of the skeletal traumatic events.

Trauma 1

This designation pertains to a circumferential fracture that translates around the skull running continuously from the left temporofrontal region, around the area superior to the external occipital protuberance, to a roughly equivalent position on the right temporofrontal region. This fracture is represented as line "1" in Figure I-3. The sides of the fracture were relatively straight edged and the absence of bevelling supported a possible propagative nature to the fracture. Four possible impact sites were identified along the trajectory of this fracture. These have been labelled as A, B, C, and D on Figure I-3 as passing from the left to the right respectively. The approximate distance between A and B is 18mm and between C and D is approximately 12mm. The approximate distance between A and C is 67mm and between B and D is 61mm. This suggests the possibility of a double impact trauma from the same double-pointed implement. The presence of internal bevelling at contact point B indicates that the implement did penetrate both diploic tables at this point only. This fracture line has been identified as the first to occur and (due to its inhibitory nature on the propagation of other fractures) passes through what is generally regarded as the thickest region of the skull and must have resulted from a trauma(s) of significant impact. It is possible that the full extent of propagation of the fracture did not occur until the second event, but it unquestionably predated the next traumatic event. The fracture dissipates anteriorly both on the right and left sides in the temporofrontal regions (Figures I-4 and I-5), confirming that the majority of the blunt force was applied to the back of the skull. This trauma coincided with some bleeding that was visible into the soft tissues of the occipital region of the scalp.

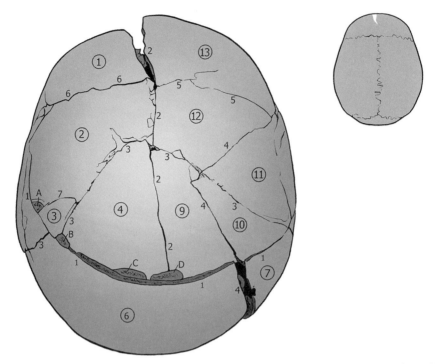

Figure I-3. Fracturing of frontal, parietal, and occipital regions. Skull fragments are indicated by the encircled numbers while fracture lines are indicated by the simple numbers. Possible impact points are labelled as A–D and are somewhat exaggerated for the purposes of this illustration.

Trauma 2

The soft tissue damage to the face was fully documented in the pathology report (Figure I-6). It is highly likely that this impact opened up the fracture line labelled "2" in Figure I-3 and the vertical fracture line that passes through the roof of the left orbit and orbital plate of the frontal bone before passing to the left of the hypophyseal fossa and terminating towards the region of the left petrous temporal bone (Figure I-7). The vault aspect of this fracture traverses a relatively para-sagittal course from the frontal to the occipital bone where it intercepts with fracture line number '1' and is halted at the location of fragment D. Therefore fracture "1" most likely predates fracture "2." All other fractures that subsequently cross the para-sagittal fracture do so in a stepped format (fractures 3, 5, and 6) and thus we surmise that they may have occurred after fracture number "2." It is not unusual for an upper face fracture to propagate through the region of the orbit and be transferred to the skull base. Although MFB was an elderly male, his bones were not overly thinned or osteoporotic but were of a healthy density given his age. The force to cause such a fracture would most likely have been substantial and may correspond

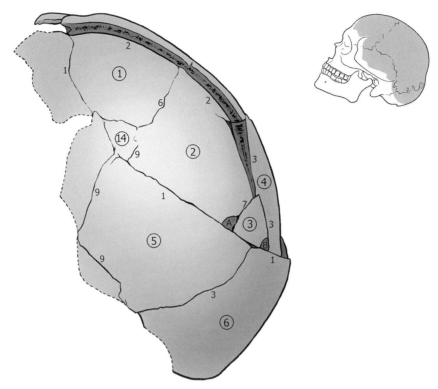

Figure I-4. Left lateral view of the vault region.

with the trauma visible to the front of his face. The nature of the soft tissue damage to the front of the face is outside the remit of the forensic anthropologist and is discussed in the pathologist's report.

Trauma 3

This third set of defects is likely to have occurred prior to the fourth event although the temporal alignment is less certain than for the previous two events. The postmortem photograph showed significant comminuted fracturing around the base of the skull, which is very similar to a ring-type fracture associated with the perimeter of the foramen magnum (Figure I-7). This type of fracture is often caused by high-impact trauma e.g., falling from a height onto the feet or some other form of significant impact, which is of sufficient force to drive the C1 vertebra up into the foramen magnum causing circumferential fracturing (see Chapter 8, this volume). These scenarios were difficult to accept given the location of the deceased and evidence from the scene of the crime. The bungalow contained no great interior heights from which the victim could have fallen.

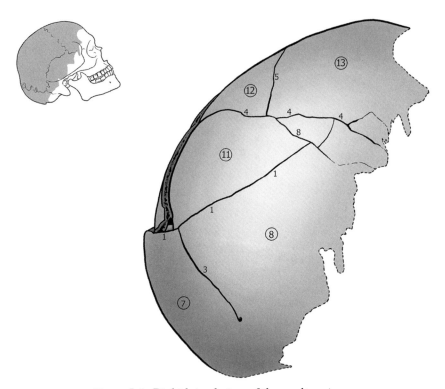

Figure I-5. Right lateral view of the vault region.

However, in an attempt to explain this fracture patterning, several other indicators of trauma needed to be considered. MFB displayed tearing to the rhomboid muscles (major and minor) on the right side of his back. These muscles act as connectors between the scapula and the neural arches of the lower cervical and upper thoracic vertebrae. Injury to these muscles generally arises from excessive movement of the upper limb causing them to tear off of their vertebral attachments. A fracture was present across the body of the sternum and also through right ribs 4–8. It is highly unlikely that MFB either fell from a great height either onto his head or onto his feet, but this does not preclude an impact trauma that would have been sufficient to drive his vertebral column upwards into the base of the occipital bone.

A mattress was propped up against one wall. It is possible that the victim was swung by his right arm (thereby ripping the rhomboids) and collided, crown first, with the mattress on the wall. This would have cushioned the actual impact point of his skull, but the momentum of the rest of his body could have been transferred up his vertebral column and into the occipital bone, thus manifesting as a comminuted, ring fracture (Figure I-7). This could have manifested in limited damage to the scalp and bones on the top of the

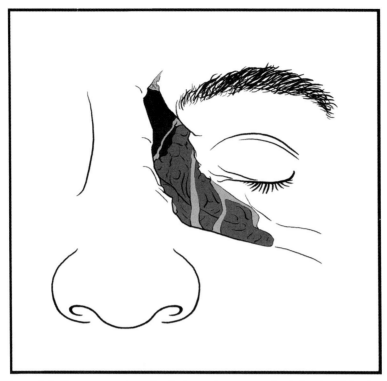

Figure I-6. Representation of soft tissue damage to the left side of the face.

head and explain the extent of cranial damage in the absence of external indicators. The fracturing seen in the sternum and ribs may support this scenario.

The impact was sufficient to propagate a further fracture from the right hand side of the ring fracture up the right side of the occipital bone as fracture line number "4" (Figures I-3 and I-7). This fracture was of significant force and was able to traverse, and propagate beyond, fracture "1." Fracture "3" predates fracture "4," but we believe that it may also emanate from the region of the ring fracture but from the left hand side. This is also a powerful fracture which runs between bone fragments 6, 2, and 4, 9 and 12, 10, and 11 and finally 7 and 8 (Figures I-3, I-4, and I-5). As fractures "3" and "4" come into approximation in the region of the upper right parietal bone, there is sufficient tension caused between the two forces of propagation that fracture "4" snapped from its trajectory and took a new right-angled route between fragments 11 and 12 (Figure I-3). Fracture "4" breaches fracture "3" on its new trajectory.

It is not clear from the postmortem photographs where fracture "3" commenced and it is highly unlikely to have been a continuation of fracture "9" which seems to have been a relatively weak fracture. Therefore it is likely that indeed fracture "9" terminated in the pre-existing fracture "3." The only

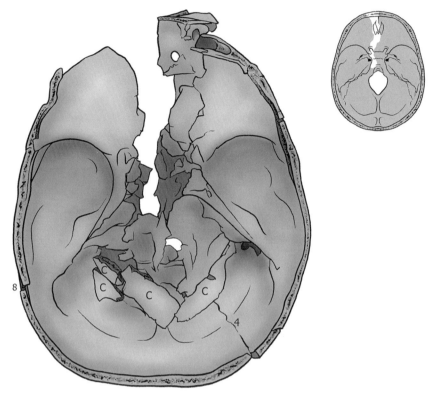

Figure I-7. Representation of fracturing at the base of the skull. The "Cs" designate comminuted-fracture fragments located around the foramen magnum.

obvious origin for this fracture is, therefore, from the comminuted region of the ring fracture around the foramen magnum, but this cannot be confirmed from the photographs. It had sufficient force to pass across fractures "1" and "2" before it terminated in what appears to be an emissary foramen on the posterolateral aspect of the right occipital bone (Figure I-5). Fracture "4" has traversed fracture "1" (Figure 3), but it did not extend as far as fracture "2" as it met with fracture "3" passing in the opposite direction. The right-angled change, of course, suggests that the stress between the two propagating forces was sufficient to alter the course of fracture "4" so that it remained on the right side of the skull.

Trauma 4

This incident does not seem to carry the same degree of force as those necessary to have caused traumas 1–3, but it should be remembered that the skull was possibly severely fragmented by this stage. There would have had to have been extensive dissipation of stress into previous fracture spaces. This trauma pertains to the proximity of the two areas of abrasion reported on the external region of the scalp. The first abrasion on the left side corresponds with bruising seen on the internal surface of the scalp and corresponds with a region of irregular fracturing that resulted in fragment 14 of the skull (Figure I-4). This fragment exhibits an upwards directed weak fracture line "6" which intersects with fracture line "2" in the para-sagittal region. A downwards fracture, number "9," passes inferiorly along the sphenotemporal junction and may have terminated in fracture number "3" on the left side of the skull.

The fracture on the right-hand side of the skull produced a fragment of bone that was bounded by fractures "4" and "8" (Figure I-5). Fracture "5" appears to have occurred in two steps (Figure I-3), suggesting possible different points of propagation. It is possible that the medial part of fracture "5" is, in fact, a continued propagation of fracture "6" across the sagittal fracture whereas the more lateral part of the fracture runs inferiorly and terminates in fracture "4."

It is difficult to define how this fracture and abrasion pattern may have arisen, but on-going investigations in relation to an object found in the room may lead to a possible solution. Our apologies that no further details can be given at this time.

Trauma 5

Additional injury likely occurred when MFB fell to his final resting position on the floor of the bedroom. It is suggested that as he came to fall face down onto the hard (not carpeted) floor, he would have bounced because he was moderately rotund. Contact with the ground might have caused reflexive flexion and extension of the cervical region. With a pre-existing basal and sagittal fracture, the left side of his skull was effectively hinged, being held in place only by soft tissue structures (Figure I-8). The force of landing might have opened and closed this vertical fracture, which may have behaved like a hinged pair of scissors. This could have cleanly cleaved the left frontal lobe and resulted in its subsequent expulsion through the tear on the skin in the region of the left orbit and in fact this "hinging" may have caused, or significantly extended, the skin tear seen on the front of his face.

CONCLUSION

This is an on-going murder investigation and for this reason, details are necessarily vague. MFB clearly died as a result of multiple traumata to his skull, and we propose that at least four traumatic events and the final adoption of the resting position could account for all the fracturing evident on the skull,

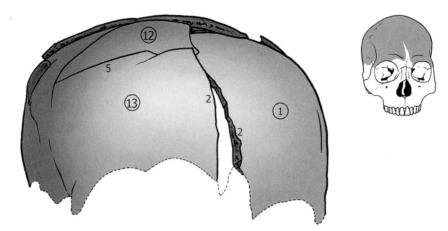

Figure I-8. Frontal view of the reconstructed vault region.

even in the absence of significant skin injury. Alternative theories are very welcome, and the authors would be happy to consider these along with advice and suggestions from experienced forensic anthropologists.

This case clearly displays the difficulties faced by the forensic expert when he or she is asked to comment on injuries in the absence of the complete skeleton but must rely only on photographs taken at the time of the post-mortem and incomplete skeletal material. It also emphasizes the importance that quality images be taken at the postmortem examination from as many different angles and aspects as possible. The results of the examination might have been better yet had the forensic anthropologist been present at the scene and autopsy.

This case illustrates that although far from ideal, the forensic anthropologist can still provide assistance even when the specialist was neither present at the scene nor had access to the remains at autopsy. At the time of writing, this case is still active and so care has been taken to disclose as little identifying information as possible as the case is extremely sensitive. Our apologies to readers if this leaves many unanswered questions or an incomplete under-standing of the situation and circumstances. However, the investigative au-thorities have permitted this communication to proceed in the hope that alternative and perhaps, as yet, unthought-of mechanisms might help explain the trauma inflicted on this elderly gentleman.

BIBLIOGRAPHY

Aare, M. and H. van Holst (2003). Injuries from motorcycle- and moped crashes in Sweden from 1987 to 1999. *Injury Control and Safety Promotion* 10(3):131–138.

Abrahams, T., L. Gallup, and F. Lincoln Avery (1994). Non-displaced shearing-type talar body fractures. *Annals of Emergency Medicine* 23:891–893.

Abrassart, S., R. Stern, and R. Peter (2009). Morbidity associated with isolated iliac wing fractures. *J Trauma* 66(1):200–203.

Adelson, L. (1974). Homicide by blunt violence: Deaths caused by manual, pedal and instrumental assault and by motor vehicle crashes. In *The Pathology of Homicide: A Vace Mecum for Pathologist, Prosecutor and Defense Counsel*, pp. 378–520. Charles C Thomas, Springfield, IL.

Adharapurapu, R., F. Jiang, and K. Vecchio (2006). Dynamic fracture of bone bone. *Materials Science and Engineering* 26:1325–1332.

Aebi, M. (2010). Classification of thoracolumbar fractures and dislocations. *European Spine Journal* 19:S2–S7.

Ahmad F., N. Kirkpatrick, J. Lynne, M. Urdang, and N. Waterhouse (2006). Buckling and hydraulic mechanisms in orbital blowout fractures: fact or fiction? *Journal of Craniofacial Surgery* 17(3):438–441.

Akaza K., Y. Bunai, M. Tsujinaka , I. Nakamura, A. Nagai, Y. Tsukata, and I. Ohya (2003). Elder abuse and neglect: Social problems revealed from 15 autopsy cases. *Legal Medicine* 5(1):7–14.

Akbarnia B. A., M. Silberstein, R. J. Rende, et al. (1986). Arthography in the diagnosis of fractures of the distal end of the humerus in infants. *Journal of Bone and Joint Surgery [Am]* 68:599.

Al Nazer R., J. Lanovaz, C. Kawalilak, J. D. Johnston, and S. Kontulainen (2012). Direct in vivo strain measurements in human bone – a systematic literature review. *Journal of Biomechanics* 45:27–40.

Al-Habdan, I. (2003). Birth-related fractures of long bones. *Indian J Pediatr* 70(12):959–960.

Albert, M. and P. Barre (1989). A scaphoid fracture associated with a displaced radial fracture in a child. *Clinical Orthopaedics* 240:233–235.

Albert, M. and D. Drvaric (1993). Injuries resulting from pathologic forces: Child abuse. In *Pediatric Fractures: A Practical Approach to Assessment and Treatment*, G. MacEwen, J. Kasser and S. Heinrich (Eds.), pp. 388. Williams and Wilkins, Baltimore.

Alexander, J., K. Leveno, J. Hauth, M. Landon, E. Thom, C. Spongy, M. Varner, A. Moawad, S. Caritis, M. Harper, R. Wapner, Y. Sorokin, M. Miodovnik, M. O'Sullivan, and B. Sibai (2006). Fetal injury associated with cesarean delivery. *Obstetrics and Gynecology* 108(4):885–890.

Alffram, P. (1964). An epidemiologic study of cervical and trochanteric fractures of the femur in an urban population: Analysis of 1,664 cases with special reference to etiologic factors. *Acta Orthop Scand Suppl* 65:1–109.

Alffram, P. and G. Bauer (1962). Epidemiology of fractures of the forearm. *Journal of Bone and Joint Surgery [Am]* 44:105–114.

Allman, F. (1967). Fractures and ligamentous injuries of the clavicle and its articulations. *Journal of Bone and Joint Surgery [Am]* 49:774–784.

Allsop D. L., C. Y. Warner, M. G. Willie, D. C. Schnieder, and A. M. Nahum (1988). Facial impact response – a comparison of the Hybrid III dummy and human cadaver. *Proceedings of the Proceedings of the 32rd Stapp Car Crash Conference.* Atlanta, GA.

Amadio, P. (1992). Scaphoid fractures. *Orthopaedic Clinics of North America* 23:7–17.

Ambade, V. and H. Godbole (2006). Comparison of wound patterns in homicide by sharp and blunt force. *Forensic Science International* 156(2):166–170.

Anderson, H. (1919). *The Medical and Surgical Aspects of Aviation.* Oxford University Press, London.

Anderson, L. (1984). Fractures of the shafts of the radius and ulna. In *Fractures in Adults,* C. Rockwood and D. Green (Eds.), pp. 511–588. J. B. Lippincott, Philadelphia.

Anderson, L. and R. D'Alonzo (1974). Fractures of the odontoid process of the axis. *Journal of Bone and Joint Surgery [Am]* 56:1663–1674.

Andreas, Z. J., L. Olivier, S. Nikola, T. Hanna, and I. Tateyuka (2011). Incidence, aetiology and pattern of mandibular fractures in central Switzerland. *Swiss Medical Weekly* 141:1–5.

Andreasen J. O. (1970). Etiology and pathogenesis of traumatic dental injuries: A clinical study of 1,298 cases. *Scandinavian Journal of Dental Research* 78:329.

———— (1981). *Traumatic Injuries of the Teeth.* W. B. Saunders, Philadelphia.

Angel, J. and P. Caldwell (1984). Death by strangulation: A forensic anthropological case from Wilmington, Delaware. In *Human Identification: Case Studies in Forensic Anthropology,* T. Rathbun and J. Buikstra (Eds.) pp. 168–175. Charles C Thomas, Springfield, IL.

Ankhrath S., P. V. Giannoudis, I. Barlow, M. C. Bellamy, S. J. Matthews, and R. M. Smith (2002). Injury patterns associated with mortality following motorcycle crashes. *Injury* 33:473–477.

Anyanechi C. E. and B. D. Saheeb (2011). Mandibular sites prone to fracture; an analysis of 174 cases in a Nigerian tertiary hospital. *Ghana Medical Journal* 45:111–114.

Arifin, M., S. Arwinder, A. Andwar, T. Djuwantono, and A. Faried (2012). Spontaneous depressed skull fracture during vaginal delivery: A report of two cases and literature review. *The Indian Journal of Neurotrauma.*

Arkader, A., J. Friedman, W. Warner, and L. Wells (2007). Complete distal femoral metaphyseal fractures: A harbinger of child abuse before walking age. *J Pediatric Orthop* 27(7):751–753.

Armour, B. S., L. Wolf, M. Mitra, and M. Brieding (2008). Differences in intimate partner violence among women with and without a disability. Paper presented at the American Public Health Association's 136th Annual Meeting.

Armstrong, P., V. Joughin, and H. Clarke (1994). Pediatric fractures of the forearm, wrist, and hand. In *Skeletal Trauma in Children*, N. Green and M. Swiointkowski (Eds.), pp 127–211. W. B. Saunders, Philadelphia.

Arneson, T., L. I. Melton, D. Lewallen, and W. O'Fallon (1988). Epidemiology of diaphyseal and distal femoral fractures in Rochester, MN. *Clinical Orthopaedics and Related Research* 234:188–194.

Arosarena, O., T. Fritsch, Y. Hsueh, B. Aynehchi, and R. Haug (2009). Maxillofacial injuries and violence against women. *Arch Facial Plast Surg* (11):1.

Asha'Ari, Z., R. Ahmad, J. Rahman, N. Kamarundin, and L. Ishlah (2011). Contrecoup injuries in patients with traumatic temporal bone fracture. *J Laryngol Otol* 125(8):781–785.

Ashhurst, D. (1992). Macromolecular synthesis and mechanical stability during fracture repair. In *Bone*, vol. 5, B Hall (Ed.). CRC Press, Boca Raton, FL.

Ashhurst, P. and R. Bromer (1992). Classification and mechanism of fractures of the leg bones involving the ankle. *AMA Archives of Surgery* 4:51–129.

Ashkenaze, D. and L. Ruby (1992). Metacarpal fractures and dislocations. *Orthopaedic Clinics of North America* 23:19–33.

Atanasijevic, T., S. Savic, S. Nikolic, and V. Djoki (2005). Frequency and severity of injuries in correlation with the height of fall. *Journal of Forensic Sciences* 50(3):608–612.

Atanasijevic T. C., V. M. Popovic, and S. D. Nikilic (2009). Characteristics of chest injury in falls from heights. *Legal Medicine* 11:S315-S317.

Athanassiadi, K., G. M., M. Moustardas, and E. Metaxas (2002). Sternal Fractures: Retrospective analysis of 100 cases. *World Journal of Surgery* 10:1243–1246.

Atkinson, P. J., H. R. (2001). Injuries produced by blunt trauma to the human patello-femoral joint vary with flexion angle of the knee. *Journal of Orthopaedic Research* 19:827–833.

Aufderheide, A. and C. Rodriguez-Martin (1998). *Encyclopedia of Human Paleopathology*. Cambridge University Press, Cambridge.

Axton, J. H. M., L. L. (1965). Congenital moulding depressions of the skull. *British Medical Journal* 1:1644–1647.

Azevado, A., R. Trent, and A. Ellis (1998). Population-based analysis of 10,766 hospitilizations for mandibular fractures in California, 1991–1993. *J Trauma* 45(6): 1084–1087.

Bado, J. (1967). The Monteggia lesion. *Clinical Orthopaedics and Related Research* 50: 71–86.

Bailey, P. (1985). Surfer's rib: Isolated first rib fracture secondary to indirect trauma. *Annals of Emergency Medicine* 14:117–120.

Bakalim, C. (1970). Fractures of the radial head and their treatment. *Acta Orthopaedica Scandinavica* 41:320–331.

Bakardjiev, A., P. P. (2007). Maxillofacial fractures in southern Bulgaria – a retrospective study of 1706 cases. *Journal of Cranio-Maxillofacial Surgery* 35:147–150.

Baker, S. and W. Spitz (1970). An evaluation of the hazard created by natural death at the wheel. *New England Journal of Medicine* 283:405.

Baker, S. P., B. J., D. F. Shanahan, and G. Li (2009). Aviation-related injury morbidity and mortality: Data from US Health Information systems. A*viation Space Environmental Medicine* 80(12):1001–1005.

Ballesteros, M. and P. Langenberg (2004). Pedestrian injuries and vehicle type in Maryland 1995–1999. *Accident Analysis and Prevention* 36:73–81.

Balthrop, P., J. Nyland, and C. Roberts (2009). Risk factors and musculoskeletal injuries associated with all-terrain vehicle accidents. *J Emerg Med* 36:121–131.

Banaszkiewicz, P., T. Scotland, and E. Myerscough (2002). Fractures in children younger than age 1 year: Importance of collaboration with child protection services. *Journal of Pediatric Orthopaedics* 22:740–744.

Banks, H. (1962). Factors influencing the result in fractures of the femoral neck. *Journal of Bone and Joint Surgery [Am]* 44:931–964.

Barancik, J. I., H. C. Thode, C. J. Kahn, J. Greensher, and S. Schechter (1992). Injuries in the Avianca Plane Crash: Aviance Flight 052–January 25, 1990. NCE Committee US Department of Energy, Mineola, NY.

Barbian, L. T. and P. S. Sledzik (2008). Healing following cranial trauma. *J Forensic Sci* 53(2):263–268.

Barei D. P. and S. E. Nork (2003). Noncontiguous fractures of the femoral neck, femoral shaft and distal femur. *Journal of Trauma* 55:80–86.

Barlow, B., M. Niemierska, R. Gandhi, and W. Leblanc (1983). Ten years of experience with falls from a height in children. *Journal of Pediatric Surgery* 18:509–511.

Barnes, R., J. Brown, R. Garden, and E. Nicoll (1976). Subcapital fractures of the femur: A prospective review. *Journal of Bone and Joint Surgery [Br]* 58:2–24.

Barry, P. and M. Hocking (1993). Infant rib fracture: Birth trauma or non-accidental injury. *Archives of Disease in Childhood* 68:250.

Barsness, K., E. Cha, D. Bernard, C. Calkins, D. Patrick, F. Karrer, and J. Strain (2003). The positive predictive value of rib fractures as an indicator of non-accidental trauma in children. *J Trauma, Injury, Infection, and Critical Care* 54(6):1107–1110.

Bassett, J., R. Gibson, and R. Wilson (1968). Blunt Injuries to the Chest. *Journal of Trauma* 8:418–429.

Bastian, H. L. (1989). Fractures of the mandible: A discussion of etiology and location. *Danish Dental Journal* 93:589–593.

Bastone, E. B., T. J. Freer, and J. R. McNamara (2000). Epidemiology of dental trauma: A review of the literature. *Australian Dental Journal* 45(1):2–9.

Battle, C. E., H. Hutchings, and P. A. Evans (2011). Risk factors that predict mortality in patients with blunt chest wall trauma: A systematic review and meta-analysis. *Injury* 43:8–17.

Bauer, G. (1960). Epidemiology of fractures in aged persons: A preliminary investigation in fracture etiology. *Clinical Orthopaedics* 17:219–225.

Beals, R. and E. Tufts (1983). Fractured femur in infancy: The role of child abuse. *J Pediatric Orthop* 3:583–586.

Beardsley, C., C. Bertsch, J. Marsh, and T. Brown (2002). Interfragmentary surface area as an index of comminution energy: Proof of concept in bone fracture surrogate. *J Biomech* 35(3):331–338.

Beaty, J. H. and J. R. Kasser (2006). The elbow: Physeal fractures, apophyseal injuries of the distal humerus, osteonecrosis of the trochlea and T-condylar fractures. In *Rockwood and Wilkins' Fractures in Children*, J. R. Kasser and J. H. Beaty (Eds.), p. 628. Lippincott, Williams and Wilkins, Philadelphia.

Beckenbaugh, R., T. Shivers, J. Dobyns, and R. Linscheid (1980). Kienbock's disease and the natural history of Kienbock's disease and consideration of lunate fractures. *Clinical Orthopaedics* 149:98–106.

Begley, A. D., D. S. Wilson, and J. Shaw (1995). Cough fracture of the first rib. *Injury* 26:565–566.

Ben-Menachem, Y. (1988). Avulsion of the innominate artery associated with fracture of the sternum. *American Journal of Roentgenology* 150:621–622.

Benedix, D. (2004). Differentiation of fragmented bone from South East Asia using histological evidence. Department of Anthropology, University of Tennessee, Knoxville.

Bensahel, H., Z. Csukonyi, O. Badelon, and S. Badaoui (1986). Fractures of the medial condyle of the humerus in children. *Journal of Pediatric Orthopaedics* 6:430–433.

Benson, E., C. Conroy, D. Hoyt, A. Eastman, S. Pacyna, K. F. Smith, T. Velky, and M. Sise (2007). Calcaneal fractures in occupants involved in severe frontal motor vehicle crashes. *Accid Anal Prev* 39(4):794–799.

Bentley, G. (1968). Impacted fractures of the neck of the femur. *Journal of Bone and Joint Surgery [Br]* 50:551–561.

Benzel, E., B. Hart, P. Ball, N. Baldwin, W. Orrison, and M. Espinosa (1994). Fractures of the C-2 vertebral body. *Journal of Neurosurgery* 81:206-212.

Bergman, G., R. Winquist, K. Mayo, and S. J. Hansen (1987). Subtrochanteric fracture of the femur: Fixation using the Zickel nail. *Journal of Bone and Joint Surgery [Am]* 69:1032–1040.

Berndt, A. and M. Harty (1959). Transchondral fractures (osteochondritis dissecans) of the talus. *Journal of Bone and Joint Surgery [Am]* 41A:988–1020.

Berrios, D. and D. Grady (1991). Domestic Violence: Risk factors and outcomes. *Western Journal of Medicine* 155(2):133–135.

Berryman, H. and S. Symes (1998). Recognizing gunshot and blunt cranial trauma from fracture interpretation. In *Forensic Osteology: Advances in the Identification of Human Remains* (2nd ed.), K. Reichs (Ed.), pp. 333–352. Charles C Thomas, Springfield, IL.

Betz, P. and W. Eisenmenger (1996). Frequency of throat-skeleton fractures in hanging. *Am J Forensic Med Pathol* 17(3):191–193.

Betz, P. and E. Liebhardt (1994). Rib fractures in children: Resuscitation or child abuse? *International Journal of Legal Medicine* 106:215–218.

Beyer, C. and M. Cabanela (1992). Unilateral facet dislocations and fracture dislocations of the cervical spine: A review. *Orthopaedics* 15:311–315.

Binford, L. (1981). *Bones: Ancient Men and Modern Myths.* Academic Press, New York.

Biroscak, B. J., P. K. Smith, and L. A. Post (2006). A practical approach to public health surveillance of violent deaths related to intimate partner relationships. *Public Health Report* 121(4):393–399.

Bjornstig, U., P. Bylund, T. Lekander, and B. Brorsson (1985). Motorcycle fatalities in Sweden. *Acta Chir Scand* 151(7):577–581.

Blacksin, M. (1993). Patterns of fracture after air bag deployment. *Journal of Trauma* 35(6):840–843.

Blake, R. B., C. M. Ursic, J. M. Clark, and S. S. Cox (1997). Alcohol and drug use in adult patients with musculoskeletal injuries. *American Journal of Orthopedics* 26(10): 709–710.

Blake, S. P. and A. M. Connors (2004). Sacral insufficiency fracture. *The British Journal of Radiology* 77:891–896.

Bloom, J., K. E. Burroughs, P. Eiff, and J. Grayzel (2012). Overview of metacarpal fractures. UptoDate.com.

Blount, W. (1955). *Fractures in Children*. Williams and Wilkins, Baltimore.

——— (1977). *Fractures in Children*. Robert E. Krieger, Huntington, NY.

Boachie-Adjei, O. (1992). Fractures of the sacrum. In *Fractures and Dislocations*, R. Gustilo, R. Kyle and D. Templeman (Eds.), pp. 717–729. Mosby, St Louis, MO.

Bode, K. and P. Newton (2007). Pediatric nonaccidental trauma: Thoracolumbar fracture-dislocation. *Spine* 32(14):E388–E392.

Bode-Jänisch, S., E. Bültmann, H. Hartmann, G. Schroeder, J. Zajaczek, and A. Debertin (2012). Serious head injury in young children: Birth trauma versus non-accidental head injury. *Forensic Sci Int* 214(1–3):e34–38.

Bogusiak, K. and P. Arbuszewski (2010). Characteristics and epidemiology of zygomaticomaxillary complex fractures. *Journal of Craniofacial Surgery* 21:1018–1023.

Bolin, H. (1961). The fibula and its relationship to the tibia and talus in injuries of the ankle due to forced external rotation. *Acta Radiologica* 56:439–448.

Bone, R. (1985). Face and facial bones: Clinical aspects. In *Biomechanics of Trauma*, A. Nahum and J. Melvin, (Eds.), pp 271–279. Appleton-Century-Croft, Norwalk, CT.

Bonneville, F., J. M., M. Runge, G. Jacquet, and J. F. Bonnefille (2004). Split atlas in a patient with odontoid fracture. *Neuroradiology* 46:450–452.

Bonnichsen, R. (1979 Pleistocene bone technology in the Beringian Refugium. *National Museum of Man Mercury Series*. Archaeological Survey of Canada Ottawa, Canada.

Bonnin, J. (1945). Sacral fractures and injuries to the cauda equine. *Journal of Bone and Joint Surgery [Br]* 27:113–127.

Bonnin, J. (1970). *Injuries to the Ankle*. Hafner, Darien, CT.

Bonnin, J. G. and W. P. Greening (1944). Fractures of the triquetrum. *British Journal of Surgery* 31:278–283.

Borgeskov, S., B. Christiansen, A. Kjaer, and I. Balslev (1966). Fractures of the carpal bones. *Acta Orthop Scand* 37:276–287.

Bormann, K. B., S. Wild, N. C. Gelrich, H. Kokemuller, C. Stuhmer, R. Schmelzeisen, and R. Schon (2009). Five-year retrospective study of mandibular fractures in Freiburg, Germany: Incidence, etiology, treatment, and complications. *Journal of Oral and Maxillofacial Surgery* 67:1251–1255.

Bostrom, A. (1972). Fractures of the patella. *Acta Orthopaedica Scandinavica* 143(Suppl):1–80.

Bosworth, D. M. (1947). Fracture dislocation of the ankle with fixed displacement of the fibula behind the talus. *J Bone and Joint Surgery [Am]* 29:130–135.

Botte, M. and R. Gelberman (1987). Fractures of the carpals, excluding the scaphoid. *Hand Clinics of North America* 3:149–161.

Botte, M., H. von Schroeder, H. Gellman, and J. Cohen (1992). Fracture of the trapezial ridge. *Clinical Orthopaedics and Related Research* 276:202–205.

Bould, M. and D. Edwards (1994). Fracture of the cervical rib: A novel seatbelt injury. *Journal of Accident and Emergency Medicine* 11:136–137.

Bowen, A. (1983). Plastic bowing of the clavicle in children: A report of two cases. *Journal of Bone and Joint Surgery [Am]* 65:403–405.

Bowen, D. (1966). Impact injuries on the railroad track: Three cases of depressed fracture of the skull. *Journal of Forensic Medicine* 13:16–22.

Bowman, S. and R. Simon (1993). Metacarpal and phalangeal fractures. *Emerg Med Clin North Am* 11(3):671–702.

Branch, T., C. Partin, P. Chamberland, E. Emeterio, and E. Sabetelle (1992). Spontaneous fractures of the humerus during pitching: A series of 12 cases. *American Journal of Sports Medicine* 20:468–470.

Brant, W. and C. Helms (2007). *Fundamentals of Diagnostic Radiology*. Lippincott Williams & Wilkins, Philadelphia.

Brasileiro, B. F. and L. A. Passeri (2006). Epidemiological analysis of maxillofacial fractures in Brazil: A 5-year prospective study. *Oral Surgery, Oral Medicine, Oral Pathology, Oral Radiology and Endodonty* 102:28–34.

Breitenecker, L. (1959). The physician and traffic accidents. *Wien Med Wochenschr* 109:861–863.

Bremke, M., H. Gedeon, J. P. Windfuhr, J. A. Werner, and A. M. Sesterhann (2009). Nasal bone fracture: Etiology, diagnostics, treatment and complications. *Laryngo-rhinotologie* 88(11):711–716.

Brinker, M. and D. O'Connor (2004). The incidence of fractures and dislocations referred for orthopaedic services in a capitated population. *The Journal of Bone & Joint Surgery [Am]* 86(2):290–297.

Britt, P. and J. Heiseman (2000). Imaging evaluation. In *Head Injury* (4th ed.). P. Cooper and J. Golfinos (Eds.). McGraw-Hill, New York.

Brogdon, B., H. Vogel, and J. McDowell (2003). *A Radiologic Atlas of Abuse, Torture, Terrorism, and Inflicted Trauma*. CRC Press, Boca Raton, FL.

Brogdon, B. G., J. M. Crotty, L. MacFeely, S. B. McCann, and M. Fitzgerald (1995). Intra-thoracic fracture-dislocation of the humerus. *Skeletal Radiology* 24: 383–385.

Brogdon, B. G. (1998). *Forensic Radiology*. CRC Press, Boca Raton, FL.

Brogdon, B. G. and J. D. McDowell (2003). Abuse of the aged. In *A Radiologic Atlas of Abuse, Torture, Terrorism, and Inflicted Trauma*, B. G. Brogdon and J. D. McDowell (Eds). CRC Press, Boca Raton, FL.

Brondum, V., C. F. Larsen, and O. Slwov, (1992). Fracture of the carpal scaphoid: Frequency and distribution in a well-defined population. *European Journal of Radiology* 15:118–122.

Brookes, J. G., R. J. Dunn, and I. R. Rogers (1993). Sternal fractures: A retrospective analysis of 272 cases. *Journal of Trauma* 35:46–54.

Brown, B. L., R. Lapinski, G. S. Berkowitz, and I. Holzman (1994). Fractured clavicle in the neonate: A retrospective three-year review. *American Journal of Perinatology* 11:331–333.

Brown, J. T. and G. Abrams (1964). Transcervical femoral fracture: A review of 195 patients treated by sliding nail-plate fixation. *Journal of Bone and Joint Surgery [Br]* 46:648–663.

Brumback, R. J. and A. L. Jones (1994). Interobserver agreement in the classification of open fractures: The results of a survey of two hundred and forty-five orthopaedic surgeons. *Journal of Bone and Joint Surgery [Am]* 76:1162–1166.

Bryan, R. and K. Dobyns (1980). Fractures of the carpal bones other than the lunate and scaphoid. *Clinical Orthopaedics and Related Research* 149:107–111.

Bryan, R. S. (1981). Fractures about the elbow in adults. *Instructional Course Lectures* 30:200–223.

Bryan, R. S. and B. F. Morrey (1985). Fractures of the distal humerus. In *The Elbow and Its Disorders*, B. F. Morrey (Ed.), pp. 302–339. W. B. Saunders, Philadelphia.

Bucholz, R., C. Court-Brown, J. Heckman, and P. I. Tornetta (Eds.) (2010). *Rockwood and Green's Fractures in Adults*, Vol. 1. Lippincott Williams and Wilkins, Philadelphia.

Bucholz, R. W. (1981). The pathological anatomy of the Malgaigne fracture dislocation of the pelvis. *Journal of Bone and Joint Surgery [Am]* 63:400–404.

_____ (1994). Lower cervical spine injuries. In *Skeletal Trauma; Fractures, Dislocations, Ligamentous Injuries*, B. D. Browner, J. B. Jupiter, A. M. Levine, and P. G. Trafton (Eds.), pp. 699–728 W. B. Saunders, Philadelphia.

Bucknill, T. M. and J. S. Blackburn (1976). Fracture dislocation of the sacrum: Report of three cases. *Journal of Bone and Joint Surgery [Br]* 58:467–470.

Buckwalter, J., M. Glimcher, R. Cooper, and R. Recker (1996a). Bone biology I: Structure, blood supply, cells, matrix, and mineralization. *Instructional Course Lectures* 45:371–386.

_____ (1996b). Bone biology II: Formation, form, modeling, remodeling and regulation of cell function. *Instructional Course Lectures* 45:387–399.

Buhr, A. and A. Cooke (1959). Fracture patterns. *Lancet* 1(7072):531–536.

Bulloch, B., C. Schubert, P. Brophy, N. Johnson, M. Reed, and R. A. Shapiro (2000). Cause and clinical characteristics of rib fractures in infants. *Pediatrics* 105(4): e48.

Burden, D. (1995). An investigation of the association between overjet lip coverage, and traumatic injury to maxillary incisors. *Eur J Orthod* 17(6):513–517.

Burke, M. (2012). *Pathology of Fractures and Mechanisms of Injury: Postmortem CT Scanning*. CRC Press, Boca Raton, FL.

Burroughs, K. E. and K. M. Walker (2012). Hip fractures in adults. UptoDate.com.

Burstein, A. H., D. T. Reilly, and M. Martens (1976). Aging of bone tissue: Mechanical properties. *Journal of Bone and Joint Surgery [Am]* 58:82–86.

Burston, G. R. (1975). Granny-beating. *British Medical Journal* 3:592.

Butt, W. E. (1962). Fractures of the hand II statistical review. *Canadian Medical Association Journal* 86:775–779.

Bux, R., S. A. Podosch, F. Ramsthaler, and P. H. Schmidt (2006). Laryngohyoid fractures after agonal falls: Not always a certain sign of strangulation. *Forensic Science International* 156:219–222.

Byard, R. W. and J. D. Gilbert (2002). Cervical fracture, decapitation, and vehicle-assisted suicide. *Journal of Forensic Sciences* 47:392–394.

Byard, R. W. and M. Tsokos (2006). Avulsion of the distal tibial shaft in aircraft crashes: A pathological feature of extreme decelerative injury. *American Journal of Forensic Medicine and Pathology* 27:337–339.

Caffey, J. (1946). Multiple fractures in the long bones of infants suffering from chronic subdural hematoma. *American Journal of Roentgenology and Radiation Therapy* 56: 163–173.

Caffey, J. (1957). Some traumatic lesions in growing bones other than fractures and dislocations: Clinical and radiological features. *Br J Radiol* 30:225–238.

Calder, J., M. Solan, S. Gidwani, S. Allen, and D. Ricketts (2002). Management of paediatric clavicle fractures – is follow-up necessary? An audit of 346 cases. *Ann R Coll Surg Engl* 84(5):331–333.

Caler, W. F. and D. R. Carter (1989). Bone creep-fatigue damage accumulation. *Journal of Biomechanics* 22:625–636.

Caliskan, M. K. and Y. Pehlivan (1996). Prognosis of root-fractured permanent incisors. *Endod Dent Traumatology* 12:129–136.

Cameron, H. U. (1980). Traumatic disruption of the manubriosternal joint in the absence of rib fractures. *Journal of Trauma* 20:892–894.

Campbell, J. and N. Glass (2009). Safety, planning, danger and lethality assessment. In *Intimate Partner Violence: A Health-Based Perspective*, C. Mitchell and D. Anglin (Eds.), pp. 319–335. Oxford University Press, New York.

Campbell, M. N. and F. S. Fairgrieve (2011). Differentiation of traumatic and heat-induced dental tissue fractures via SEM analysis. *Journal of Forensic Sciences* 56(3): 715–719.

Campman, S. C. and S. A. Luzi (2007). The sensitivity and specificity of control surface injuries in aircraft accident fatalities. *American Journal of Forensic Medicine and Pathology* 28:111–115.

Canale, S. T. (1992). Physeal injuries. In *Skeletal Trauma Fractures, Dislocations, Ligamentous Injuries*, B. Browner, J. Jupiter, A. Levine, and F. Trafton (Eds.), pp. 15–55. W. B. Saunders, Philadelphia.

Canale, S. T. and F. B. Kelly, Jr. (1976). Fractures of the neck of the talus: Long-term evaluation of 71 cases. *Journal of Bone and Joint Surgery [Am]* 60:143–156.

Canale, S. T. and R. H. Belding (1980). Osteochondral lesions of the talux. *Journal of Bone and Joint Surgery [Am]* 62:97–102.

Capaldo, S. D. and R. J. Blumenschine (1994). A quantitative diagnosis of notches made by hammerstone percussion and carnivore gnawing on bovid long bones. *American Antiquity* 59(4):724–748.

Carli, A., C. De Jesus, and P. Martineau (2012). Isolated axillary artery injury due to blunt trauma in ice hockey. *Clin J Sport Med* 22(5):446–447.

Carpenter, M. (1991). *Core Text of Neuroanatomy* (4th ed.). Williams and Wilkins, Baltimore.

Carr, J. B., J. J. Hamilton, and L. S. Bear (1989). Experimental intra-articular calcaneal fractures: Anatomic basis for a new classification. *Foot and Ankle* 10:81–87.

Carson, S., D. P. Woolridge, J. Colletti, and K. Kilgore (2006). Pediatric upper extremity injuries. *Pediatric Clinics of North America* 53:41.

Carter, D. R., W. C. Hayes, and D. J. Schurman (1976). Fatigue life of compact bone: II. Effects of microstructure and density. *Journal of Biomechanics* 9:211–218.

_____ (1976). Bone compressive strength: The influence of density and strain rate. *Science* 194:1174–1176.

Carter, D. R. (1983). The relationship between in vivo strains and cortical bone remodeling. *CRC Critical Reviews in Biomedical Engineering* 8:1–28.

Carter, D. R., W. C. Hayes, and D. J. Schurman (1985). Biomechanics of bone. In *The Biomechanics of Trauma*, A.M. Nahum and J. Melvin (Eds.), pp. 135–165 Appleton-Century-Crofts, Norwalk, CT.

Catalano, S. (2006). *Intimate Partner Violence In The United States.* Bureau of Justice Statistics, NCJ 210675.

Catalano, S., E. Smith, H. Snyder, and M. Rand (2009). *Female Victims of Violence.* Bureau of Justice Statistics, NCJ 228356.

Cave, E. F. (1963). Fractures of the os calcis – the problem in general. *Clinical Orthopaedics* 30:64–66.

Cedell, C. A. (1974). Rupture of the posterior talotibial ligament with avulsion of a bone fragment from the talus. *Acta Orthopaedica Scandinavica* 45:454–461.

Cerny, M. (1983). Our experience with estimation of an individual's age from skeletal remains of the degree of thyroid cartilage ossification. *Acta Universitatis Palackianae Olomucensis* 3:121–124.

Cezayirlioglu, H. B., E. Bahniuk, D. T. Dovy, and K. G. Heiple (1985). Anisotropic yield behavior of bone under combined axial force and torque. *Journal of Biomechanics* 18:61–69.

Chadwick, R. and R. F. Kyle (1992). Fractures and dislocations of the proximal humerus, scapula, sternoclavicular joint, acromioclavicular joint and clavicle. In *Fractures and Dislocations,* R. B. Gustilo, R. F. Kyle, and D. C. Templeman (Eds.), pp. 255–340. Mosby, St Louis, MO.

Chakkalakal, D. A. (2005). Alcohol-induced bone loss and deficient bone repair. *Alcohol Clin Exp Res* 29(12):2077–2090.

Chalmers, D. J., D. P. A. O'Hare, and D. I. McBride (2000). The incidence, nature, and severity of injuries in New Zealand civil aviation. *Aviation Space Environmental Medicine* 71:388–395.

Chamay, A. and P. Tschantz (1972). Mechanical influence in bone remodeling: Experimental research on Wolff's law. *Journal of Biomechanics* 5:173–180.

Chan, G. and D. Yoshida (2003). Fracture of the lateral process of the talus associated with snowboarding. *Annals of Emergency Medicine* 41(6):854–858.

Chan, M. C. K., P. Fenton, and A. A. Conlan (1994). Unusual site of spontaneous first-rib fracture: Case report. *Canadian Journal of Surgery* 37:425–427.

Chance, G. Q. (1948). Note on a type of flexion fracture of the spine. *British Journal of Radiology* 21:452–453.

Chandra, J., T. D. Dogra, and P. C. Dikshit (1979). Pattern of cranio-intracranial injuries in fatal vehicular accidents in Delhi, 1866–76. *Medicine, Science and the Law* 19: 186–194.

Chapman, M. W. (1978). Fractures and fracture-dislocations of the ankle and foot. In *DuVries' Surgery of the Foot* (4th ed.), R. A. Mann (Ed.). Mosby, St Louis, MO.

Chase, J. M., T. R. Light, and L. S. Benson (1997). Coronal fracture of the hamate body. *American Journal of Orthopedics* 26:568–571.

Chattopadhyay, S. and C. Tripathi (2010). Skull fracture and haemorrhage pattern among fatal and nonfatal head injury assault victims – a critical analysis. *J Inj Violence Res* 2(2):99–103.

Cheatham, J. (1983). Physical abuse of the elderly. *Psychiatr Hosp* 14(2):102–103.

Chen, C. H., T. Y. Wang, P. K. Tsay, J. B. Lai, C. T. Chen, H. T. Liao, C. H. Lin, and Y. R. Chen (2008). A 162-case review of palatal fracture: Management strategy from a 10-year experience. *Plastic and Reconstructive Surgery Journal* 121:2065–2073.

Chi, M. J., M. Ku, K. H. Shin, and S. Baek (2010). An analysis of 733 surgically treated blowout fractures. *Ophthalmologica* 224:167–175.

Choi, B. J., S. Park, D. W. Lee, J. Y. Ohe, and Y. D. Kwon (2011). Effects of lower third molars on the incidence of mandibular angle and condylar fractures. *J Craniofac Surg* 22(4):1521–1525.

Christensen, A. M. (2004). The influence of behavior on free-fall injury patterns: Possible implications for forensic anthropological investigations. *J Forensic Sci* 49(1): 5–10.

Christiansen, B. A. and M. L. Bouxsein (2010). Biomechanics of vertebral fractures and the vertebral fracture cascade. *Current Osteoporosis Reports* 8:198–204.

Chu, S., J. L. Kelsey, T. H. Keegan, et al. (2004). Risk factors for proximal humerus fracture. *American Journal of Epidemiology* 160(360).

Chung, K. C. and S. V. Spilson (2001). The frequency and epidemiology of hand and forearm fractures in the United States. *Journal of Hand Surgery (American)* 26:908.

Cina, S. J., J. L. Koelpin, C. A. Nichols, and S. E. Conradi (1994). A decade of train-pedestrian fatalities: The Charleston experience. *Journal of Forensic Sciences* 39:668–673.

Claes, L., M. Reusch, M. Gockelman, M. Ohnmaacht, T. Wehner, M. Amling, F. T. Bell, and A. Ignatius (2011). Metaphyseal fracture healing follows similar biomechanical rules as diaphyseal healing. *Journal of Orthopedic Research* 29:425–432.

Claes, L., S. Recknagel, and A. Ignatius (2012). Fracture healing under healthy inflammatory conditions. *National Review of Rheumatology* 8:133–143.

Clark, C. (Ed.) (2009). *The Cervical Spine.* Wolters Kluwer Health.

Clark, E. G. and K. L. Sperry (1992). Distinctive blunt force injuries caused by a crescent wrench. *Journal of Forensic Sciences* 37(4):1172–1178.

Clarke, N. M., F. R. Shelton, C. C. Taylor, T. Khan, and S. Needhirajan (2012). The incidence of fractures in children under the age of 24 months – in relation to non-accidental injury. *Injury* 43(6):762–765.

Clarke, P., E. M. Braunstein, B. N. Weissman, and J. L. Sosman (1983). Sesamoid fracture of the thumb. *British Journal of Radiology* 56:485.

Clyburn, T. A., D. R. Lionberger, and H. S. Tullos (1982). Bilateral fracture of the transverse process of the atlas. *Journal of Bone and Joint Surgery* 64(6):948.

Cochran, G. V. B., R. E. Zickel, and J. W. Fielding (1980). Stress analysis of subtrochanteric fractures: Effect of muscle forces and internal fixation devices. In *Current Concepts of Internal Fixation of Fractures*, H. K. Uhthoff (Ed.), pp. 211–227. Springer, Berlin.

Codman, E. A. (1934). *The Shoulder: Rupture of the Supraspinatus Tendon and Other Lesions in or about the Subacromial Bursa.* T Todd, Boston.

Coelho, L., T. Ribeiro, R. Dias, A. Santos, and T. Magalhaes (2010). Elder homicide in the north of Portugal. *Journal of Forensic and Legal Medicine,* 17:383–387.

Coffey, C., K. Haley, J. Hayes, and J. Groner (2005). The risk of child abuse in infants and toddlers with lower extremity injuries. *J Pediatric Surgery* 40:120–123.

Coimbra, R., C. Conroy, G. T. Tominaga, V. Bansal, and A. Schwartz (2010). Causes of scapula fractures differ from other shoulder injuries in occupants seriously injured during motor vehicle crashes. *Injury* 41:151–155.

Cokluk, C., M. Takayasu, J. Yoshida (2005). Pedicle fracture of the axis: Report of two cases and a review of the literature. *Clinical Neurology and Neurosurgery* 107:136–139.

Cole, R. J., H. P. Brown, R. E. Stein, and R. G. Pearce (1995). Avulsion fracture of the tubersotiy of the calcaneus in children: A report of four cases and review of the literature. *Journal of Bone and Joint Surgery [Am]* 77:1568–1571.

Collins, J. (2000). Chest wall trauma. *J Thoracic Imaging* 15(2):112–119.

Collins, K. A. (2006). Elder maltreatment. *Archives of Pathology and Laboratory Medicine* 130:1290–1296.

Collins, K. A. and S. E. Presnell (2006). Elder homicide: A 20-year study. *American Journal of Forensic Medicine and Pathology* 27:183–187.

Coltart, W. D. (1952). Aviator's astragulus. *Journal of Bone and Joint Surgery [Br]* 34:545–566.

Conn, J. and P. Wade (1961). Injuries of the elbow: A ten year review. *Journal of Trauma* 1:248–268.

Connor, M. (2007). *Forensic Methods: Excavation for the Archaeologist and Investigator.* Littlefield, Lanham, MD.

Cook, D., P. Walker, and P. Lambert (1997). Skeletal evidence for child abuse: A physical anthropology perspective. *J For Sci* 42(2):196–207.

Cook, G. C. and J. C. Bjelland (1979). Acute bowing fracture of the fibula in an adult. *Radiology* 131:637–638.

Cooney, W. P., R. L. Linscheid, and J. H. Dobyns (1996). Fractures and dislocations of the wrist. In *Rockwood and Green's Fractures in Adults, Vol 1* (4th ed.). C. A. Rockwood, R. W. Bucholz, and J. D. Heckman (Eds.). Lippincott-Raven, Philadelphia.

Cooper, A. and E. L. Smith (2011). *Homicide Trends in the United States, 1980–2008.* US Bureau of Justice Statistics.

Cooper, C., T. O'Neill, and A. Silman (1993). Epidemiology of vertebral fractures. *Bone* 14:S89–97.

Cooper, P. and J. Golfinos (Eds.) (2000). *Head Injury* (4th ed.). McGraw-Hill, New York.

Cooper, S. (1822). *The First Lines of the Practice of Surgery: Designed as an Introduction for Students, and a Concise Book of Reference for Practitioners.* J. V. Seaman, New York.

Coote, J. M., C. G. Sterard, and D. J. Grier (2000). Bilateral acromial fractures in an infant with malignant osteopetrosis. *Clinical Radiology* 55(1):70–72.

Copeland, A. R. (1986). True vehicular homicide. *American Journal of Forensic Medicine and Pathology* 7:305–307.

Cormier, J., S. Manoogian, S. Rowson, A. Santiago, C. McNally, S. Duma, and I. J. Bolte (2010). The tolerance of the nasal bone to blunt impact. *Ann Adv Automot Med* 54:3–14.

Cormier, J. and S. Duma (2009). The epidemiology of facial fractures in automotive collisions. *Proceedings of the Annals of Advances in Automotive Medicine* 53:169–176.

Cormier, J., S. Manoogian, J. Bisplinghoff, S. Rowson, A. Santago, C. McNally, S. Duma, and J. Bolte (2011). The tolerance of the frontal bone to blunt impact. *Journal of Biomechanical Engineering* 133(2):021004.

Cosker, T. D. A., A. Ghanour, S. K. Gupta, K. J. J. Tayton(2005). Pelvic ramus fracture in the elderly: 50 patients studied with MRI. *Acta Orthopaedica* 76:513–516.

Cossio, P. I., F. E. Galvez, J. L. G. Perez, J. L. G., A. Garcia-Peria, and J. M. H. Cuisado (1994). Mandibular fractures in children: A retrospective study of 99 fractures in 59 patients. *International Journal of Oral and Maxillofacial Surgery* 23:329–331.

Court-Brown, C. M., A. Garg, M. M. McQueen (2001). The epidemiology of proximal humeral fractures. *Acta Orthop Scand* 72:365.

Cowin, S. C. (1989a). Mechanics of materials. In *Bone Mechanics*, S. C. Cowin (Ed.), pp. 15–42. CRC Press, Boca Raton, FL.

_____ (1989b). The mechanical properties of cortical bone tissue. In *Bone Mechanics*, S. C. Cowin (Ed.), pp. 97–128. CRC Press, Boca Raton, FL.

Craig, E. (1990). Fractures of the clavicle. In *The Shoulder*, 1, pp. 367–401.

Crandall, M. L., A. B. Nathens, and F. P. Rivara (2004). Injury patterns among female trauma patients: Recognizing intentional injury. *Journal of Trauma Injury, Infection, and Critical Care* 57:42–45.

Crestanello, J. A., L. E. Samuels, M. S. Kaufman, M. P. Thomas, and R. Talucci (1999). Sternal fracture with mediastinal hematoma: Delayed cardiopulonary sequelae. *Journal of Trauma* 47(1):161–164.

Crosby, L. A. and T. Fitzgibbons (1990). Computerized tomography scanning of acute intra-articular fractures of the calcaneus: A new classification system. *Journal of Bone and Joint Surgery [Am]* 72:852–859.

Cross, P. and T. Simmons (2010). The Influence of penetrative trauma on the rate of decomposition. *J Forensic Sci* 55(2):295–301.

Cruz, A. A. V. and G. C. D. Eichenberger (2004). Epidemiology and management of orbital fractures. *Current Opinion in Ophthalmology* 15:416–421.

Cumming, R. G., M. C. Nevitt, and S. R. Cummings (1997). Epidemiology of hip fractures. *Epidemiologic Reviews* 19:244–257.

Cummings, S. and L. Melton (2002). Epidemiology and outcomes of osteoporotic fractures. *The Lancet* 359(9319):1761–1767.

Cummings, S. R., J. L. Kelsey, M. C. Nevitt, and K. J. O'Dowd (1985). Epidemiology of osteoporosis and osteoporotic fractures. *Epidemiologic Reviews* 7:178–208.

Currey, J. (2002). *Bones: Structure and Mechanics.* Princeton University Press, Princeton, NJ.

Currey, J. D. (1970). The mechanical properties of bone. *Clinical Orthopaedics* 73:210–231.

_____ (1984). *The Mechanical Adaptations of Bone.* Princeton University Press, Princeton, NJ.

Currey, J. D. and G. Butler (1975). The mechanical properties of bone tissue in children. *Journal of Bone and Joint Surgery* 57-A(6):810–814.

D'Souza, D. H., S. S. Harish, and J. Kiran (2010). Fusion in the hyoid bone: Usefulness and implications. *Med Sci Law* 50(4):197–199.

Dalati, T. (2005). Isolated hyoid bone fracture: Review of an unusual case. *Int J Oral Maxillofac Surg* 34(4):449–452.

Daniels, T. R. and J. W. Smith (1993). Talar neck fractures. *Foot and Ankle* 14:225–234.

Dastgeer, B. M. and D. J. Mikolich (1987). Fracture-dislocation of manubriosternal joint: An unusual complication of seizures. *Journal of Trauma* 27:91–93.

Davidson, M., J. Lindsey, and J. Davis (1987). Requirements and selection of animal models. Israel J Med Sci 23:551–555.

Davis, K. (1985). *A Taphonomic Approach to Bone Fracturing and Applications to Several South African Pleistocene Sites.* Binghamton: State University of New York.

de Barros, J. W. and D. J. Oliveira (1995). Fractures of the humerus in arm wrestling. *International Orthopaedics* 19:390–391.

De Boeck, H. P., P. P. Casteleyn, and P. Opdecam (1986). Fracture of the medial humeral condyle: Report of a case in an infant. *J Bone and Joint Surgery [Am]* 69: 1442–1444.

De Jonge, J. J., J. Kingma, B. van der Lei, and H. J. Klasen (1994). Phalangeal fractures of the hand: An analysis of gender and age-related incidence and aetiology. *Journal of Hand Surgery [Br & Europe]* 19B:168–170.

Dedjientcheu, V., A. Niamshi, P. Ongolo-Zogo, M. Kobela, B. Rillet, A. Essomba, and M. Sosso (2006). Growing skull fractures. *Child's Nervous System* 22(7):721–725.

DeFriend, D. and K. Franklin (2001). Isolated sgernal fracture: A swing-related injury in two children. *Pediatric Radiology* 31:200–202.

Degan, T., B. Morrey, and D. Braun (1982). Surgical excision for anterior process fractures of the calcaneus. *Journal of Bone and Joint Surgery [Am]* 64:519–524.

Degan, T. J., B. F. Morrey, and D. P. Braun (1982). Surgical excision for anterior-process fractures of the calcaneus. *Journal of Bone and Joint Surgery [Am]* 64:519–523.

Dehner, J. R. (1971). Seatbelt injuries of the spine and abdomen. *American Journal of Roentgenology* 111:833–843.

Dejeammes, M. (1984). Lower abdomen and pelvis: Kinematics, tolerance levels and injury criteria. In *Biomechanics of Impact Trauma*, B. Aldman and A. Chapon (Eds.), pp. 289–307. Elsevier Science, Amsterdam.

Delabarde, T. (2008). Multiple healed rib fractures – timing of injuries in regard to death. In *Skeletal Trauma: Identification of Injuries Resulting from Human Rights Abuse and Armed Conflict*, E. H. Kimmerle and J. P. Baraybar (Eds.), pp. 236–244. CRC Press, Boca Raton, FL.

Delannoy, Y., A. Becart, T. Colard, R. Delille, G. Tournel, V. Hedouin, and D. Gosset (2012). Skull wounds linked with blunt force trauma (hammer example): A report of two depressed skull fractures – Elements of biomechanical explanation. *Legal Medicine* 14:258–262.

DeLee, J. C., D. P. Green, and K. E. Wilkins (1984). Fractures and dislocations of the elbow. In *Fractures in Adults*, C. A. Rockwood and D. P. Green (Eds.), pp. 559–652. J. B. Lippincott, Philadelphia.

DeLee, J. C. (1984). Fractures and dislocations of the hip. In *Fractures in Adults*, C. A. Rockwood and D. P. Green (Eds.), pp. 1211–1356. J. B. Lippincott, Philadelphia.

DeLee J. C., K. E. Wilkins, L. F. Rogers, and C. A. Rockwood (1980). Fracture-separation of the distal humeral epiphysis. *Journal of Bone and Joint Surgery (American)* 62:46.

DeLee, J. D. (1986). Fractures and dislocations of the foot. In *Surgery of the Foot*, R. A. Mann (Ed.), Mosby, St Louis, MO.

Della-Giustina, K. and D. A. Della-Gustina (1999). Emergency department evaluation and treatment of pediatric orthopedic injuries. *Emergency Medical Cinics North America* 17:895.

Demetriades, D., M. J. Martin, G. Velmahos, A. Salim, K. Alo, and P. Rhee (2004). Pedestrians injured by automobiles: Relationship of age to injury type and severity. *Journal of the American College of Surgeons* 199:382–387.

Denham, A. F., P. Y. Frasier, E. G. Hooten, L. Belton, W. Newton, et al. (2007). Intimate partner violence among Latinas in Eastern North Carolina. *Violence Against Women* 13(2):123–140.

Denis, F. (1982). Updated classification of thoracolumbar fractures. *Orthopaedic Transactions* 6:8

_____ (1984). Spinal instability as defined by the three-column spine concept in acute spinal trauma. *Clinical Orthopaedics and Related Research* 189:65–76.

Denis, F., S. David, T. Comfort (1988). Sacral fractures: An important problem: Retrospective analysis of 236 cases. *Clinical Orthopaedics and Related Research* 227: 67–81.

deSouza, I. J. (1992a). Fractures and dislocations about the ankle. In *Fractures and Dislocations*, R. B. Gustilo, R. F. Kyle, and D. C. Templeman (Eds.), pp. 997–1118. Mosby, St. Louis, MO.

_____ (1992b). Fractures and dislocations of the foot. In *Fractures and Dislocations*, R. B. Gustilo, R. F. Kyle, and D. C. Templeman (Eds.), pp. 1119–1221. Mosby, St Louis, MO.

Di Maio, V. (1999). *Gunshot Wounds: Practical Aspects of Firearms, Ballistics, and Forensic Techniques*. CRC Press, Boca Raton, FL.

Diamond, P., C. M. Hansen, and M. R. Christoferson (1994). Child abuse presenting as a thoracolumbar spinal fracture dislocation: A case report. *Pediatric Emergency Care* 10:83–86.

Diangelis, A., J. Andreason, K. Ebeleseder, D. Kenny, M. Trope, A. Sigurdsson, L. Anderson, C. Bourguignon, M. Flores, M. Hicks, A. Lenzi, B. Malmgren, A. Moule, Y. Pohl, and M. Tsukiboshi (2012). International Association of Dental Traumatology guidelines for the management of traumatic dental injuries: Fractures and luxations of permanent teeth. *Dent Traumatol* 28(1):2–12.

Dias, J. J. and Gregg, P. J. (1991). Acromioclavicular joint injuries in sports. *Sports Medicine* 11:125–132.

Dickenson, A. J. (1991). Fracture of the hyoid bone following minimal trauma. *Injury: The British Journal of Accident Surgery* 22:420–421.

DiMaio, D. J. and V. J. M. DiMaio (1989). *Forensic Pathology*. Elsevier Science, New York.

DiMaio, V. (2000). Homicidal asphyxia. *American Journal of Forensic Medicine and Pathology* 21(1):1–4.

Dirkmaat, D., L. Cabo, S. Ousley, and S. Symes (2008). New perspectives in forensic anthropology. *Yearbook Phys Anthropol* 51:33–52.

Doblare M., J. M. Garcia, and M. J. Gomez (2004). Modelling bone tissue fracture and healing: A review. *Engineering Fracture Mechanics* 71:1809–1840.

Dobyns, J. (1990). *Yearbook of Hand Surgery*. Year Book Medical, Chicago.

Dobyns, J. D., R. L. Linscheid, and W. P. J. Cooney (1983). Fractures and dislocations of the wrist and hand, then and now. *Journal of Hand Surgery* 8:651–656.

Dobyns, J. H., F. H. Sim, and R. L. Linscheid (1978). Sports stress syndromes of the hand and wrist. *American Journal of Sports Medicine* 6:236.

Dobyns, J. H. and R. L. Linscheid (1984). Fractures and dislocations of the wrist. In *Fractures in Adults*, C. A. Rockwood and D. P. Green (Eds.), pp. 411–509. J. B. Lippincott, Philadelphia.

Dobyns, J. H., R. D. Beckerbaugh, F. S. Bryon, et al. (1982). Fractures of the hand and wrist. In *Hand Surgery* (3rd ed.), J. E. Flynn (Ed.). Williams and Wilkins, Baltimore.

Dóczi, J. and A. Renner (1994). Epidemiology of distal radius fractures in Budapest. *Acta Orthopaedica Scandinavica* 65:432–433.

Doerr, T. and R. Mathog (2009). Le Forte Fractures (Maxillary Fractures). In *Facial Plastic and Reconstructive Surgery*, I. Papel and J. Frodel (Eds.), pp. 991–1000 Thieme, Stuttgart.

Dolinak, D. (2007). Rib fractures in infants due to cardiopulmonary resuscitation efforts. *American Journal of Forensic Med Pathol* 28(2):107–110.

Donahue, W., N. Harkey, K. Modaniou, L. Sequeira, and R. Martin (2000). Bone strain and micro-cracks as stress fracture sites in human metatarsals. *Bone* 27(6):827–833.

Doumouchtsis, S. K. and S. Arulkumaran (2008). Head trauma after instrumental births. *Clinics in Perinatology* 35(1):69–83.

Dovey, J. and J. Heerfordt (1971). Tibial condyle fractures. *Acta Chirurgica Scandinavica* 137:521–531.

Drakos, M. C., B. T. Feeley, R. Barnes, M. Muller, T. P. Burruss, and R. F. Warren (2011). Lower cervical posterior element fractures in the National Football League: A report of 2 cases and a review of the literature. *Neurosurgery* 68(6):E1743–E1749.

Drew, L. B. and W. E. Drew (2004). The contre-coup phenomenon: A new understanding of the mechanism of closed head injury. *Neurocrit Care* 1(3):385–390.

Duan, D. and Y. Zhang. Does the presence of mandibular third molars increase the risk of angle fracture and simultaneously decrease the risk of condylar fracture? *International Journal of Oral and Maxillofacial Surgery* 37:25–28.

Dulchavsky, S. A., E. R. Geller, and D. A. Iorio (1993). Analysis of injuries following the crash of Avianca Flight 52. *Journal of Trauma* 34:282–284.

Duma, S. M. and M. V. Jernigan (2003). The effects of airbags on orbital fracture patterns in automobile crashes. *Ophthalmic Plastic and Reconstructive Surgery* 19(2):107–111

Dumas, J. L. and N. Walker (1992). Bilateral scapular fractures secondary to electrical shock. *Archives of Orthopaedic and Trauma Surgery* 111:287–288.

Dummit, E. S. and R. L. Reid (1969). Unique tibial shaft fractures resulting from helicopter crashes. *Clinical Orthopaedics and Related Research* 66:155–158.

Duncan, C. C. (1993). Skull fractures in infancy and childhood. *Pediatrics in Review* 14:389–390.

Dupras, T. L., J. J. Schultz, S. M. Wheeler, and L. J. Williams (2006). *Forensic Recovery of Human Remains: Archaeological Approaches.* CRC Press, Boca Raton, FL.

Duprey, S., K. Bruyere, and J. Verriest (2008). Influence of geometrical personalization on the simulation of clavicle fractures. *J Biomech* 41(1):200–207.

Dupuis, O., R. Silveira, C. Dupont, C. Mottolese, P. Kahn, A. Dittmar, and R. Rudigoz (2005). Comparison of "instrument associated" and "spontaneous" obstetric depressed skull fractures in a cohort of 68 neonates. *Am J Obstetrics and Gynecology* 192(1):165–170.

Dupuis, O., R. Silveira, C. Dupont C. Mottolese, P. Kahn, A. Dittmar, and R. C. Rudigoz (2005). Comparison of "instrument-associated" and "spontaenous" obstetric depressed skull fractures in a cohort of 68 neonates. *American Journal of Obstetrics and Gynecology* 192:165–170.

Edwards, T. J., D. J. David, D. A. Simpson, and A. A. Abbott (1994). Patterns of mandibular fracture in Adelaide, South Australia. *Australian and New Zealand Journal of Surgery* 64:307–311.

Effendi, B., D. Roy, B. Cornish, R. G. Dussault, and C. A. Laurin (1981). Fractures of the ring of the axis: A classification based on the analysis of 131 cases. *Journal of Bone and Joint Surgery* 63B:319–327.

Eggensperger Wymann, N. M., A. Holzle, Z. Zachariou, and T. Iizuka (2008). Pediatic craniofacial trauma. *Journal of Oral and Maxillofacial Surgeons* 66:58–64.

Ehrlich, E., A. Tischler, and H. Maxeiner (2009). Lethal pedestrian – passenger car collisions in Berlin: Changed injury patterns in two different time intervals. *Legal Medicine* 11:S324–S326.

Eichenholtz, S. M. and D. B. Levine (1964). Fractures of the tarsal navicular bone. *Clinical Orthopaedics and Related Research* 34:142–157.

Eisele, J. W., H. J. Bonnell, and D. T. Reay (1983). Boot top fractures in pedestrians: A forensic masquerade. *Am J of Forensic Med* 4:181–184.

Eismont, F. J., S. R. Garfin, and J. J. Abitol (1994). Thoracic and upper lumbar spine injuries. In *Skeletal Trauma: Fractures, Dislocations, Ligamentous Injuries*, B. D. Browner, J. B. Jupiter, A. M. Levine, and P. G. Trafton (Eds.), pp. 729–803. W. B. Saunders, Philadelphia.

El-Khoury, G. Y., C. R. Clark, and A. W. Gravett (1984). Acute traumatic rotary atlanto-axial dislocation in children: A report of three cases. *Journal of Bone and Joint Surgery [Am]* 66:774–777.

Ellis, E., K. F. Moos, and A. El-Attar (1985). Ten years of mandibular fractures: An analysis of 2137 cases. *Oral Surgery, Oral Medicine and Oral Pathology* 59:120–129.

Ellis, J. (1965). Smith's and Barton's fractures: A method of treatment. *Journal of Bone and Joint Surgery [Br]* 47:724–727.

Ellis, R. G. (1970). *The Classification and Treatment of Injuries to the Teeth of Children* (5th ed.). Year Book Medical, Chicago.

Enlow, D. and S. Brown (1958). A comparative histological study of fossil and recent bone tissue III. *Texas J Sci* 10:187–230.

Epps, C. H., Jr. (1984). Fractures of the shaft of the humerus In *Fractures in Adults*, C. A. Rockwood and D. P. Green (Eds.), pp. 653–674. J. B. Lippincott, Philadelphia.

Erdmann, D., K. E. Follmar, M. DeBruijn, A. D. Bruno, S. H. Jung, D. Edelman, S. Mukundan, and J. R. Marcus (2008). A retrospective analysis of facial fracture etiologies. *Annals of Plastic Surgery* 60:398–403

Eren, O. T. and R. Hotby (1998). Straddle pelvic stress fracture in a female marathon runner: A case report. *Am J Sports Med* 26(6):850–851.

Eriksson, C. (1976). Electrical properties of bone. In *Biochemistry and Physiology of Bone*, G. H. Bourne (Ed.), pp. 329–384. Academic Press, New York.

Escher, F. (1969). Fronto-basal fractures. *Rev Otoneuroopthalmol* 41(7):412–413.

———— (1970). Diagnostic and therapeutic problems of open fronto-basal fractures. *Schweiz Rundsch Med Prax* 59(13):484–485.

———— (1973). The trauma of the basis of the skull in the view of the otorhinolaryngology. *HNO* 21(5):129–144.

Eski, M., I. Sahin, M. Deveci, M. Turegun, S. Isik, and M. Sengezer (2006). A retrospective analysis of 101 zygomatico-orbital fractures. *Journal of Craniofacial Surgery* 17(6):1059–1064.

Eskola, A., S. Vainionpaeae, P. Myllynes, et al. (1986). Outcome of clavicular fracture in 89 patients. *Archives of Orthopaedic and Traumatic Surgery*, 105:337–338.

Essex-Lopresti, P. (1952). The mechanism, reduction technique and results in fractures of the os calcis. *British Journal of Surgery* 39:395–419.

Evans, A. W. (2011). Fatal train accidents on Europe's railways: 1980–2009. *Accident Analysis and Prevention* 43:391–401.

Evans, D. C. (1982). Biomechanics of spinal injury. In *The Biomechanics of Musculoskeletal Injury*, E. R. Gonza and I. J. Harrington (Eds.), pp. 163–224. Williams and Wilkins, Baltimore.

Evans, E. M. (1949a). Pronation injuries of the forearm with special reference to the anterior Monteggia fracture. *Journal of Bone and Joint Surgery [Br]* 31:578–588.

––––––– (1949b). The treatment of trochanteric fractures of the femur. *Journal of Bone and Joint Surgery [Br]* 31:190–203.

––––––– (1951). Trochanteric fractures. *Journal of Bone and Joint Surgery [Br]* 33:192–204.

Evans, F. G. (1975). Mechanical properties and histology of cortical bone from younger and older men. *Anatomical Record* 185:1–12.

Evans, L. (1986). The effectiveness of safety belts in preventing fatalities. *Accident Analysis and Prevention* 18:229–241.

Eyers, P. S. G. and P. H. Roberts (1993). Association of seating arrangements and multiple pelvic fractures in a road traffic accident. *Injury* 24:682–683.

Failinger, M. and P. I. J. McGanity (1992). Unstable fractures of the pelvic ring. *Journal of Bone and Joint Surgery [Am]* 72:781–791.

Falzon, A. L. and G. G. Davis (1996). A 15 year retrospective review of homicide in the elderly. *Journal of Forensic Sciences* 43(2):371–374.

Fanslow, J., R. Norton, and C. Spinola (1998). Indicators of assault-related injuries among women presenting to the emergency department. *Ann Emerg Med* 32(3 Pt 1): 341–348.

Feldman, K. and D. Brewer (1984). Child abuse, cardopulmonary resusciation, and rib fractures. *Pediatrics* 73(3):339–342.

Fenton, T., W. Birkby, and J. Conelison (2003). A fast and safe non-bleaching method for forensic skeletal preparation. *Journal of Forensic Sciences* 48(2):277–281.

Ferguson, L., A. Wilkinson, and T. Beattie (2003). Fracture of the sternum in children. *Emerg Med J* 20:518–520.

Ferguson, G. and B. L. Allen (1984). A mechanistic classification of thoracolumbar spine fractures. *Clinical Orthopaedics and Related Research* 189:77–88.

Fermanis, G., S. A. Deane, and P. M. Fitzgerald (1985). The significance of first and second rib fractures. *Australian and New Zealand Journal of Surgery* 55:383–386.

Fielding, J. W. and H. J. Magliato (1966). Subtrochanteric fractures. *Surgery, Gynecology and Obstetrics* 122:555–560.

Finegan, O. (2008). The interpretation of skeletal trauma resulting from injuries sustained prior to, and as a direct result of, free-fall. In *Skeletal Trauma: Identification of Injuries Resulting from Human Rights Abuse and Armed Conflict*, E. H. Kimmerle and J. P. Baraybar (Eds.), pp. 181–195. CRC Press, Boca Raton, FL.

Fischer, J., W. J. Kleeman, and H. D. Troger (1994). Types of trauma in cases of homicide. *Forensic Science International* 68:161–167.

Fisk, G. F. (1984). The wrist. *Journal of Bone and Joint Surgery [Br]* 66:396–407.

Fleege, M. A., P. J. Jacobson, D. L. Renfrew, C. M. Steyers, and G. Y. El-Khoury (1991). Pisiform fractures. *Skeletal Radiology* 20:169–172.

Fletcher, B. and B. G. Brogdon (1967). Seat-belt fractures of the spine and sternum. *JAMA* 200:167.

Fowler, A. W. (1957). Flexion-compression injury of the sternum. *Journal of Bone and Joint Surgery [Br]* 68:478–497.

Fox, J. and M. Zawitz (2007). Homicide trends in the United States. Bureau of Juatice Statistics, Washington, DC.

Fracasso, T., S. Schmidt, and A. Schmeling (2011). [Commentary on Kremer et al. 2008, Kremer and Saubageau 2009, and Guyomarc'h et al 2010]. *Journal of Forensic Sciences* 56(6):1662.

Freeman, M. A. R., R. C. Todd, and C. J. Pirie (1974). The role of fatigue in the pathogenesis of senile femoral neck fractures. *Journal of Bone and Joint Surgery [Br]* 56:698–702.

Fridrich, K. L., G. Pena-Valasco, and R. A. Olson (1992). Changing trends with mandibular fracture: A review of 1067 cases. *Journal of Oral and Maxillofacial Surgery* 50:586–589.

Friedman, L. S., S. Avilla, K. Tanouye, and K. Joseph (2011). A case-control study of severe physical abuse of older adults. *Journal of the American Geriatric Society* 59(3):417–422.

Fuhrman, G., F. I. Stieg, and C. Buerk (1990). Blunt laryngeal trauma: Classification and management protocol. *J Trauma* 30(1):87–92.

Fujiwara, S., Y. Yanagida, and Y. Mizoi (1989). Impact-induced intracranial pressure caused by an accelerated motion of the head or by skull deformation – an experimental study using physical models of the head and neck, and ones of the skull. *Forensic Science International* 43:159–169.

Fulginiti, L. C., M. H. Czuzak, and K. M. Taylor (1999). Scatter versus impact during aircraft crashes: Implications for forensic anthropologists. In *Broken Bones: Anthropological Analysis of Blunt Force Trauma*, A. Galloway (Ed.). Charles C Thomas, Springfield, IL.

Gadd, C. W., A. M. Nahum, J. Gatts, and J. P. Danford (1968). A study of head and facial bone impact tolerances. *Proceedings of the Proceedings of the GM Auto Safety Seminar* Detroit, MI.

Gage, J. R. and R. Premer (1971). Os calcis fractures: An analysis of 37. *Minnesota Medicine* 54:169–176.

Galeazzi, R. (1934). Di una particolare sindrome traumatica dello sheletro dell avambroccio. *Atti Memorie Societe Lombardi Chirurgia* 2:12.

Galloway, A., R. A. Stini, S. C. Fox, and P. Stein (1990b). Stature loss among an older United States population and its relation to bone mineral status. *American Journal of Physical Anthropology* 83:467–476.

Galloway, A. (1996). Personal Communication.

Galloway, A., P. Willey, and L. Snyder (1997). Human bone mineral densities and survival of bone elements: A contemporary sample. In *Forensic Taphonomy: The Post-Mortem Fate of Human Remains*, W. Haglund and M. Sorg, (Eds.), pp. 295–317. CRC Press, Boca Raton, FL.

Galloway, A. and J. J. Snodgrass (1998). Biological and chemical hazards of forensic skeletal material. *Journal of Forensic Sciences* 43:940–948.

Galloway, A. (Ed.) (1999). *Broken Bones: Anthropological Analysis of Blunt Force Trauma.* Charles C Thomas, Springfield, IL.

Galloway, A. and L. Zephro (2005). Skeletal trauma analysis of the lower extremity. In *Forensic Medicine of the Lower Extremity: Human Identification and Trauma Analysis of the Thigh, Leg, and Foot,* J. Rich, D. E. Dean, and R. H. Powers (Eds.). Humana Press, New Jersey.

Galloway, A. and L. Zephro (2004). Skeletal evidence of homicidal compression. *Proceedings of the American Academy of Forensic Sciences,* V.

Ganhdi, R. K., P. Wilson, J. J. Bason Brown, and W. MacLeod (1963). Spontaneous correction of deformity flowing fracture of the forearm in children. *British Journal of Surgery* 50:5–10.

Garcia, V., C. Gotschall, M. Eichelberger, and L. Lowman (1990). Rib fractures in children: A marker a severe trauma. *J of Trauma* 30(6):695–700.

Garcia-Elias, M. (1987). Dorsal fractures of the triquetrum – avulsion or compression fractures? *Journal of Hand Surgery (Am)* 12:266–268.

_____ (2001). Carpal bone fractures (excluding scaphoid fractures). In *The Wrist,* H. K. Watson and J. Weinberg (Eds.), p. 174. Lippincott Williams & Wilkins, Philadelphia.

Garcia-Godoy, F. (1981). A classification for traumatic injuries to primay and permanent teeth. *Journal of Pedodontology* 5:295–297.

Garza-Mercado, R. (1982). Intrauterine depressed skull fractures of the newborn. *Neurosurgery* 10(6):694–697.

Gatliff, B. (2001). Skull protection and preparation for reconstruction. In *Forensic Art and Illustration,* K. Taylor (Ed.), pp. 333–334. CRC Press, Boca Raton, FL.

Gauthier, D. K. and W. B. Brankston (2004). "Who kills whom" revisited: A sociological study of variation in the sex ratio of spouse killings. *Homicide Studies* 8(2): 96–122.

Gebauer, M., F. Barvenci, M. Mumme, F. T. Bell, E. Vettorazzi, J. M. Rueger, K. Pueschel, and M. Arnling (2010). Microarchitecture of the radial head and its changes in aging. *Calcified Tissue International* 86:14–22.

Gedda, K. O. and E. Moberg (1953). Open reduction and osteosynthesis of the so-called Bennett's fracture in the carpometacarpal joint of the thumb. *Acta Orthopaedica Scandinavica* 22:249–256.

Gedda, K. O. (1954). Studies on Bennett fractures: Anatomy, roentgenology, and therapy. *Acta Chirurgica Scandinavica* 193 (Suppl):5–114.

Gehweiler, J. A., D. Duff, S. Martinez, M. D. Miller, and W. M. Clark (1976). Fractures of the atlas vertebra. *Skeletal Radiology* 1:97–102.

Gentry, L. R., W. F. Manor, P. A. Turski, and C. M. Strother (1983). High-resolution CT analysis of facial struts in trauma 2 normal anatomy. *American Journal of Roentgenology* 140:523–532.

George, R. (2007). *Facial Geometry: Graphic Facial Analysis for Forensic Artists.* Charles C Thomas, Springfield, IL.

Gerber, P. and K. Coffman (2007). Non-accidental head trauma in infants. *Child's Nervous System* 23:499–507.

Gershuni, D. H. (1985). Clinical aspects of extremity fractures. In *Biomechanics of Trauma*, A. M. Nahum and J. Melvin (Eds.), pp. 413–446 Appleton-Century-Crofts, Norwalk, CT.

Giannoudis, P., M. Grotz, C. Tzioupis, H. Dinopoulos, G. Wells, O. Bouamra, and F. Lecky (2007). Prevalence of pelvic fractures, associated injuries, and mortality: The United Kingdom perspective. *J Trauma-Injury Infection and Critical Care* 63(4):875–883.

Gifford, D. (1981). *Taphonomy and Paleoecology: A critical Review of Archaeology's sister disciplines. Advances in Archaeological Method and Theory.* Academic Press, New York.

Gifford-Gonzalez, D. (1989). Ethnographic analogues for interpreting modified bones: Some cases from East Africa. In *Bone Modification*, R. Bonnichsen and M. Sorg (Eds.), pp. 179–224. Center for the Study of the First Americans, Orono.

Gilliland, M. G. F. and R. Folberg (1996). Shaken babies – some have no impact injuries. *Journal of Forensic Sciences* 41:114–116.

Gladwell, M. and C. Viozzi (2008). Temporal bone fractures: A review for the oral and maxillofacial surgeon. 66(3):513-522.

Goedkoop, A. Y., E. B. H. van Onselen, R. B. Karim, et al. (2000). The 'mirrored' Bennett fracture of the base of the fifth metacarpal. *Archives of Orthopaedic and Trauma Surgery* 120(10):592–593.

Goldsmith, W. (1984). Mechanical aspects involving trauma to the human neck. In *The Biomechanics of Impact Trauma*, B. Aldman and A. Chapon (Eds.), pp. 139–147. Elsevier Science, Amsterdam.

Golob, J. F., J. A. Claridge, C. J. Yowler, J. J. Como, and J. R. Peerless (2008). Isolated cervical spine fractures in the elderly: A deadly injury. *Journal of Trauma* 64:311–315.

Gomes, P. P., L. A. Passeri, and J. R. Barbosa (2006). A 5-year retrospective study of zygomatico-orbital complex and zygomatic arch fractures in Sao Paulo State, Brazil. *Journal of Oral and Maxillofacial Surgery* 64:63–67.

Gonza, E. R. (1982). Biomechanics of long bone injuries. In *Biomechanics of Musculo-skeletal Injuries*, E. Gonza (Ed.), pp. 1–24. Williams and Wilkins, Baltimore.

Gonzalez, T. A. (1933). Manual strangulation. *Archives of Pathology* 15:55–66.

Gonzalez, T. A., M. Vance, M. Helpern, and C. I. Umberger (1954). *Legal Medicine Pathology, and Toxicology.* Appleton-Century-Crofts, New York.

Goonetilleke, U. K. (1980). Injuries caused by falls from heights. *Medicine, Science and the Law* 20:262–275.

Goss, T. P. (1996). The scapula: Coracoid, acromial and avulsion fractures. *American Journal of Orthopedics* 25:106–115.

Gotis-Graham, I., L. McGuigan, T. Diamond, I. Portek, and R. Quinn (1994). Sacral insufficiency fractures in the elderly. *J Bone Joint Surg* 76(6):882–886.

Granek, E., S. P. Baker, H. Abbey, E. Robinson, A. H. Myeres, J. S. Samdofff, and L. E. Klein (1987). Medications and diagnoses in relation to falls in long-term care facility. *Journal of the American Geriatric Society* 35:503–511.

Granhed, P. and A. Karladani (1997). Bilateral acetabular fracture as a result of epileptic seizure: a report of two cases. *Injury* 26:65–68.

Green, D. P. and S. A. Rowland (1984). Fractures and dislocations in the hand. In *Fractures in Adults*, C. A. Rockwood and D. P. Green, (Eds.), pp. 313–409. J. B. Lippincott, Philadelphia.

Green, H., R. James, J. Gilbert, and R. Byard (2000). Fractures of the hyoid and laryngeal cartilages in suicidal hangings. *J Clin Forensic Med* 7(3):123–126.

Green, M. A. (1973). Morbid anatomical findings in strangulation. *Forensic Science* 2:317–323.

Green, N. E. and M. F. Swiontkowski (1994). *Child Abuse: Skeletal Trauma in Children.* W. B. Saunders, Philadelphia.

Greene, D., C. Maas, G. Carvallho, and R. Raven (1999). Epidemiology of facial injury in female blunt assault trauma cases. *Arch Facial Plastic Surg* 1(4):288–291.

Greenes, D. and S. Schutzman (1997). Infants with isolated skull fracture: What are their clinical characteristics and do they require hospitalization? *Annals of Emergency Medicine* 30(3):253–259.

Greenfield, L., M. Rand, D. Craven, P. Klaus, C. Perkins, and C. Ringel (1998). *Violence by intimates: Analysis of data on crimes by current or former spouses, boyfriend, and girlfriends.* Bureau of Justice Statistics NCJ-167237.

Gregerson, H. N. (1971). Fracture of the humerus from muscular violence. *Acta Orthopaedica Scandinavica* 42:506–512.

Griffin, N. and B. Richmond (2005). Cross-sectional geometry of the human forefoot. *Bone* 37(2):253–260.

Gruss, J. (1982). Fronto-naso-orbital trauma. *Clin Plast Surg* 9(4):577–589.

Grynpas, M. D. (2003). The role of bone quality on bone loss and bone fragility. In *Bone Loss and Osteoporosis: An Anthropological Perspective*, S. Stout and S. C. Agarwal (Eds.), pp. 33–44. Kluwer Academic, New York.

Guiral, J. J., L. Real, and J. M. Curto (1996). Isolated fracture of the coracoid process of the scapula. *Acta Orthopaedica Belgica* 62:60–61.

Gunther, D., F. W. Ast, H. D. Troger, and W. J. Kleeman (1999). Unexpected findings in the investigation of an airplane crash. *Forensic Science International,* 104:189–194.

Gunther, W., S. Symes, and H. Berryman (2000). Characteristics of child abuse by anteroposterior manual compression versus cardiopulmonary resuscitation. *Am J Forensic Med and Path* 21(1):5–10.

Gupta, R., D. Clarke, and P. Wyer (1995). Stress fracture of the hyoid bone caused by induced vomiting. *Ann Emerg Med* 26(4):518–521.

Gupta, S. M., J. Chandra, and T. D. Dogra (1982). Blunt force lesions related to the heights of fall. *American Journal of Forensic Medicine and Pathology* 3:35–43.

Gurdian, E. S. and H. R. Lissner (1947). Deformation of the skull in head injury as studied by the "stress-coat" technique. *American Journal of Surgery* 73:269–281.

Gurdjian, E. S., J. E. Webster, and H. R. Lissner (1953). Observation on prediction of fracture site. *Radiology* 60:226–235.

Gurdjian, E. S. (1975). *Impact Head Injury, Mechanistic, Clinical and Preventive Correlations.* Charles C Thomas, Springfield, IL.

Gustilo, R. B., L. Simpson, R. Nixon, et al. (1969). Analysis of 511 bone fractures. *Clinical Orthopaedics* 66:148–154.

Gustilo, R. B. (1990). *The Classification Manual.* Mosby Year Book, St Louis, MO.

Gustilo, R. B., R. F. Kyle, and D. C. Templeman (1992). Fractures of the tibial plateau. In *Fractures and Dislocations*, R. B. Gustilo, R. F. Kyle, and D. C. Templeman (Eds.), pp. 945–979. Mosby, St Louis, MO.

Gustilo, R. B. (1992). Fractures of the tibia and fibula. In *Fractures and Dislocations*, R. B. Gustilo, R. F. Kyle, and D. C. Templeman (Eds.), pp. 901–944. Mosby, St Louis, MO.

Guyomarch'h, P., M. Campagna-Villancourt, C. Kremer, and A. Sauvageau (2010). Discrimination of falls and blows in blunt head trauma: A multi-criteria approach. *Journal of Forensic Sciences* 55(2):423–427.

Habermeyer, P., P. Magosch, and S. Lichtenberg (2006). Classifications of fractures of the clavicle. In *Classifications and Scores of the Shoulder*, pp. 105–117. Springer, Germany.

Haddad, G. H. and R. Zickel (1967). Instestinal performation and fracture of the lumbar spine caused by lap-type seatbelts. *New York Journal of Medicine* 67:930–932.

Haddon, W., P. Valien, J. R. McCarroll, and C. J. Umberger (1961). A controlled investigation of the characteristics of adult pedestrians fatally injured by motor vehicles in Manhattan. *Journal of Chronic Diseases* 14:655–678.

Hadley, M. N., C. A. Dickman, C. M. Browner, and V. K. H. Sonntag (1988). Acute traumatic atlas fractures: management and long-term outcome. *Neurosurgery* 23:31–35.

Hadley, M. N., B. C. Fitzpatrick, V. K. H. Sonntag, and C. M. Browner (1992). Facet fracture-dislocation injuries of the cervical spine. *Neurosurgery* 30:661–666.

Hadley, M. N., C. M. Browner, S. S. Liu, and V. K. Sonntag (1988). New subtype of acute odontoid fractures (Type IIA). *Neurosurgery* 22:67–71.

Hagan, W. (1983). Pharyngoesophageal perforations after blunt trauma to the neck. *Otolaryngology* 91(6):620–626.

Haglund, W. D. (1997a). Rodents and human remains. In *Forensic Taphonomy: The Postmortem Fate of Human Remains*, W. D. Haglund and M. H. Sorg (Eds.), pp. 405–414. CRC Press, Boca Raton, FL.

———— (1997b). Dogs and coyotes: Postmortem involvement with human remains. In *The Postmortem Fate of Human Remains*, W. D. Haglund and M. H. Sorg (Eds.), pp. 367–381. CRC Press, Boca Raton, FL.

Hall, S. (2006). *Basic Biomechanics* (5th ed.). McGraw-Hill, New York.

Hamilton, W. C. (Ed.) (1984). *Traumatic Disorders of the Ankle*. Springer-Verlag, New York.

Hanafi, M., N. Al-Sarraf, S. Hazem, and A. Abdelaziz (2011). Pattern and presentation of blunt chest trauma among different age groups. *Asian Cardiovasc Thorac Ann* 19:48–51.

Hand, W. L., C. R. Hand, and A. W. Dunn (1971). Avulsion fractures of the tibial tubercle. *Journal of Bone and Joint Surgery [Am]* 53:1579–1583.

Hannon, M., P. Hadjizacharia, L. Chan, D. Plurad, and D. Demetriades (2009). Prognostic significance of lower extremity long bone fractures after automobile versus pedestrian injuries. *Journal of Trauma* 67:1384–1388.

Hansch, C. F. (1977). Throat-skeleton fractures by strangulation. *Zeitschrift fur Rechtzmedizin* 79:143–149.

Hansen, S. T. (1992). Foot injuries. In *Skeletal Trauma: Fractures, Dislocations, Ligamentous Injuries*, B. D. Browner, J. B. Jupiter, A. M. Levine, and P. G. Trafton (Eds.), pp. 1959–1991. W. B. Saunders, Philadelphia.

Hanson, B., P. Cummings, F. Rivara, and M. John (2004). Impact of impacted mandibular third molars in mandibular angle and condylar fractures. *J Can Dent Assoc* (70):1.

Hardcastle, P. H., R. Reschauer, E. Kutscha-Lissberg, and W. Schoffmann (1982). Injuries to the tarsometatarsal joint: incidence, classification and treatment. *Journal of Bone and Joint Surgery [Br]* 64:349–356.

Hardt, N. and J. Kuttenberger (2009). *Craniofacial Trauma: Diagnosis and Management.* Springer, Dusseldorf.

Harington, I. J. (1982). Biomechanics of joint injuries. In *Biomechanics of Musculoskeletal Injury*, E. R. Gozna (Ed.), pp 31–82. Williams and Wilkins, Baltimore.

Harkess, J. and W. Ramsey (1991). Principles of fractures and dislocations. In *Rockwood and Green's Fractures in Adults*, (3rd ed.), C. A. Rockwood, R. W. Bucholz, and J. D. Heckman (Eds.). J. B. Lippincott, Philadelphia.

Harkess, J. W., W. C. Ramsey, and J. W. Harkess (1991). Principles of fractures and dislocations. In *Fractures in Adults*, (3rd ed.). C. A. Rockwood and D. P. Green (Eds.), pp. 1–20. J. B. Lippincott, Philadelphia.

Harm, T. and J. Raja (1981). Types of injuries and interrelated conditions of victims and assailants in attempted and homicidal strangulation. *Forensic Science International* 18:101–123.

Hart, C. L. and J. D. Griffith (2003). Rise in landing-related skydiving fatalities. *Perceptual and Motor Skills* 97:390–392.

Hart, E., M. Albrignth, G. Rebello, and B. Grottkau (2006). Broken bones: Common pediatric fractures. *Orthopaedic Nursing* 25(4):251–256.

Hart, G. (2005). Fracture pattern interpretation in the skull: Differentiating blunt force from ballistics trauma using concentric fractures. *J For Sci* 50:1276–1281.

Harvey, C., S. Allen, and D. O'Regan (2006). Interpretation of hand radiographs. *British Journal of Hospital Medicine* 67(3):48–52.

Harvey, F. H. and A. M. Jones (1980). "Typical" basal skull fracture of both petrous bones: An unreliable indicator of head impact site. *Journal of Forensic Sciences* 25:280–285.

Harwood-Nash, D., E. Hendrick, and A. Hudson (1971). The significance of skull fractures in children. *Radiology* 10(1):151–156.

Hasselman, C., M. Vogt, K. Stone, J. Cauley, and S. F. Conti (2003). Foot and ankle fractures in elderly white women: Incidence and risk factors. *J Bone and Joint Surgery [Am]* 85-A(5):820–824.

Hatton M. P., L. M. Walkins, and P. A. D. Rubin (2001). Orbital fractures in children. *Ophthalmic Plastic and Reconstructive Surgery* 17(3):174–179.

Haug, R. H., J. D. Savage, M. U. Likavec, and P. J. Conforti (1992). A review of 100 closed head injuries associated with facial fractures. *Journal of Oral and Maxillofacial Surgeons* 50(3):218–222.

Haug R. H., J. E. Van Sickels, and W. S. Jenkins (2002). Demographics and treatment options for orbital roof fractures. *Oral Surgery, Oral Medicine, Oral Pathology, Oral Radiology and Endodonty* 93:238–245.

Hawkins, L. G. (1965). Fracture of the lateral process of the talus. *Journal of Bone and Joint Surgery [Am]* 47:1170–1173.

———— (1970). Fractures of the neck of the talus. *Journal of Bone and Joint Surgery [Am]* 52:991–1002.

Hawley, D. A., M. A. Clark, and J. E. Pless (1995). Fatalities involving bicycles: A non-random population. *Journal of Forensic Sciences* 40:205–207.

Haynes, G. (1983). Frequencies of spiral and green-bone fractures on ungulate limb bones in modern surface assemblages. *Amer Antiquity* 48(1):102–114.

Hays, M. B. and A. M. Bernhang (1992). Fractures of the atlas vertebra: A three-part fracture not previously classified. *Spine* 17:240–242.

Heaney, R. P. (1989). Osteoporotic fracture space: A hypothesis. *Bone and Mineral* 6: 1–13.

Heary, R., C. Hunt, A. Krieger, J. Schulder, and C. Vaid (1993). Nonsurgical treatment of compound depressed skull fractures. *J Trauma* 35(3):441–447.

Hechter, S., D. Huyer, and D. Manson (2002). Sternal fractures as a manifestation of abusive injury in children. *Pediatric Radiology* 32:902–906.

Heckman, J. D. (1984). Fractures ad dislocations of the foot. In *Fractures in Adults*, C. A. Rockwood and D. P. Green (Eds.), pp. 1703–1832. J. B. Lippincott, Philadelphia.

Hecova, H., V. Tzigjounadis, V. Merglova, and J. Netolicky (2010). A retrospective study of 889 injured permanent teeth. *Dental Traumatology* 26:466–475.

Hegenbarth, R. and K. Ebel (1976). Roentgen findings in fractures of the vertebral column in childhood: An examination of 35 patients and its results. *Pediatric Radiology* 5:34–39

Heise, R. H., P. J. Srivatsa, and P. R. Karsell (1996). Spontaneous intrauterine linear skull fracture: A rare complication of spontaneous vaginal delivery. *Obstetrics and Gynecology* 87(5):851–854.

Helfer, R. E., T. L. Slovis, and M. Black (1977). Injuries resulting when small children fall out of bed. *Pediatrics* 60:533–535.

Helfet, D. L. (1992). Fractures of the distal femur. In *Skeletal Trauma: Fractures, Dislocations, Ligamentous Injuries*, B. D. Browner, J. B. Jupiter, A. M. Levine, and P. G. Trafton (Eds.), pp. 1643–1683. W. B. Saunders, Philadelphia.

Hellier, C. and R. Connelly (2009). Cause of death in judicial hanging: A review and case study. *Medicine, Science and the Law* 49(1):18–26.

Henrikson, B. (1966). Supracondylar fracture of the humerus in children. *Acta Chirurgica Scandinavica* 369 (Suppl):5–45.

Henrys, P., E. D. Lyne, C. Lifton, and G. Salciccioli (1977). Clinical review of cervical spine injuries in children. *Clinical Orthopaedics* 129:172–176.

Hermel, M. B. and J. Gershjon-Cohen (1953). The nutcracker fracture of the cuboid by indirect violence. *Radiology* 60:850–854.

Hernandez, M. A. (1994). Fracture of the posterior process of the talus: A discussion and case presentation. *Texas Medicine* 90:57–50.

Hess, T. R., S. Rupp, T. Hopf, M. Gleitz, and J. Liebler (1994). Lateral tibial avulsion fractures and disruptions to the anterior cruciate ligament. *Clinical Orthopaedics and Related Research* 303:193–197.

Hickey, K. and P. McKenna (1996). Skull fracture caused by vacuum extraction. *Obstetrics and Gynecology* 88(4):671–673.

Higuera, S., E. I. Lee, P. Cole, L. H. Hollier, and S. Stal (2007). Nasal trauma and the deviated nose. *Plastic and Reconstructive Surgery Journal* 120(Suppl 2):64S–75S.

Hinds, J. D., G. Allen, and C. G. Morris (2007). Trauma and motorcyclists: Born to be wild, bound to be injured? *Injury* 38:1131–1138.

Hipp, J. A., E. J. Cheal, and W. C. Hayes (1992). Biomechanics of fractures. In *Skeletal Trauma: Fractures, Dislocations, Ligamentous Injuries*, B. D. Browner, J. B. Jupiter, A. M. Levine, and P. G. Trafton (Eds.), pp. 95–125. W. B. Saunders, Philadelphia.

Hirano, K. and G. Inoue (2005). Classification and treatment of hamate fractures. *Hand Surgery* 10:151–157.

Hiss, J., T. Kahana, and C. Kugel (1996). Beaten to death: Why do they die? *Journal of Trauma, Injury, Infection, and Critical Care* 40(1):27–30.

Hitosugi, M., K. Mizuno, T. Nagai, and S. Tokudome (2011). Analysis of maxillofacial injuries of vehicle passengers involved in frontal collisions. *Journal of Oral and Maxillofacial Surgeons* 69:1146–1151.

Hocker, K. and A. Menschik (1994). Chip fractures of the triquetrum: Mechanisms, classification and results. *Journal of Hand Surgery [Br]* 19:584.

Hodgson, V. R. (1967). Tolerance of facial bones to impact. *American Journal of Anatomy* 120:113–122.

Hogg, N. J. V., T. C. Stewart, J. E. A. Armstrong, and M. J. Girotti (2000). Epidemiology of maxillofacial injuries at trauma hospitals in Ontario, Canada, between 1992 and 1997. *Journal of Trauma* 49:425–432.

Hohl, M., E. E. Johnson, and D. A. Wiss (1974). Tibial condylar fractures: Long term follow-up. *Texas Medicine* 70:46–56.

Hohl, M., R. L. Larson, and D. C. Jones (1984). Fractures and dislocations of the knee. In *Fractures in Adults*, C. A. Rockwood and D. P. Green (Eds.), pp. 1429–1591. J. B. Lippincott, Philadelphia.

Hohl, M., E. E. Johnson, and D. A. Wiss (1992). Fractures of the knee. In *Fractures*, C. A. Rockwood and D. P. Green (Eds.), pp. 1725–1797. J. B. Lippincott, Philadelphia.

Hokan, R., G. M. Bryce, and N. J. Cobb (1993). Dislocation of scaphoid and fractured capitate in a child. *Injury* 24:496–497.

Holdsworth, F. W. (1963). Fractures, dislocations, and fracture-dislocations of the spine. *Journal of Bone and Joint Surgery [Br]* 45:6–35.

———— (1970). Fractures, dislocations, and fracture-dislocations of the spine. *Journal of Bone and Joint Surgery [Am]* 52:1534–1551.

Holmes, P., J. Koehler, G. McGwin, Jr., and L. W. Rue, III (2004). Frequency of maxillofacial injuries in all-terrain vehicle collisions. *J Oral and Maxillofac Surg* 62: 697.

Horak, J. and B. E. Nilsson (1975). Epidemiology of fracture of the upper end of the humerus. *Clinical Orthopaedics and Related Research* 112:250–253.

Horal, J., A. Nachemson, and S. Scheller (1972). Clinical and radiological long-term follow-up of vertebral fractures in children. *Acta Orthopaedica Scandinavica* 43:491–503.

Horii, E., R. Nakamura, K. Watenabe, and K. Tsunoda (1994). Scaphoid fracture as a "puncher's fracture." *Journal of Orthopaedic Trauma* 6:107–110.

Horn, J. S. (1954). The traumatic anatomy and treatment of the acute acromioclavicular dislocations. *Journal of Bone and Joint Surgery* 36:194–201.

Hoshi, K., S. Tsukikaea, M. Oowada, K. Igabashi, and A. Sato (1994). Calcaneus and vertebrae bone mineral density values and fracture threshold. *Tohoku Journal of Experimental Medicine* 174:333–341.

Hovland, E. (1992). Horizontal root fractures: Treatment and repair. *Dental Clinics of North America* 36(2):509–525.

Hoyer, C. B., T. S. Nielssen, L. L. Nagel, L. Uhrenhold, and L. W. T. Boel (2012). Investigation of a fatal airplane crash: Autopsy, computed tomography, and injury pattern analysis used to determine who was steering the plane at the time of the accident: A case report. *Forensic Science, Medicine and Pathology* 8:179–188.

Hoyt, W.A. (1967). Etiology of shoulder injuries in athletes. *Journal of Bone and Joint Surgery [Am]* 49:755–756.

Hsu, J., T. Joseph, and A. Ellis (2003). Thoracolumbar fracture in blunt trauma patients: Guidelines for diagnosis and imaging. *Injury* 34(6):426–433

Hubbard, D. D. (1976). Fractures of the dorsal and lumbar spine. *Orthopaedic Clinics of North America* 7:605–614.

Hubbard, K. A., B. L. Klein, M. Hernandez, D. Forrester, and J. M. Chamberlain (1995). Mandibular fractures in children with chin lacerations. *Pediatric Emergency Care* 11:83–85.

Hughes, C. E. and C. A. White (2009). Crack propagation in teeth: A comparison of perimortem and postmortem behavior of dental materials and cracks. *J Forensic Sci* 54(2):263–266.

Hughston, J. C. (1957). Fractures of the forearm. *Journal of Bone and Joint Surgery [Am]* 44:1664–1667.

Huisman, T. A., J. Fischer, U. V. Willi, G. F. Eich, and E. Martin (1999). "Growing fontanelle": A serious complication of difficult vacuum extraction. *Neuroradiology* 41(5):381–383.

Hunsaker, D. M. and L. B. Thorne (2002). Suicide by blunt force trauma. *Am J Forensic Med Pathol* 23(4):355–359.

Hunt, D. D. (1970). Compensation fracture of the anterior articular surface of the calcaneus. *Journal of Bone and Joint Surgery [Am]* 52:1637–1642.

Hunter, J. M. and N. J. Cowan (1970). Fifth metacarpal fractures in a compensation clinic population. *Journal of Bone and Joint Surgery [Am]* 52:1159–1165.

Hunter, L. Y. (1981). Stress fracture of the tarsal navicular. *American Journal of Sports Medicine* 9:217–219.

Hwang, K. and D. Kim (2011). Assessment of zygomatic fractures. *J Craniofac Surg* 22(4):1416–1421.

Ideberg, R. (1984). Fractures of the scapula involving the glenoid fossa. In *Surgery of the Shoulder,* J. E. Bateman and R. P. Welsh (Eds.), pp. 63–66. B.D. Decker, Philadelphia.

———— (1987). Unusual glenoid fractures: A report on 92 cases. *Acta Orthopaedica Scandinavica,* 58:191–192.

Ideberg, R., S. Grevsten, and S. Larsson (1995). Epidemiology of scapular fractures: Incidence and classification of 338 fractures. *Acta Orthopaedica Scandinavica* 66:395–397.

Iida, S., S. Hassfeld, T. Reuther, H. G. Schweigert, C. Haag, J. Klein, and J. Muhling (2003). Maxillofacial fractures resulting from falls. *Journal of Cranio-Maxillo-Facial Surgery* 31:278–283.

Iizuka, H., T. Shimizu, W. Hasegawa, and K. Takagishi (2001). Fractures of the posterior part of the body and unilateral spinous process of the axis. *Spine* 26(22):E528–530.

Inaoka, S., S. Carneiro, B. Vasconcelos, and J. Leal (2009). Relationship between mandibular fracture and impacted third molar. *Med Oral Pathol Oral Cir Buccal* 14(7):E249–254.

Iscan, M. (2001). Global forensic anthropology in the 21st. *Forensic Science International* 117:1–6.

Itani, M., G. A. Evans, and W. M. Park (1982). Spontaneous sternal collapse. *Journal of Bone and Joint Surgery [Br]* 64:178–181.

Jacob, H. A. C. and T. Suezawa (1985). On the initiation of spondylolysis through mechanical factors. In *Biomechanics: Current Interdisciplinary Research*, S. M. Perren and E. Schneider (Eds.), pp. 519–524 Martinus Nijhoff, Dordrecht.

Jahss, M. H. and B. S. Kay (1983). An anatomic study of the anterior superior process of the *os calcis* and its clinical application. *Foot and Ankle* 3:268–281.

Jakob, R. P., T. Kristiansen, K. Mayo, et al. (1984). Classification and aspects of treatment of fractures of the proximal humerus. In *Surgery of the Shoulder*, J. E. Bateman and R. P. Welsh (Eds.), pp. 330–343. B. C. Decker, Philadelphia.

Jansen, M. (1926). March foot. *Journal of Bone and Joint Surgery [Br]* 8:202.

Jarrett, P. J. and T. E. Whitesides (1994). Injuries of the cervicocranium. In *Skeletal Trauma: Fractures, Dislocations, Ligamentous Injuries*, B. D. Browner, J. B. Jupiter, A. M. Levine, and P. G. Trafton (Eds.), pp. 665–697 W. B. Saunders, Philadelphia.

Jarry, L. and H. K. Uhthoff (1971). Differences in healing of metaphyseal and diaphyseal fractures. *Canadian Journal of Surgery* 14:127–135.

Jarvis, J. and P. Moroz (2006). Fractures and dislocations of the foot. In *Rockwood and Wilkins' Fractures in Children* (6th ed.), J. Beaty and J. Kasser (Eds.). Lippincott Williams and Wilkins, Philadelphia.

Jatla, K. and R. Enzenauer (2004). Orbital fractures: A review of current literature. *Curr Surg* 61(1):25.

Jeffers, R. F., H. Boon Tan, C. Nicolopoulos, R. Kamath, and P. V. Giannoudis (2003). Prevalence and patterns of foot injuries following motorcycle trauma. *Journal of Orthopaedic Trauma* 18(2):87–91.

Jefferson, G. (1920). Fractures of the atlas vertebra. *British Journal of Surgery* 7:407–422.

———— (1927–28). Discussion on spinal injuries. *Proceedings of the Royal Society of Medicine* 21:625–648.

Jensen, J. S. (1980a). Classification of trochanteric fractures. *Acta Orthopaedica Scandinavica* 51:803–810.

———— (1980b). Mechanical strength of sliding-screw hip implants. *Acta Orthopaedica Scandinavica*, 51:625–632.

———— (1981). Trochanteric fractures: An epidemiological, clinical and biomechanical study. *Acta Orthopaedica Scandinavica* 188(Suppl):1–100.

Jobe, M. T. (1993). Fractures and dislocations of the hand. In *Fractures and Dislocations*, R. B. Gustilo, R. F. Kyle, and D. C. Templeman (Eds.), pp. 611–644. Mosby, St. Louis, MO.

John, S. D., C. S. Moorthy, and L. E. Swischuk (1997). Expanding the concept of the toddler's fracture. *Radiographics* 17:367–376.

John, S. M., P. Kelly, and A. Vincent (2012). Patterns of structural head injury in children younger than 3 years: A ten-year review of 519 patients. *Journal of Trauma Acute Care Surgery* 74(1):276–281.

Johner, R. and O. Wruhs (1983). Classification of tibial shaft fractures and correlation with results after rigid internal fixation. *Clinical Orthopaedics and Related Research* 178:7–25.

Johnson, K. (2009). Skeletal aspects of non-accidental injury. In *Calcium and Bone Disorders in Children and Adolescents*, J. Allgrove and N. Shaw (Eds.), pp. 233–245. Karger, Basel.

Johnson, K. D. (1992). Femoral shaft fractures. In *Skeletal Trauma: Fractures, Dislocations, Ligamentous Injuries*. B. D. Browner, J. B. Jupiter, A. M. Levine, and P. G. Trafton (Eds.), pp. 1525–1641. W. B. Saunders, Philadelphia.

Johnson, N. (1985). Current developments in bone technology. *Advances in Archaeological Method and Theory*, Vol. 8. Academic Press, Orlando.

Johnston, G. (1962). Follow-up of one hundred cases of fracture of the head of the radius with a review of the literature. *Ulster Medical Journal* 31:51–56.

Johnston, G. W. (1962). Follow-up of one hundred cases of fracture of head of the radius with a review of literature. *Ulster Medical Journal* 31:51–56.

Johnston, I. and T. Branfoot (1992). Sternal fracture: A modern review. *Archives of Emergency Medicine* 10:24–28.

Johnstone, D. J., W. J. P. Radford, and E. J. Parnell (1993). Inter-observer variation using the AO/ASIF classification of long bone fractures *Injury* 24:163–165.

Jones, E. (1994). Skeletal growth and development as related to trauma. In *Skeletal Trauma in Children*, N. E. Gree and M. F. Swiotokowski, (Eds.), pp. 1–13. W. B. Saunders, Philadelphia.

Jones, H., G. McBride, and R. Mumby (1989). Sternal fractures associated with spinal injury. *Journal of Trauma* 29(3):360–364.

Jones, R. P. and R. Leach (1902). Fracture of the base of the fifth metatarsal bone by indirect violence. *Ann Surg*, 35:697–700.

_____ (1980). Fracture of the ulnar sesamoid bone of the thumb. *American Journal of Sports Medicine* 8:446–447.

Jones, R. S. and S. Kutty (1993). Intra-articular fractures of the hamate. *Injury* 24: 272–273.

Judd, M. (2008). The parry problem. *Journal of Archaeological Science* 35(6):1658–1666.

Judet, R., J. Judet, and E. Letournel (1964). Fractures of the acetabulum: Classification and surgical approaches to open reduction. *Journal of Bone and Joint Surgery [Am]* 46:1615–1646.

Jumbelic, M. I. (1995). Fatal injuries in a minor traffic collision. *Journal of Forensic Sciences* 40:492–494.

Jupiter, J. B. and M. R. Belsky (1992a). Trauma to the adult elbow and fractures of the distal humerus. In *Skeletal Trauma: Fractures, Dislocations, Ligamentous Injuries*, B. D. Browner, J. B. Jupiter, A. M. Levine, and P. G. Trafton (Eds.), pp. 1125–1176. W. B. Saunders, Philadelphia.

Juszczyk, M., L. Cristolfolini, and M. Viceconti (2011). The human proximal femur behaves linearly elastic up to failure under loading physiological loading conditions. *J Biomech* 44(12):2259–2266.

Kalideen, J. and K. Setyapal (1994). Fractures of the acromion in tetanus neonatorum. *Clinical Radiology* 49:563–565.

Kalla, T. P. and S. J. Kaminski (1992). A calcaneal fracture from a fall or a fall from a calcaneal fracture? *Journal of Foot Surgery* 31:446–449.

Kam, A. C. A. and P. C. A. Kam (1994). Scapular and proximal humeral head fractures: An unusual complication of cardiopulmonary resuscitation. *Anesthesia* 49:1055–1057.

Kane, W. J. (1984). Fractures of the pelvis. In *Fractures in Adults*, C. A. Rockwood and D. P. Green (Eds.), pp. 1093–1209. J. B. Lippincott, Philadelphia.

Kaplan, E. B. (1965). *Functional and Surgical Anatomy of the Hand* (2nd ed.). J. B. Lippincott, Philadelphia.

Kaplan, L. (1940). The treatment of fractures and dislocations of the hand and fingers: Technic of unpadded casts for carpal, metacarpal, and phalangeal fractures. *Surgical Clinics of North America* 20:1695–1720.

Karger, G., T. K. Teige, M. Fuchs, B. Brinkman (2001). Was the pedestrian hit in an erect position before being run over? *Forensic Science International* 119:217–220.

Karlsson, M. K., P. Herbertsson, A. Nordqvist, J. Besjakov, P. O. Josefsson, and R. Hasserlus (2010). Comminuted fractures of the radial heal: Favorable outcome after 15–25 years of follow-up in 19 patients. *Acta Orthopaedica* 81:224–227.

Kasser, J. R. and J. H. Beaty (2001). Supracondylar fractures of the distal humerus. In *Rockwood and Wilkins' Fractures in Children* (5th ed.). J. R. Kasser and J. H. Beaty (Eds.), p. 577. Lippincott, Williams & Wilkins, Philadelphia.

Katzen, J., R. Jarrahn, J. Eby, R. Mathiasen, D. Marguiles, and H. K. Shahinian (2003). Craniofacial and skull base trauma. *Journal of Trauma, Injury, Infection and Critical Care* 54(5):1026–1034.

Kaushal, L., J. Rai, and S. P. P. Singh (1994). Comminuted intra-articular fractures of the distal humerus. *International Orthopaedics* 18:276–279.

Kavanaugh, J. H., T. D. Brower, and R. V. Mann (1978). The Jones fracture revisited. *Journal of Bone and Joint Surgery [Am]* 60:776–782.

Keaveny, T. M. and W. C. Hayes (1993). Mechanical properties of cortical and trabecular bone. In *Bone*, Vol. 7, B.K. Hall (Ed.), pp. 285–344. CRC Press, Boca Raton, FL.

Kelamis, J. A., G. S. Mundinger, J. M. Feiner, A. H. Dorafshar, P. N. Manson, and E. D. Rodriguez (2011). Isolated bilateral zygomatic arch fractures of the facial skeleton are associated with skull base fractures. *Plastic and Reconstructive Surgery Journal* 128:962–970.

Kelikian, H. (1965). *Hallux Vulgus: Allied Deformities of the Forefoot and Metatarsalgia.* W. B. Saunders, Philadelphia.

Kellam, J. F. and J. B. Jupiter (1992). Diaphyseal fractures of the forearm. In *Skeletal Trauma: Fractures, Dislocations, Ligamentous Injuries*, B. D. Browner, J. B. Jupiter, A. M. Levine, and P. G. Trafton (Eds.), pp. 1095–1124. W. B. Saunders, Philadelphia.

Kellam, J. F. and B. D. Browner (1992). Fractures of the pelvic ring. In *Skeletal Trauma: Fractures, Dislocations, Ligamentous Injuries*, B. D. Browner, J. B. Jupiter, A. M. Levine, and P. G. Trafton (Eds.), pp. 849–897. W. B. Saunders, Philadelphia.

Kellman, R. M. and C. Schmidt (2009). The paranasal sinuses as a protective crumple zone for the orbit. *The Laryngoscope* 119:1682–1690.

Kelsey, J., T. Keegan, M. Prill, C. Quesenberry, and S. Sidney (2006). Risk factors for fracture of the shafts of the tibia and fibula in older individuals. *Osteoporosis International* 17(1):143–149.

Kelsey, J. L., W. S. Browner, D. G. Seeley, M. C. Nevitt, and S. R. Cummings (1992). Risk factors for fractures of the distal forearm and proximal humerus. *American Journal of Epidemiology* 135:477–489.

Kemp, A., A. Joshi, M. Mann, V. Tempest, A. Lui, S. Holden, and S. Maguire (2010). What are the clinical and radiological characteristic of spinal injuries for physical abuse: A systematic review. Arch Dis Child 95:355–360.

Kemp, A. M., F. Dunstan, S. Harrison, S. Morris, M. Mann, K. Rolfe, S. Datta, D. P. Thomas, J. R. Sibert, and S. Maguire (2008). Patterns of skeletal fractures in child abuse: A systematic review. *BMJ* 377(a1518).

Kemp, A. M., F. Dunstan, S. Harrison, S. Morris, M. Mann, K. Rolfe, S. Datta, D. P. Thomas, J. R. Sibert, and S. Maguire (2008). Patterns of skeletal fractures in child abuse: Systematic review. *British Medical Journal* 337:1518–1525.

Kempe, C. (1962). The battered-child syndrome. *JAMA* 181(1):17–24.

Kemper, A. R., E. A. Kennedy, C. McNally, S. J. Manoogian, J. D. Stitzel, and S. M. Duma (2011). Reducing chest injuries in automobile collisions: Rib fracture timing and implications for thoracic injury criteria. *Journal of Biomechanical Engineering* 39(8):2141–2151.

Kennedy, J. and W. Bailey (1968). Experimental tibial-plateau fractures: Studies of the mechanism and a classification. *Journal of Bone and Joint Surgery* 50(8):1522–1534.

Kennedy, J. C., R. W. Grainger, and R. W. McGraw (1966). Osteochondral fractures of the femoral condyles. *Journal of Bone and Joint Surgery [Br]* 48:437–440.

Kerley, E. R. (1978). The identification of battered infant skeletons. *Journal of Forensic Sciences* 223:164–168.

Kerr, H. D. (1992). Hamate-metacarpal fracture dislocation. *Journal of Emergency Medicine* 10:565–568.

Khokhlov, V. (1997). Injuries to the hyoid bone and laryngeal cartilages: Effectiveness of different methods of medicolegal investigation. *Forensic Sci Int*, 88(3):173–183.

Kim, D., M. Berkowitz, and D. Pressman (2003). Avulsion fractures of the medial tubercle of the posterior process of the talus. *Foot and Ankle International* 24(2):172–175.

Kim, M., Y. Park, S. Kim, Y. S. Yoon, K. R. Lee, T. H. Lim, H. Lim, H. Y. Park, J. M. Park, and S. P. Chung (2013). Chest injury following cardipulmonary resuscitation: A prospective computed tomography evaluation. *Resuscitation* 84(3):361–364.

Kim, M. Y., D. P. Reidy, P. C. Nolan, and J. A. Finkelstein (2001). Transverse sacral fractures: Case series and literature review. *Canadian Journal of Surgery* 44(5):359–363.

Kimmerle, E. H. and J. P. Baraybar (2008). Skeletal evidence of torture. In *Skeletal Trauma: Identification of Injuries Resulting from Human Rights Abuse and Armed Conflict*, E. H. Kimmerle and J. P. Baraybar (Eds.), pp. 201–233. CRC Press, Boca Raton FL.

King, A., D. Diefendorf, J. Apthorp, V. Negrete, and M. Carlson (1988). Analysis of 429 fractures in 189 battered children. *J Pediatric Orthopaedics* 8:585–589.

King, A. I. (1984). The spine: Its anatomy, kinematics, injury mechanisms and tolerance to impact. In *Biomechanics of Impact Trauma*, B. Aldman and A. Chapon (Eds.), pp. 191–226. Elsevier Science, Amsterdam.

Kingston, P. and C. Phillipson (1994). Elder abuse and neglect. *Br J Nurs* 3(22):1171–1172, 1189–1190.

Kleinman, P. (1998). Shaken babies. *Lancet* 352(9130):815–816.

Kleinman, P. and S. J. Marks, Jr. (1992). Vertebral body fractures in child abuse: Radiologic-histolopathologic correlates. *Invest Radiol* 27:715–722.

_____ (1996). A regional approach to classic metaphyseal lesions in abused infants: The distal tibia. *American Journal of Roentgenol* 166:1207–1212.

Kleinman, P., S. J. Marks, and B. Blackbourne (1985). The metaphyseal lesion in abused infants: A radiological-histopathological study. *AJR* 146:895–905.

Kleinman, P., S. J. Marks, K. Nimkin, S. Raydar, and S. Kessler (1996). Rib fractures in 31 abused infants: Postmortem radiologic-histopathologic study. *Radiology* 200:807–810.

Kleinman, P., S. J. Marks, J. Richmond, and B. Blackbourne (1995). Inflicted skeletal injury: A postnortem radiologic-histopothalogic study in 31 infants *AJR* 165:775–779.

Kleinman, P. and A. Schlesinger (1997). Mechanical factors associated with posterior rib fractures: Laboratory and case studies. *Pediatric Radiology* 27:87–91.

Kleinman, P. and Y. Shelton (1997). Hangman's fracture in an abused infant: Imaging features. *Pediatric Radiology* 27:776–777.

Klepinger, L. (2006). *Fundamentals of Forensic Anthropology.* John Wiley and Sons, New Jersey.

Knight, B. (1991). *Forensic Pathology.* Oxford University Press, New York.

Ko, R. (1953). The tension test upon compact substance in the long bone of human extremities. *Journal of the Kyoto Prefecture Medical University* 53:505.

Kocher, T. (1896). *Beitrage zur kenntniss eineger tisch wichtiger frakturformen.* Sallman, Basil.

Kohr, R. M. (1992). Car surfing in Indiana: An unusual form of motor vehicle fatality. *Journal of Forensic Sciences* 37:1693–1696.

Korres, D. S., K. Stamos, A. Andreakos, S. Spyridonos, and K. Kavadias (1994). The anterior inferior angle fracture of the lower cervical vertebrae. *European Spine Journal* 3:202–205.

Koval, K. and J. Zuckerman (2002). *Handbook of Fractures.* Lippincott Williams and Wilkins, Philadelphia.

Kratter, J. (1921). *Lehrbuch der Gerichtlichen Medizin mit Zugrundelegung der deutschen und osterreichischen Gesetzgebung und ihrer Neuordnung Band 2.* Enke, Stuttgart.

Kraus, J., T. Rice, C. Peek-Asa, and D. McArthur (2003). Facial trauma and the risk of intracranial injury in motorcycle riders. *Ann Emerg Med* 41(1):18–26.

Krefft, S. (1970). Who was at the controls when the fatal accident occurred? *Aerospace Medicine* 41:785–789.

Kremer, C., S. Racette, C. A. Dionne, and A. Sauvageau (2008). Discrimination of falls and blows in blunt head trauma: A systematic study of the hat brim rule in relation to skull fractures. *J Forensic Sci* 53(3):716–719.

Kremer, C. and A. Sauvageau (2009). Discrimination of falls and blows in blunt head trauma: Assessment of predictability through combined criteria. *J Forensic Sci* 54(4):923–926.

Kricun, M. E., R. Kricun (1992). Fractures of the lumbar spine. *Seminars in Roentgenology* 27:262–270.

Krogman, W. (1962). *The Human Skeleton in Forensic Medicine.* Charles C Thomas, Springfield, IL.

Kroman, A. (2004). Experimental study of fracture propogation in the human skull: A re-testing of popular theories. *Proceedings of the American Academy of Forensic Sciences* 10:314.

Kroman, A., T. Kress, and D. Porta (2011). Fracture propogation in the human cranium: A re-testing of popular theories. *Clinical Anatomy* 24:309–318.

Krueger, M. A., D. A. Green, D. Hoyt, and S. R. Garfin (1996). Overlooked spine injuries associated with lumbar transverse process fractures. *Clinical Orthopaedics and Related Research* 327:191–195.

Kuhn, J. E., D. S. Louis, and R. T. Loder (1995). Divergent single-column fractures of the distal part of the humerus. *Journal of Bone and Joint Surgery [Am]* 77:538–542.

Kulowski, J. (1961). Interconnected motorist injuries of the hip, femoral shaft and knee. *5th Stapp Car Crash Conference,*105–124

Kulvatunyou, N., R. S. Friese, B. Joseph, T. O'Keeffe, J. L. Wynne, A. L. Tang, and P. Rhee (2012). Incidence and pattern of cervical spine injury in blunt assault: It is not how they are hit, but how they fall. *Journal of Trauma* 72:271–275.

Kyle, R. F. (1992). Fractures of the hip. In *Fractures and Dislocations*, R. B. Gustilo, R. F. Kyle, and D. C. Templeman (Eds.), pp. 783–854. Mosby, St Louis, MO.

Lachman, E. (1972). Anatomy of judicial hanging. *Resident and Staff Physician* July:46–54.

Laliotis, M., B. H. Pennie, H. Carty, and L. Klenerman (1993). Toddler's fracture of the calcaneum. *Injury* 24:169–170.

Lam, M., G. Wong, and T. Lao (2002). Reappraisal of neonatal clavicular fracture: Relationship between infant size and risk factors. *J Reprod Med* 47(11):903–908.

Landells, C. D. and P. K. Van Peteghem (1988). Fractures of the atlas: Classification, treatment and morbidity. *Spine* 13:450–452.

Lane, N. and P. Sambrook (2006). Osteoporosis and the *Osteoporosis of Rheumatic Diseases* (3rd ed.). Mosby, St. Louis, MO.

Lansinger, O. (1977). Fractures of the acetabulum: A clinical, radiological and experimental study. *Acta Orthopaedica Scandinavica* 165:1–125.

Larsen, C. F., V. Brondum, and O. Skov (1992). Epidemiology of scaphoid fractures in Odense, Denmark. *Acta Orthopaedica Scandinavica* 63:216–218.

Lauge-Hansen, N. (1948). Fractures of the ankle: Analytic historic survey as basis of new experimental roentgenologic and clinical investigations. *Archives of Surgery* 56:269–317.

Lauge-Hansen, N. (1950). Fractures of the ankle. II. Combined experimental-surgical and experimental roentgenologic investigation. *Archives of Surgery* 60:957–985.

Lauridsen, E., N. Hermann, T. Gerds, S. Kreiborg, and J. Andreason (2012). Pattern of traumatic dental injuries in the permanent dentition among children, adolescents, and adults. *Dent Traumatol* 28(5):358–363.

Law, S. (1993). Thickness and resistivity variations over the upper surface of the human skull. *Brain Topography* 62(2):909–1009.

Lawrence, S. J. and M. J. Botte (1993). Jones' fractures and related fractures of the proximal fifth metatarsal. *Foot and Ankle* 14:358–365.

Lawson, G. M., C. Hajduca, and M. M. McQueen (1995). Sports fractures of the distal radius – epidemiology and outcome. *Injury* 26:33.

Le, B., E. Dierks, I. Ueeck-Homer, and B. Potter (2001). Maxillofacial injuries associated with domestic violence. *J Oral and Maxillofac Surg* 59:1277–1283.

Le Fort, R. (1901). Etude experimentale sur les fractures de la machoire superieure. *Revue de Chirurgie.*

Leach, R. (1984). Fractures of the tibia and fibula. In *Fractures in Adults,* C. A. Rockwood and D. P. Green, (Eds.), pp. 1593–1663. J. B. Lippincott, Philadelphia.

LeCount, E. R. and C. W. Apfelbach (1920). Pathologic anatomy of traumatic fractures of the cranial bones and concomitant brain injuries. *JAMA* 74:501–511.

Lederer, W., D. Mair, W. Rabi, and W. Baubin (2004). Frequency of rib and sternum fractures associated with out-of-hospital resuscitation is underestimated by conventional chest x-ray. *Resuscitation* 60(2):157–162.

Lee, K. (2009). Interpersonal violence and facial fractures. *Journal of Oral and Maxillofacial Surgery* 67:1878–1883.

Lee, S. H., P. Darent-Molina, and G. Breart (2002). Risk factors for fractures of the proximal humerus: Results from the EPIDOS prospective study. *Journal of Bone and Mineral Research* 17:817.

Leffers, D. (1992). Dislocations and soft tissue injuries of the knee. In *Skeletal Trauma: Fractures, Dislocations, Ligamentous Injuries,* B. D. Browner, J. B. Jupiter, A. M. Levine, and P. G. Trafton (Eds.), pp. 1717–1743. W. B. Saunders, Philadelphia.

LeFort, R. (1886). Étude expérimentale sur les fractures de la mâchoire supérieure.

Leone, A., A. Cerase, C. Colosimo, L. Lauro, A. Puca, P. Marano (2000). Occipital condylar fractures: A review. *Radiology* 216:635–644.

Leonidas, J. (1983). Skeletal trauma in the child abuse syndrome. *Pediatric Annals* 12(12):875–881.

Letournel, E. (1980). Acetabulum fractures: Classification and management. *Clinical Orthopaedics and Related Research* 151:81–106.

Leung, Y., S. Ip, W. Ip, W. Kam, and Y. Wai (2005). The criss-cross injury mechanism in forearm injuries. *Acta Orthop Trauma Surg* 125:298–303.

Leventhal, J., S. Thomas, S. Rosenfeld, and R. Markowitz (1993). Fractures in young children: Distinguishing child abuse from unintentional injuries. *Am J Diseases in Children* 147(1):87–92.

Levin, T., W. Berndon, I. Cassell, and N. Blitman (2003). Thoracolumbar fracture with listhesis: An uncommon manifestation of child abuse. *Pediatric Radiology* 33:305–310.

Levine, A. M. and C .C. Edwards (1989). Traumatic lesions of the occipito-atlanto-axial complex. *Clinical Orthopaedics and Related Research* 239:53–68.

———— (1992). Lumbar and sacral spine trauma. In *Skeletal Trauma: Fractures, Dislocations, Ligamentous Injuries,* B. D. Browner, J. B. Jupiter, A. M. Levine, and P. G. Trafton, (Eds.), pp. 805–848. W. B. Saunders, Philadelphia.

Levy, M., R. Fischel, G. Stern, and E. Goldberg (1979). Chip fractures of the triquetrum, the mechanism of injury. *Journal of Bone and Joint Surgery [Am]* 61:355–357.

Levy, R. N., J. D. Capozzi, and M. A. Mont (1992). Intertrochanteric hip fractures. In *Skeletal Trauma: Fractures, Dislocations, Ligamentous Injuries,* B. D. Browner, J. B. Jupiter, A. M. Levine, and P. G. Trafton (Eds.), pp. 1443–1484. W. B. Saunders, Philadelphia.

Li, G. and S. P. Baker (1997). Injury patterns in aviation-related fatalities: Implications for preventive strategies. *American Journal of Forensic Medicine and Pathology* 18(3):265–270.

Li, L. (2012). Forensic pathology. In *Injury Research: Theories, Methods, and Approaches,* G. Li and S. Baker (Eds.). Springer, New York.

Liao, W. and K. Hsu (2011). Traumatic first costosternal joint subluxation complicated with occult pneumothorax: An unusual case. *Eur J Emerg Med* 18(6):365–366.

Liaw, Y. H. and A. Pollack (1996). Bilateral scapular fractures from electrical injury. *Australian and New Zealand Journal of Surgery* 66:189–190.

Lieberman, D. E., J. D. Polk, and B. Demes (2004). Predicting long bone loading from cross-sectional geometry. *Am J of Phys Anthropol* 123:156–171.

Liebschner, M. A. K. (2004). Biomechanical considerations of animal models in tissue engineering of bone. *Biomaterials* 25(9):1697–1714.

Lillehei, K. O. and M. N. Robinson (1994). A critical analysis of the fatal injuries resulting from the Continental Flight 1713 airline disaster: Evidence in favor of improved passenger restraint Systems. *Journal of Trauma* 37(5):826–830.

Lin, P. T. and J. R. Gill (2009). Subway train-related fatalities in New York City: Accident versus suicide. *J Forensic Sci* 54(6):1414–1418.

Lindahl, L. (1977). Condylar fractures of the mandible. I: Classification and relation to age, occlusion and concomitant injuries of teeth and teeth-supporting structures, and fractures of the mandibular body. *International Journal of Oral Surgery* 6:12–21.

Line, Jr. W., R. B. Stanley, Jr., and J. H. Choi (1985). Strangulation: A full spectrum of blunt neck trauma. *Annals of Otology, Rhinology and Laryngology* 94:542–546.

Lips, P. (1997). Epidemiology and predictors of fractures associated with osteoporosis. *American Journal of Medicine* 103:3S–11S.

Liu, B., R. Ivers, R. Norton, S. Blows, and S. K. Lo (2003). Helmets for preventing injury in motorcycle riders. *Cochrane Database System Review* 4:CD004333.

Lo Casto, A., G. D. Priolo, A. Garufi, P. Purpura, S. Salerno, G. La Tona, and F. Coppolino (2012). Imaging evaluation of facial complex strut fractures. *Seminars in Ultrasound, CT and MRI* 33:396–409.

Loder, R. and J. Feinberg (2007). Orthopaedic injuries in children with non-accidental trauma: Demographic and incidence from the 2000 Kids' Inpatient Database. *J Pediatric Orthop* 27(4):421–426.

Lombardi, D. A., G. S. Smith, T. K. Courtney, M. J. Brennan, J. Y. Kim, and M. J. Perry (2011). Work-related falls from ladders: A follow-back study of US emergency department cases. *Scandinavian Journal of Work Environment, Health* 37(6):525–532.

Lonergan, G., A. Baker, M. Morey, and S. Boos (2003). Child abuse: Radiologic-pathologic correlation. *AFIP Archives* 23(4):811–845.

Loo, G. T., J. H. Siegel, P. C. Dischinger, D. Rixen, A. R. Burgess, M. D. Addis, T. O'Quinn, L. McCammon, C. B. Schmidhauser, P. Marsh, P. A. Hodge, and F. Bents (1996). Airbag protection versus compartment intrusion effect determines the pattern of injuries in multiple trauma motor vehicle crashes. *Journal of Trauma* 41:935.

Looser, K. G. and H. D. Crombie (1976). Pelvic fractures: An anatomic guide to severity of injury: Review of 100 cases. *American Journal of Surgery* 132:638–642.

Lorentzen, J. E. and M. Movin (1976). Fracture of the first rib. *Acta Orthop Scand* 47:632–634.

Love, J. (2011). Maceration: A search for a magical potion. *Newsletter of the Society of Forensic Anthropology* 3:3.

Love, J. and L. Sanchez (2009). Recognition of skeletal fractures in infants: An autopsy technique. *Journal of Forensic Sciences* 54(6):1443–1446.

Love, J. and S. Symes (2004). Understanding rib fracture patterns: Incomplete and buckle fractures. *Journal of Forensic Sciences* 49(6):1153–1158.

Lowdon, I. M. R. (1986). Fractures of the metacarpal neck of the little finger. *Injury* 17:189–192.

Lowenstein, S. R., M. Yaron, R. Carrera, D. Devereux, and L. M. Jacobs (1989). Vertical trauma: Injuries to patients who fall and land on their feet. *Annals of Emergency Medicine* 18:161–165.

Lowy, M. (1969). Avulsion fractures of the calcaneus. *Journal of Bone and Joint Surgery [Br]* 51:492–494.

Lucas, G. M., J. E. Hutton, R. C. Lim, and C. Mathewson (1981). Injuries sustained from high velocity impact with water: An experience from the Golden Gate Bridge. *Journal of Trauma* 21:612–618.

Luke, J. L., D. T. Reay, J. E. Eisele, and H. J. Bonnell (1985). Correlation of circumstances with pathological findings in asphyxial deaths by hanging: a prospective study of 61 cases from Seattle, WA. *J Forensic Sci* 30:1140–1147.

Lukhele, M. (1994). Fractures of the vertebral lamina associated with unifacet and bifacet cervical spine dislocations. *South African Journal of Surgery* 32(3):112–114.

Lustman, J. and I. Milhem (1994). Mandibular fractures in infants: Review of the literature and report of seven cases. *Journal of Oral and Maxillofacial Surgery* 52:240–245.

Lüthje, P., I. Nurmi, M. Takaja, M. Heliovaara, and S. Santavirta (1995). Incidence of pelvic fractures in Finland in 1988. *Acta Orthopaedica Scandinavica* 66:245–248.

Ly, P. and L. Fallat (1993). Transchondral fractures of the talus: A review of 64 surgical cases. *Journal of Foot and Ankle Surgery* 32:352–374.

Lyman, R. L. (1994). *Vertebrate Taphonomy.* Cambridge University Press, Cambridge, MA.

Lynch, T. C., J. V. Crues, F. W. Morgan, W. E. Sheehan. W. E., L. P. Harter, R. Ryu, et al. (1989). Bone abnormalities of the knee: Prevalence and significance at MR imaging. *Radiology* 171:761–766.

Lynnerup, N., J. G. Astrup, and B. Sejrsen (2005). Thickness of the human cranial diploe in relation to age, sex and general body build. *Head and Face Medicine* 1:13–19.

Maat, G. J. R. (2008). Dating of fractures in human dry tissue – the Berisha case. In *Skeletal Trauma: Identification of Injuries Resulting from Human Rights Abuse and Armed Conflict*, E. H. Kimmerle and B. J. Baraybar (Eds.), pp. 245–254. CRC Press, Boca Raton, FL.

Mabrey, J. D. and M. D. Fitch (1989). Plastic deformation in pediatric fractures: Mechanism and treatment. *Journal of Pediatric Orthopaedics* 9:310–314.

Mackey, M. (1984). Injuries to the face and to skin. In *Biomechanics of Impact Trauma*, B. Aldman and A. Chapon (Eds.), pp. 335–340. Elsevier Science, Amsterdam.

MacLean, J. G. B. and J. Hutchinson (2012). Serious neck injuries in U19 rugby union players: An audit of admissions to spinal injury units in Great Britain and Ireland. *British Journal of Sports Medicine* 46:591–594.

Maeda, H., T. Higuchi, M. Imura, and K. Noguchi (1993). Ring fracture of the base of the skull and atlanto-occipital avulsion due to anteroflexion on motorcycle riders in a head-on collision accident. *Medicine, Science and the Law* 33:266–269.

Maguire, J. K. and S. T. Canale (1993). Fractures of the patella in children in adolescents. *Journal of Pediatric Orthopaedics* 13:567–571.

Maguire, S., M. Mann, N. John, B. Ellaway, J. Sibert, and A. Kemp (2006). Does cardio-pulmonary resuscitation cause rib fractures in children? A systematic review. *Child Abuse and Neglect* 30:739–751.

Main, B. J. and R. L. Jowett (1975). Injuries of the midtarsal joint. *Journal of Bone and Joint Surgery [Br]* 57:89–97.

Maissonneuve, M. J. G. (1840). Recherches sur la fracture du perone. *Archives Generales de Medecine*, 7:165.

Makhdoomi, K. R., J. Doyle, and M. Malony (1993). Transverse fracture of the patella in children. *Archives of Orthopaedic and Trauma Surgery* 112:302–303.

Malberg, M. I. (2001). A new system of classification for spinal injuries. *Spine Journal* 1:18–25.

Malgaigne, J. F. (1859). *Treatise on Fractures.* J. B. Lippincott, Philadelphia.

Malhotra, N., M. Kundabala, and S. Acharaya (2011). A review of root fractures: Diagnosis, treatment and prognosis. *Dent Update* 38(9):615–619, 623–624.

Manaster, B. J. and C. L. Andrews (1994). Fractures and dislocations of the knee and proximal tibia and fibula. *Seminars in Roentgenology* 29:113–133.

Mandalia, V. and J. Henson (2008). Traumatic bone bruising-a review article. *European Journal of Radiology* 67(1):54–61.

Mandelstam, S., D. Cook, M. Fitzgerald, and M. Ditchfield (2003). Complementary use of radiological skeletal survey and bone scintography in detection of bony injuries in suspected child abuse. *Arch Dis Child* 88:387–390.

Manolidis, S., B. Weeks, M. Kirby, M. Scarlett, and L. Hollier (2002). Classification and surgical management of orbital fractures: Experience with 111 orbital reconstructions. *J Craniofac Surg* 13(6):726.

Manson, P. N., M. G. Stanwix, M. J. Yaremchuk, H. Hui-Chou, and E. D. Rodriguez (2009). Frontobasal fractures: Anatomical classification and clinical significance. *Plastic and Reconstructive Surgery Journal* 124:2096–2106.

Many, A., S. H. Brenner, Y. Yaron, A. Lusky, M. R. Peyser, and J. B. Lessing (1996). Prospective study of incidence and predisposing factors for clavicular fracture in the newborn. *Acta Obstetrica et Gynecologica Scandinavica* 75:378–381.

Maples, W. (1986). Trauma analysis by the forensic anthropologist. In *Forensic Osteology: Advances in the Identification of Human Remains* (1st ed.), K. Reichs (Ed.), pp. 218–228. Charles C Thomas, Springrield, IL.

Maravic, M., A. Ostertag, and M. Cohen-Solal (2012). Subrochanteric / femoral shaft versus hip fractures: Incidences and identification of risk factors. *Journal of Bone and Mineral Research* 27:130–137.

Marchessault, J., M. Conti, and M. E. Baratz (2009). Carpal fractures in athletes excluding the scaphoid. *Hand Clinics* 25:371.

Marean, C., Y. Abe, C. Frey, and R. Randall (2000). Zooarchaeological and taphonomic analysis of the Die Kelders Cave 1 layers 10 and 1: Middle stone age larger mammal fauna. *J Human Evolution* 38(1):197–233.

Margerl, F., M. Aebi, S. Gertzbein, J. Harms, and S. Nazarian (1994). A comprehensive classification of thoracic and lumbar injuries. *Eur Spine J* 3:184–291.

Marker P., A. Nielsen, and H. L. Bastian (2000). Fractures of the mandibular condyle. *British Journal of Oral and Maxillofacial Surgery* 38:417–421.

Marks, M., J. Hudson, and S. Elkins (1999). Craniofacial fractures: Collaboration spells success. In *Broken Bones: Anthropological Analysis of Blunt Force Trauma*, A. Galloway (Ed.). Charles C Thomas, Springfield, IL.

Marlin, D., M. Clark, and S. Standish (1991). Identification of human remains by comparison of frontal sinus radiographs: A series of four cases. *J Forensic Sci* 36(6):1765–1772.

Marshall, S., F. Mueller, D. Kirby, and J. Yang (2003). Evaluation of safety belts and faceguards for prevention of injuries for prevention of injuries in youth baseball. *JAMA* 289:568.

Martin, R. (1991). Determinants of the mechanical properties of bones. *Journal of Biomechanics* 24(1):79–88.

Martin, R. B. and D. B. Burr (1998). *Skeletal Tissue Mechanics.* Springer, New York.

Martin, W., III and H. O. Riddervold (1979). Acute plastic bowing fractures of the fibula. *Radiology* 131:639–640.

Martiniakova, M., B. Grosskopf, M. Vondrakova, R. Omelka, and M. Fabis (2006). Differences in femoral contact bone tissue microscopic structure between adult cows (Bos taurus) and pigs (Sus scrofa domestica). *J Veterinary Medicine Anatomia, Histologia, Embrologia* 35(3):167–170.

Martins M. M. S., N. Homsi, C. C. S. Pereira, E. C. G. Jardim, and I. R. Garcia (2011). Epidemiologic evaluation of mandibular fractures in the Rio de Janeiro high-complexity hospital. *Journal of Craniofacial Surgery* 22(6):2026–2030.

Martos, V. and C. Jackowski (2012). Bilateral fractures of the transverse processus: A diagnostic sign of overrun? *Forensic Science International* 219:244–247.

Mason, M. (1954). Some observations on fractures of the head of the radius with a review of one hundred cases. *British Journal of Surgery* 42:123–132.

Matsubara, S., A. Izumi, T. Nagai, I. Kikkawa, and M. Suzuki (2008). Femur fracture during abdominal breech delivery. *Archives of Gynecology and Obstetrics* 278:195–197.

Matsui, Y. (2005). Effects of vehicle bumper height and impact velocity on type of lower-extremity injury in vehicle-pedestrian accidents. *Accident Analysis and Prevention* 37:633–640.

Matsui, Y., M. Hitosugi, and K. Mizuno (2011). Severity of vehicle bumper location in vehicle-to-pedestrian impact accidents. *Forensic Science International* 212:205–209.

Matsui, Y., G. Schroeder, U. Bosch (2004). Injury pattern and response of human thigh under lateral loading simulating car-pedestrian impact. *Proceedings of the Proceedings of the SP-1878 Vehicle Aggressivity and Compatibility, Structural Crashworthiness, and Pedestrian Safety*, 01-1603.

Matta, J. (1992). Surgical treatment of acetabulum fractures. In *Skeletal Trauma: Fractures, Dislocations, Ligamentous Injuries*, B. D. Browner, J. B. Jupiter, A. M. Levine, and P. G. Trafton (Eds.), pp. 899–924. W. B. Saunders, Philadelphia.

Matthes, G., U. Shmucker, E. Lignitz, M. Huth, A. Ekkenkamp, and J. Seifert (2006). Does the frontal airbag avoid thoracic injury? *Arch Orthop Trauma Surg* 126(8):541–544.

Mayer, T., M. L. Walker, D. G. Johnson, and M. E. Matlak (1981). Causes of morbidity and mortality in severe pediatric trauma. *JAMA* 245:719–721.

Mazess, R. B. (1987). Bone density in diagnosis of osteoporosis: Thresholds and breakpoints. *Calcified Tissue International* 41:117–118.

McCord, C. D., M. Tanenbaum, and W. R. Nunery (Eds.) (1995). Acute orbital trauma: Diagnosis and treatment. In *Oculoplastic Surgery*, pp. 515–551. Raven Press, New York.

McCormack, T., E. Karaikovic, and R. W. Gaines (1994). The load sharing classification of acute thoracolumbar spinal injuries. *Spine* 19(15):1157–1169.

McCoy, G. F., R. A. Johnstone, and J. Kenwright (1989). Biomechanics aspects of pelvic and hip injuries in road traffic accidents. *Journal of Orthopaedic Trauma* 3:118–123.

McCrory, P. and C. Bladin (1996). Fractures of the lateral process of the talus: A clinical review of "Snowboarder's ankle." *Clinical Journal of Sports Medicine* 6:124–128.

McCue, F. C., III, W. H. Baugher, D. N. Kulund, and J. H. Gleck (1979). Hand and wrist injuries in the athlete. *American Journal of Sports Medicine* 7:275–286.

McElfresh, E. C. and J. H. Dobyns (1983). Intra-articular metacarpal head fractures. *Journal of Hand Surgery* 8:383–393.

McElhaney, J. E., V. L. Reynolds, and J. F. Hilyard (1976). *Handbook of Human Tolerance.* Japan Automobile Research Institute, Inc, Tokyo.

McGee, M. B. (1991). Unusual blunt force wound patterns due to a hexagonal steel bar. *American Journal of Forensic Medicine and Pathology* 12:149–152.

McGrory, B. J., R. A. Klassen, E. Y. S. Chao, J. W. Staehell, and A. L. Weaver (1993). Acute fractures and dislocations of the cervical spine in children and adolescents. *Journal of Bone and Joint Surgery [Am]* 75:988–995.

McGwin, G., J. Metzger, J. E. Alonso, et al. (2003). The association between occupant restraint systems and risk of injury in frontal motor vehicle collisions. *Journal of Trauma* 54:1182.

McKerrell, J., V. Bowen, G. Johnston, and J. Zondervan (1987). Boxer's fractures – conservative or operative management? *Journal of Trauma* 27:486–490.

McMinn, D. J. W. (1981). Mallet finger and fractures. *Injury* 12:477–479.

McMurtry, R. Y. and J. B. Jupiter (1992). Fractures of the distal radius. In *Skeletal Trauma: Fractures, Dislocations, Ligamentous Injuries*, B. D. Browner, J. B. Jupiter, A. M. Levine, and P. G. Trafton (Eds.), pp. 1063–1094. W. B. Saunders, Philadelphia.

Meek, R. N. (1992). Fractures of the pelvis. In *Fractures and Dislocations*, R. B. Gustilo, R. F. Kyle, and D. C. Templeman (Eds.), pp. 733–755. Mosby, St. Louis, MO.

Megyesi, M. S., S. P. Nawrocki, and N. H. Haskell (2005). Using accumulated degree-days to estimate the postmortem interval from decomposed human remains. *Journal of Forensic Sciences* 50:618–626.

Meldon, S. and L. Moettus (1995). Thoracolumbar spine fractures: Clinical presentation and the effect of altered sensorium and major injury. *J Trauma* 39(6):1110–1114.

Melick, L. and K. Ressor (1990). Spiral tibial fractures of children: Commonly accidental spiral long bone fractures. *Am J Emerg Med* 8:234–237.

Melick, R. A. and D. R. Miller (1966). Variations of tensile strength of human cortical bone with age. *Clinical Science* 30:243–248.

Melton, L. J., III and S. R. Cummings (1987). Heterogeneity of age-related fractures: Implications for epidemiology. *Bone and Mineral* 2:321–331.

Melton, L. J., III (1993). Epidemiology of age-related fractures. In *The Osteoporotic Syndrome: Detection, Prevention, and Treatment* (3rd ed.). L. V. Avioli (Ed.), pp. 17–35. Wiley-Liss, New York.

Melton, L. J., III (1995). Epidemiology of fractures In *Osteoporosis: Etiology, Diagnosis and Management* (2nd ed.). B. L. Riggs and L. J. Melton III (Eds.), pp. 225–247. Lippincott-Raven, Philadelphia.

Melvin, J. W. and E. G. Evans (1971). A strain energy approach to the mechanics of skull fracture. *Proceedings of the 15th Stapp Conference*, pp. 666–685.

Merbs, C. F. (1995). Incomplete spondylolysis and healing: A study of ancient Canadian Eskimo skeletons. *Spine* 20:2328–2334.

Merrill, K. D. (1993). The Maisonneuve fracture of the fibula. *Clinical Orthopaedics and Related Research* 287:218–223.

Merten, D. F., M. A. Radlowski, and J. C. Leonidas (1983). The abused child: A radiological reappraisal. *Radiology* 146:377–381.

Meservy, C., T. Towbin, R. McLaurin, P. Myers, and W. Ball (1987). Radiographic characteristics of skull fractures resulting. *Am J Roentgenology* 149(1):173–175.

Meurman, K. O. A. (1981). Less common stress fractures in the foot. *British Journal of Radiology* 54:1–7.

Meyers, M. and F. McKeever (1959). Fractures of the intercondylar eminence of the tibia. *Journal of Bone and Joint Surgery [Am]* 41:209–222.

Mikhail, J. and D. Huelke (1997). Air bags: An update. *J Emerg Nurs* 5:439–445.

Mikić, Z. (1975). Galeazzi fracture-dislocations. *J Bone and Joint Surgery [Am]* 57(8): 1071–1080.

Milch, H. (1931). Unusual fractures of the capitulum humeri and the capitulum radii. *Journal of Bone and Joint Surgery* 13:882–886.

Milch, H. (1934). Fracture of the hamate bone. *Journal of Bone and Joint Surgery* 16:459.

Miller, K., P. Walker, and R. O'Halloran (1998). Age and sex-related variation in hyoid bone morphology. *J Forensic Sciences* 43(6):1138–1143.

Miller, M. E. and J. R. Ada (1992). Injuries to the shoulder girdle. In *Skeletal Trauma: Fractures, Dislocations, Ligamentous Injuries*, B. D. Browner, J. B. Jupiter, A. M. Levine, and P. G. Trafton (Eds.), pp. 1291–1310. W. B. Saunders, Philadelphia.

Miller, W. E. (1964). Comminuted fractures of the distal end of the humerus in the adult. *Journal of Bone and Joint Surgery [Am]* 46:644–657.

Miranda, P., M. Villa, J. A. Alvarez-Garijo, and A. Perez-Nunez (2007). Birth trauma and development of growing fracture after coronol suture disruption. *Child's Nervous System* 23(3):355–358.

Mithani, S. K., H. St. Hiliare, B. S. Brooke, I. M. Smith, R. Bluebond-Langner, and E. D. Rodriguez (2009). Predictable patterns of intra-cranial and cervical spine injury in craniomaxillofacial trauma: Analysis of 4,786 patients. *Plastic and Reconstructive Surgery Journal* 123:1293–1301.

Moczygemba, C., P. Paramsothy, S. Meikle, A. Kourtis, W. Barfield, E. Kuklina, S. Posner, M. Whiteman, and D. J. Jamieson (2010). Route of delivery and neonatal birth trauma. *Am J Obstetrics and Gynecology* 202(4):361.

Mohanty, M., M. Panigrahi, S. Maohanty, J. Dash, and S. Dash (2007). Self-defense injuries in homicidal deaths. *J Forensic and Legal Medicine* 14(4):213–215.

Mohit, A. A., J. A. Schuster, S. K. Mirza, and F. A. Mann (2003). "Plough" fractures: Shear fracture of the anterior arch of the atlas. *American Journal of Roentgenology* 181:770.

Mondin, V., A. Rinaldo, and A. Ferlito (2005). Management of nasal bone fractures. *American Journal of Otolaryngology – Head and Neck Medicine and Surgery* 26:181–185.

Monjok, E. (2008). Clavicle fractures during birth. *Am Fam Physician* 15(78):697.

Monkhouse, S. and M. Kelly (2008). Airbag-related chest wall burn as a marker of underlying injury: A case report. *J Med Case Rep* 24(2):91.

Monteggia, G. B. (1814). *Instituzione Chirurgiche* (2nd ed.). Maspero, Milan.

Montovani, J. C., E. Noguiera, F. D. Ferreira, A. C. L. Neto, and V. Nakajima (2006). Surgery of frontal sinus fractures: Epidemiologic study and evaluation of techniques. *Rev Bras Otorrinolaringol* 72(2):204–209.

Mooney, V. and B. F. Claudi (1984). Fractures of the shaft of the femur. In *Fractures in Adults*, C. A. Rockwood and D. P. Green (Eds.), pp. 1357–1427. J. B. Lippincott, Philadelphia.

Morild, I. and P. K. Lilleng (2012). Different mechanisms of decapitation: Three classics and one unique case history. *Journal of Forensic Sciences* 57(6):1659–1664.

Morlan, R. (1980). *Taphonomy and archaeology in the upper pleistocene of the Northern Yokon Territory: A glimpse of the peopling of the New World.* National Museum of Man, Ottowa.

———— (1984). Toward the definition of criteria for the recognition of artificial bone alterations. *Quaternary Research* 22(2):160–171.

Morrey, B. F. and T. Stormont (1988). Force transmission through the radial head. *Journal of Bone and Joint Surgery [Am]* 70:250–256.

Morrey, B. F. (1993). Fractures and dislocations of the elbow. In *Fractures and Dislocations*, R. B. Gustilo, R. F. Kyle, and D. C. Templeman (Eds.), pp. 387–497. Mosby, St. Louis, MO.

Morris, F. (1989). Do head-restraints protect the neck from whiplash injuries? *Archives of Emergency Medicine* 6:17–21.

Mourad, L. (1996). Bosworth fracture. *Orthopaedic Nursing* 15:22.

Muelleman, R. L., J. Reuwer, T. G. Sanson, L. Gerson, B. Woolard, A. H. Yancy, and E. Bernstein (1996). An emergency medicine approach to violence throughout the life cycle. *SAEM Public Health and Education Committee, Academy of Emergency Medicine* 3(7):705–715.

Müller, M. E., M. Allgower, M. R. Schneider, and H. Willenegger (1991). *Manual of Internal Fixation.* Springer-Verlag, New York.

Mullich, S. (1977). The lateral Monteggia fracture. *Journal of Bone and Joint Surgery [Am]* 59:543–545.

Mulligan, R. and R. Mahabir (2010). The prevalence of cervical spine injury, head injury, or both with isolated and multiple craniomaxillofacial fractures. *Plastic Reconstr Surg* 126:1647.

Munante-Cardenas, J., L. Asprino, M. DeMoraes, J. Algergaria-Barbosa, and R. Moreira (2010). Mandibular fractures in a group of Brazilian subjects under 18 years of age: An epidemiological analysis. *Int J Pediatr Otorhinolaryngol* 74(11):1267–1280.

Muralikuttan, K. P. and M. Sankarari-Kuty (1999). Supracondylar stress fracture of the femur. *Injury* 30:66–67.

Murphy, G. (1976). Death on the railway. *Journal of Forensic Sciences* 21:218–226.

Murphy, G. K. (1989). The Podmore case. *American Journal of Forensic Medicine and Pathology* 10(3):247–250.

Murphy, J., J. Nyland, J. Lantry, and C. Roberts (2009). Motorcyclist "biker couples"; A descriptive analysis of orthopaedic and non-orthopaedic injuries. *Injury* 40:1195–1199.

Murphy, K., S. Waa, H. Jaffer, A. Sauter, and A. Chan (2013). A literature review of findings in physical elder abuse. *Canadian Association of Radiologists Journal* 64(1):10–14.

Murphy, R. X., K. Birmingham, W. J. Okunski, et al. (2000). The influence of airbag and restraining devices on the patterns of facial trauma in motor vehicle collisions. *Plastic and Reconstructive Surgery Journal* 105:516.

Murphy, S. P., P. S. Sledzik, R. W. Mann, and M. A. Kelley (1990). Macroscopic bone remodeling following trauma: Reconsidering the term perimortem. Paper presented at the American Academy of Forensic Sciences, Cincinnati.

Murray, J. A. M. and A. G. D. Maran (1986). A pathological classification of nasal fractures. *Injury* 17:338–344.

Nagata, T., H. Uno, and M. J. Perry (2010). Clinical consequences of road traffic injuries among the elderly in Japan. *BMC Public Health* 10:375–382.

Nahum, A. M. (1976). The prediction of maxillofacial trauma. *Transactions of the American Academy of Ophthamology and Otology* 84:932–933.

Naim-Ur, R., Z. Jamjoon, A. Jamjoon, and W. R. Murshid (1994). Growing skull fractures: Classification and management. *British Journal of Neurosurgery* 8:667–679.

Nance, E. P., Jr. and J. J. Kaye (1982). Injuuries of the quadriceps mechanism. *Radiology* 142:301–307.

Natu, S. S., H. Pradhan, H. Gupta, S. Alam, S. Gupta, R. Pradhan, S. Mohammad, M. Kohli, V. P. Sinha, R. Shankar, and A. Agarwal (2012). An epidemiological study on pattern and incidence of mandibular fractures. In *Plastic Surgery International*, p. 7. Hindawi Publishing Corporation.

Neer, C. S. (1984). Fractures and dislocations of the shoulder part I: Fractures about the shoulder In *Fractures in Adults*, C. A. Rockwood and D. P. Green, (Eds.), pp. 675–721. J. B. Lippincott, Philadelphia.

Neyt, J. (1998). Use of animal models in musculoskeletal research. *The Iowa Orthopaedic Journal* 18:118–123.

Ng, C. and C. Hall (1998). Costochondral junction fractures and intra-abdominal trauma in non-accidental injury (child abuse). *Pediatric Radiology* 28:671–676.

Nicholas, R., J. Hadley, C. Paul, and P. Janes (1994). "Snowboarder's fracture": Fracture of the lateral process of the talus. *Journal of the American Board of Family Practitioners* 7:130–133.

Nicoll, E. A. (1949). Fractures of the dorso-lumbar spine. *Journal of Bone and Joint Surgery [Br]* 31:376–394.

Nikolik, S., J. Micic, T. C. Atanasijevic, V. Djokic, and D. Djonic (2003). Analysis of neck injuries in hanging. *Am J Forensic Med Pathol* 24(2):179–182.

Noe-Nygaard, N. (1977). Butchering and marrow fracturing as a taphonomic factor in archaeological deposits. *Paleobiology* 3:218–237.

Nordqvist, A. and C. Petersson (1994). The incidence of fractures of the clavicle. *Clinical Orthopaedics and Related Research* 300:127–132.

Norfray, J., L. Rogers, and G. Adams (1980). Common calcaneal avulsion fracture. *Am J Roentgenol* 134:119–123.

Norris, T. R. (1992). Fractures of the proximal humerus and dislocations of the shoulder. In *Skeletal Trauma: Fractures, Dislocations, Ligamentous Injuries*, B. D. Browner, J. B. Jupiter, A. M. Levine, and P. G. Trafton (Eds.), pp. 1201–1290. W. B. Saunders, Philadelphia.

Norton, W. L. (1962). Fractures and dislocations of the cervical spine. *Journal of Bone and Joint Surgery [Am]* 44:115–139.

Nusse, G. (2003). Mold making of the skull. *Journal of Forensic Identification* 6:666–689.

Nyqvist, G. W., J. Cavanaugh, S. J. Goldberg, and A. I. King(1986). Facial impact tolerance and response. *Proceedings of the Proceedings of the 30th Stapp Car Crash Conference*. San Diego, CA.

O'Brien, J. J., W. L. Butterfield, and H. R. Gossling (1977). Jefferson fracture with disruption of the transverse ligament. *Clinical Orthopaedics and Related Research* 126: 135–138.

O'Connor, E. and J. Walsham (2009). Review article: Indications for thoracolumbar imaging in blunt trauma patients: A review of current literature. *Emergency Medicine Australasia* 21:94–101.

O'Halloran, R. L. and L. K. Lundy (1987). Age and ossification of the hyoid bone: Forensic implications. *Journal of Forensic Sciences* 32:1655–1659.

O'Neill, B. (1985). The statistics of trauma. In *The Biomechanics of Trauma*, A. M. Nahum and J. Melvin (Eds.), pp. 17–30. Appleton-Century-Crofts, Norwalk, CT.

Oehmichem, M., R. Auer, and H. Konig (2005). *Forensic Neuropathology and Associated Neurology*. Springer, New York.

Ogawa, K. and A. Yashida (1998). Throwing fracture of the humeral shaft: An analysis of 90 patients. *American Journal of Sports Medicine* 26:242.

Ogden, J. A., R. B. Tross, and M. J. Murphy (1980). Fractures of the tibial tuberosity in adolescents. *Journal of Bone and Joint Surgery [Am]* 62:205–215.

Oginni, F. O., V. I. Ugboko, O. Ogundipe, and B. O. Adegbebingbe (2006). Motorcycle-related maxillofacial injuries among Nigerian intracity road users. *Journal of Oral and Maxillofacial Surgery* 64:56–62.

Oh, J., H. Min, T. Park, S. Lee, and S. Kim (2007). Isolated cricoid fracture associated with blunt neck trauma. *Emerg Med J* 24(7):505–506.

Old, J. and M. Calvert (2004). Vertebral compression fractures in the elderly. *Am Family Physician* 69(1):111–116.

Ortner, D. J. and W. G. J. Putschar (1981). *Identification of Pathological Conditions in Human Skeletal Remains*. Smithsonian Contributions to Anthropology Smithsonian Institution Press, Washington, DC.

Outram, A. (2001). A new approach to identifying bone marrow and grease exploitation: Why the indeterminate fragments should not be ignored. *J Archaeological Sci* 28:401–410.

_____ (2002). Bone fracture and within-bone nutrients: An experimentally-based method for investigating levels of marrow extraction. In *Consuming Passions and*

Patterns of Consumption, P. Miracle and N. Milner (Eds.), pp. 51–53. McDonald Institute for Archaeological Research, Cambridge, MA.

Palmer, A. K. (1981). Trapezial ridge fractures. *Journal of Hand Surgery* 6:561–564.

Palmer, I. (1948). Mechanism and treatment of fractures of the calcaneus. *Journal of Bone and Joint Surgery [Am]* 30:2–8.

Palvanen, M., P. Kannus, S. Niemi, and J. Kakkari (2006). Update in the epidemiology of proximal humeral fractures. *Clinical Orthopaedics and Related Research* pp. 442–487.

Pandya, N., K. Baldwin, H. Wolfgruber, C. Christian, D. Drummond, and H. Hosalkar (2009). Child abuse and orthopaedic injury patterns: Analysis at a level 1 pediatric trauma center. *J Pediatric Orthop* 29(6):618–625.

Pankovich, A. M. (1979). Fractures of the fibula at the distal tibiofibular syndesmoses. *Clinical Orthopaedics and Related Research* 143:138–147.

Paparo, G. and H. Siegel (1984). Neck markings and fractures in suicidal hangings *Forensic Sci Int* 24(1):27–35.

Papp, S. (2010). Carpal bone fractures. *Hand Clinics* 26:119–127.

Paster, S. B., F. W. Van Houten, and D. F. Adams (1974). Percutaneous balloon catherization: A technique for the control of arterial hemorrhage caused by pelvic trauma. *JAMA* 230:573.

Patonay, B. C. and W. R. Oliver (2010). Can birth trauma be confused for abuse? *Journal of Forensic Sciences* 55(4):1123–1125.

Patrick, L., D. Van Kirk, and G. Nyquist (1968). *Vehicle accelerator crash simulator: Proceedings of the 12th Stapp Car Crash Conference.* Society of Automotive Engineers, Warrendale, PA.

Pauweis, F. (1935). *De Schenkenholsbruck, em mechanisches problem Grundlagen des Heilungsvorganges Prognose und kausale Therapie. Zeitschrift fur Orthopadische Chirurgie Suppl,* 63:54–78.

Pavel, A., J. M. Pitman, E. M. Lance, and P. A. Wade (1965). The posterior Monteggia fracture: A clinical study. *Journal of Trauma* 5:185–199.

Pavlov, H. and R. H. Freiberger (1978). Fractures and dislocations about the shoulder. *Seminars in Roentgenology* 13:85–96.

Paza, A., A. Abuabara, and L. Passeri (2008). Analysis of 115 mandibular angle fractures. *Journal of Oral and Maxillofacial Surgery* 66:73–76.

Pedram H., Z. M. Reza, R. M. Reza, A. R. Vaccaro, and R. M. Vafa (2010). Spinal fractures resulting from traumatic injuries. *Chinese Journal of Traumatology* 13(1):3–9.

Peek, G. J. and R. K. Firmin (1995). Isolated sternal fracture: An audit of 10 years' experience. *Injury* 26:385–388.

Peh, W. C. G. and N. S. Evans (1993). Pelvic insufficiency fractures in the elderly. *Annals of the Academy of Medicine* 22:818–822.

Pellegrini, V. D., Jr. (1988). Fractures at the base of the thumb. *Hand Clinics of North America* 4:87–102.

Pennel, G. F. and G. Sutherland (1961). Fractures of the pelvis. In *Americann Academy of Orthopedic Surgeons Film Library.*

Pennel, G. F., G. A. McDonald, and C. A. Dale (1966). Stress studies of the lumbar spine. *Journal of Bone and Joint Surgery [Br]* 46:786.

Penny, J. N. and L. A. Davis (1980). Fractures and fracture-dislocations of the neck of the talus. *Journal of Trauma* 20:1029–1037.

Penrose, J. H. (1951). The Monteggia fracture with posterior dislocation of the radial head. *Journal of Bone and Joint Surgery [Br]* 633:65–73.

Perciaccante, V., H. Ochs, and T. Dotson (1999). Head, neck and facial injuries as markers for domestic violence in women. *J of Oral and Maxillofacial Surgery* 57:760–763.

Perdikis, G., T. Schmitt, D. Chait, and A. Richards (2000). Blunt laryngeal fracture: Another airbag injury. *Journal of Trauma* 48:544–546.

Perkins, S., S. Dayan, E. Sklarew, M. Hamilton, and G. Bussell (2000). The incidence of sports-related facial trauma in children. *Ear Nose Throat J* 79(8):632–634, 636, 638.

Perren, S. M. (2002). Evolution of the internal fixation of long bone fractures: The scientific basis of biological internal fixation choosing a new balance between stability and biology. *Journal of Bone and Joint Surgery [Br]* 84-B:1093–1110.

Perry, J. F. (1980). Pelvic open fractures. *Clinical Orthopaedics* 151:41–45.

Peterson, L., B. Romanus, and E. Dahlberg (1976). Fracture of the collum tali: An experimental study. *Journal of Biomechanics* 9(4):277–279.

Petridou, E., B. Browne, E. Lichter, X. Dedoukou, D. Alexe, and N. Dessypris (2002). What distinguishes unintentional injuries from injuries due to intimate partner violence: A study in a Greek ambulatory care settings. *Injury Prevention* 8:197–201.

Petrucelli, E. (1984). Limbs: Anatomy, types of injuries and future priorities In *The Biomechanics of Impact Trauma*, B. Aldman and A. Chapon (Eds.), pp. 311–326. Elsevier Science, Amsterdam.

Pickering, R. B. (2009). *The Use of Forensic Anthropology* (2nd ed.). CRC Press, Boca Raton, FL.

Pickering, T., M. Dominguez-Rodrigo, C. Egeland, and C. Brain (2005). The contribution of limb bone fracture patterns to reconstructing early hominid behavior at Swartkrans cave (South Africa): Archaeological application of a new analytical method. *International J of Osteoarchaeology* 15(4):247–260.

Pierce, M., G. Bertocci, E. Vogeley, and M. Moreland (2004). Evaluating long bone fractures in children: A biomechanical approach with illustrative cases. *Child Abuse and Neglect* 28:505–524.

Pipkin, G. (1957). Treatment of grade IV fracture-dislocation of the hip. *Journal of Bone and Joint Surgery [Am]* 39:1027–1042.

Plezbert, J. A. and A. T. Oestreich (1994). Fracture of a lamina in the cervical spine. *Journal of Manipulation and Physiological Therapeutics* 17:552–557.

Plueckhahn, V. D. and S. M. Cordner (1991). *Ethics, Legal Medicine and Forensic Pathology*. Melbourne University Press, Melbourne.

Pollanen, M. and D. A. Chiasson (1996). Fracture of the hyoid bone in strangulation: Comparison of fractured and unfractured hyoids from victims of strangulation. *Journal of Forensic Sciences* 41:110–113.

Pollanen, M. and D. H. Ubelaker (1997). Forensic significance of the polymorphism of hyoid bone shape. *Journal of Forensic Sciences* 42:890–892.

Poole, G. V., Jr. and R. T. Myers (1981). Morbidity and mortality rates in major blunt trauma to the upper chest. *Annals of Surgery* 193:70–75.

Poole, G. V., E. F. Ward, J. A. Griswold, F. F. Muakkassa, and H. S. H. Hau (1992). Complications of pelvic fractures from blunt trauma. *The American Surgeon* 58:225–231.

Pope, E. (2012 Fatal fire death course notes. San Luis Obispo Fire Department, San Luis Obispo, CA.

Pope, E., H. Davis, and A. Shidner (2010). Differentiating peri- and postmortem fractures in burned postcranial remains. *Proceedings of the American Academy of Forensic Sciences* 16:352.

Porta, D. (2005). Biomechanics of impact injury. In *Forensic Medicine of the Lower Extremity*, J. Rich, D. Dean, and R. Powers (Eds.), pp. 279–310. Humana Press, Ottowa.

Porta, D., S. Frick, T. Kress, and P. Fuller (1999). Transverse, oblique, and wedge fracture patterns: Variation on the bending theme. *Clinical Anatomy* 12:208.

Postacchini, F., S. Gumina, P. De Santis, and F. Alba (2002). Epidemiology of clavicle fractures. *Journal of Shoulder and Elbow Surgery* 16:452–456.

Poston, H. (1921–1922). Traction fracture of the lesser trochanter of the femur. *British Journal of Surgery* 9:256–258.

Pratt, H., E. Davies, and L. King (2008). Traumatic injuries of the C1/C2 complex: Computed tomographic imaging appearances. *Current Problems in Diagnostic Radiology* 37:26–38.

Pull ter Gunne, A. F., R. L. Skolasky, and D. B. Cohen (2010). Fracture characteristics predict patient mortality after blunt force cervical trauma. *Eur J Emerg Med* 17(2):107–109; discussion 126–127.

Purkiss, S. and T. Graham (1993). Sternal fractures. *Br J Hosp Med* 50(2-3):107–112.

Purkiss, S. F. and T. R. Graham (1993). Sternal fractures. *British Journal of Hospital Medicine* 50:108–112.

Putnam, M. D. and M. Fischer (1993). Forearm fractures. In *Fractures and Dislocations*, R. B. Gustilo, R. F. Kyle, and D. C. Templeman (Eds.), pp. 499–552. Mosby, St. Louis, MO.

Putnam, M. D. (1993). Fractures and dislocations of the carpus including the distal radius. In *Fractures and Dislocations*, R. B. Gustilo, R. F. Kyle, and D. C. Templeman (Eds.), pp. 553–610. Mosby, St. Louis, MO.

Puzzanchera, C., G. Chamberlin, and W. Kang (2012). Easy Access to the FBI's Supplementary Homicide Reports: 1980–2010. http://www.ojjdp.gov/ojstatbb/ezashr/asp/vic_display.asp?row_var=v05. Downloaded June, 2012.

Quaday, K. A. (1995). Morbidity and mortality of rib fractures. *Journal of Trauma* 39(617).

Raasch, F. D., Jr. (1985). Forensic analysis of trauma. In *The Biomechanics of Impact Trauma*, B. Aldman and A. Chapon (Eds.), pp. 167–179. Elsevier Science, Amsterdam.

Rabl, W., C. Haid, and M. Krismer (1996). Biomechanical properties of the human tibia: Fracture benavior and morphology. *Forensic Science International* 83(1):39.

Raffa, J. and N. M. Christensen (1976). Compound fractures of the pelvis. *American Journal of Surgery* 132:282–286.

Ragnarsson, B. and B. Jacobsson (1992). Epidemiology of pelvic fractures in a Swedish county. *Acta Orthopaedica Scandinavica* 63:297–300.

Rand, M. (1997). Violence-related injuries treated in the emergency department. U.S. Department of Justice, Office of Justice Programs, Washington, D.C.

Rang, M. (1974). *Children's Fractures.* J. B. Lippencott, Philadelphia.

Ranjith, R., H. Mullett, and T. Burke (2002). Hangman's fracture caused by suspected child abuse: A case report. *J Pediatric Orthop* 11(4):329–348.

Rankin, L. M. (1937). Fractures of the pelvis. *Annals of Surgery* 106:266–277.

Rash, W. (2012). Hyoid/hyoid fracture. *J Emergency Nursing* 37(2):182–183.

Rawes, M. L., J. Roberts, and J. J. Dias (1995). Bilateral fibula head fractures complicating an epileptic seizure. *Injury* 26:562.

Raymond, D., C. Van Ee, G. Crawford, and C. Bir (2009). Tolerance of the skull to blunt ballistic temporo-parietal impact. *Journal of Biomechanics* 42(15):2479–2485.

Recinos, G., K. Inaba, J. Dubose, G. Barmparas, P. G. Teixeira, P. Talving, D. Plurad, D. Green, and D. Demetriades (2009). Epidemiology of sternal fractures. *American Surgery* 75(5):401–404.

Recker, R. and R. Heaney (1993). Peak bone mineral density in young women. *JAMA* 270(24):2926–2927.

Recker, R. R. (1993). Architecture and vertebral fracture. *Calcified Tissue International,* 53(Suppl):S139–142.

Reckling, F. W. (1982). Unstable fracture dislocations of the forearm. *Archives of Surgery* 96:99–1007.

Reed, M. H. (1976). Pelvic fractures in children. *Journal of the Canadian Association of Radiology* 27:255–261.

Reehal, P. (2010). Facial injury in sport. *Curr Sports Med Rep* 9:27.

Regan, W. and B. Morrey (1989). Fractures of the coronoid process of the ulna. *Journal of Bone and Joint Surgery [Am]* 71:1348–1354.

Reibel, D. B. and P. A. Wade (1962). Fractures of the tibial plateau. *Journal of Trauma* 2:337–352.

Reichard, R. (2008). Birth injury of the cranium and central nervous system. *Brain Pathology* 16:565–570.

Reid, M. R. (1997). *Violence-Related Injuries Treated in Hospital Emergency Departments.* Bureau of Justice Statistics.

Reilly, D. T. and A. H. Burstein (1974). The mechanical properties of cortical bone. *Journal of Bone and Joint Surgery [Am]* 56:1001–1022.

Rennison, C. M. and S. Welchans (2000). *Intimate partner violence.* Office of Justice Programs, NCJ 178247.

Restifo, K. M. and G. D. Kelen (1993). Case report: Sternal fracture from a seatbelt. *Journal of Emergency Medicine* 12:321–323.

Rewers, A., H. Hedegaard, D. Lezotte, K. Meng, K. Battan, K. Emery, and R. Hamman (2005). Childhood femur fractures, associated injuries, and sociodemographic risk fractures: A population-based study. *Pediatrics* 115(5):543–552.

Rex, C. and P. Kay (2000). Features of femoral fractures in non-accidental injury. *Journal of Pediatric Orthopaedics* 20(3):411–413.

Rezende, F. M. do C, C. Gaujac, A. C. Rocha, and M. P. S. de M Peres (2007). A prospective study of dentoalveolar trama at the *Hospital das Clinicas,* Sao Paulo University Medical School. *Clinics* 62(2):133–138.

Rhee, P., E. Kuncir, L. Johnson, C. Brown, G. Velmahos, M. Martin, D. Wang, A. Salim, J. Doucet, S. Kennedy, and D. Demetriades (2006). Cervical spine injury is highly dependent on the mechanism of injury following blunt and penetrating assault. *Journal of Trauma* 61:1166–1170.

Rhine, J. S. (1998). *Bone Voyage: A Journey in Forensic Anthropology.* University of New Mexico Press, Albuquerque, NM.

Richards, D. and J. Carroll (2012). Relationship between types of head injury and age of pedestrian. *Accident Analysis and Prevention* 47:16–23.

Richardson, J. D., J. Harty, M. Amin, and L. M. Flint (1982). Open pelvic fractures. *Journal of Trauma* 22:533–538.

Richardson, J. D., R. McElvein, and J. K. Trinkle (1975). First rib fracture: A hallmark of severe trauma. *Annals of Surgery* 181(3):251–254.

Richli, W. R. and D. I. Rosenthal (1984). Avulsion fracture of the fifth metatarsal: Experimental study of pathomechanics. *American Journal of Radiology* 143:889–891.

Richter, D., M. Hahn, P. Ostermann, A. Ekkernkamp, and G. Muhr (1996). Vertical deceleration injuries: A comparative studies of the injury patterns of 101 patients after accidental and intentional high falls. *Injury* 27(9):655–659.

Rider, D. L. (1937). Fractures of the metacarpals, metatarsals and phalanges. *American Journal of Surgery* 38:549–559.

Rieth, P. L. (1948). Fractures of the radial head. *South Surg* 14:154–159.

Riggs, B. L. and L. J. Melton III (1988). Osteoporosis and age-related fracture syndromes. *Ciba Foundation Symposium* 134:129–142.

_____ (1995). The worldwide problem of osteoporosis: Insights afforded by epidemiology. *Bone* 17:505S–511S.

Riseborough, E. J. and E. L. Radin (1969). Intracondylar T-fractures of the humerus in the adult. *Journal of Bone and Joint Surgery [Am]* 51:130–141.

Rivara, F. P., T. D. Koepsell, and D. C. Grossman, et al. (2000). Effectiveness of automatic shoulder belt systems in motor vehicle crashes. *JAMA* 283:2826.

Riviello, R. (2010). *Manual of Forensic Emergency: A Guide for Clinicians.* Jones and Bartlett.

Roberts, S. W., C. Hernandez, M. C. Maberry, M. D. Adams, K. J. Leveno, and G. D. Wendel (1995). Obstetric clavicular fracture: The enigma of normal birth. *Obstetrics and Gynecology* 86:978–981.

Robertson, A., T. Branfoot, I. F. Barlow, and P. V. Giannoudis (2002). Spinal injury patterns resulting from car and motorcycle accidents. *Spine* 27(24):2825–2830.

Robinson, C. M. (1998). Fractures of the clavicle in the adult: Epidemiology and classification. *J Bone and Joint Surgery [Br]* 80(3):476–484.

Rockswold, G. L. (1996). Head injury. In *Emergency Medicine: A Comprehensive Study Guide* (4th ed.), J. Tintinalli (Ed.). McGraw-Hill, New York.

Rockwood, C. A. and D. P. Green (2009). *Rockwood & Green's Fractures in Adults* (7th ed.). Wolters/Kluwer/Lippincott Williams and Wilkins, Philadelphia.

Rockwood, C. A. and F. A. Matson (1990). *The Shoulder.* W. B. Saunders, Philadelphia.

Rodge, S., H. Hougen, and K. Poulsen (2003). Homicide by blunt force in 2 Scandinavian capitals. *American Journal of Forensic Medicine and Pathology* 24:288–291.

Rodgers, J. A., T. C. Fitzgibbons, and L. A. Crosby (1995). Intra-articular fracture of the calcaneus. *Nebraska Medical Journal* 80:140–148.

Roesen, H. M. and I. O. Kanat (1993). Anterior process fracture of the calcaneus. *The Journal of Foot and Ankle Surgery* 32:424–429.

Rogers, L. F., S. Malave, Jr, H. White, and M. O. Tachdijian (1978). Plastic bowing, torus and greenstick supracondylar fractures of the humerus: Radiographic clues to obscure fractures of the elbow in children. *Radiology* 128:145–150.

Rogers, L. F. (1992). *Radiology of Skeletal Trauma* (2nd ed.). Churchill Livingstone, New York.

Ross, A. and S. Abel (2011). *The Juvenile Skeleton in Forensic Abuse Investigations.* Humana Press, Totowa, NJ.

Ross, A. H., R. L. Jantz, and W. F. McCormick (1998). Cranial thickness in American females and males. *Journal of Forensic Sciences* 43(2):267–272.

Rothenberger, D. A., R. Velasco, R. Strate, R. P. Fischer, and J. F. Perry (1978). Open pelvic fracture: A lethal injury. *Journal of Trauma* 18:184–187.

Roudsari, B., C. Mock, R. Kaufman, D. Grossman, B. Henary, and J. Crandall (2004). Pedestrian crashes: Higher injury severity and mortality rate for light truck vehicles compared with passenger vehicles. *Injury Prevention* 10:154–158.

Rowe, A., M. S. Socher, K. S. Staples, W. L. Wahl, and S. C. Wang (2004). Pelvic ring fractures: Implications of vehicle design, crash type, and occupant characteristics. *Surgery* 136:842–847.

Rowe, C. R., H. T. Sakellarides, P. A. Freeman, and C. Sorbie (1963). Fractures of the os calcis: A long-term follow-up study of 146 patients. *Journal of the American Medical Association* 184:920–923.

Rowe, C. R. (1968). An atlas of anatomy and treatment of midclavicular fractures. *Clinical Orthopaedics* 58:29–42.

Roy-Camile, R., G. Saillant, G. Gagna, et al. (1985). Transverse fracture of the upper sacrum: Suicidal jumper's fracture. *Spine* 10:838–845.

Rubin, A. (1964). Birth injuries: Incidence, mechanisms and end results. *Obstetrics and Gynecology* 23:218–221.

Ruby, L. (1992). Fractures and dislocation of the carpus. In *Skeletal Trauma: Fractures, Dislocations, Ligamentous Injuries,* B. D. Browner, J. B. Jupiter, A. M. Levine, and P. G. Trafton (Eds.), pp. 1025–1062. W. B. Saunders, Philadelphia.

Rüedi, T. P. and M. Allgower (1969). Fractures of the lower end of the tibia into the ankle-joint. *Injury* 1:92.

Runner, M., M. Yoshihama, and S. Novick (2009). *Intimate Partner Violence in Immigrant and Refugee Communities: Challenges, Promising Practices and Recommendations.* Bureau of Justice Statistics.

Russel, T. A. and J. C. Taylor (1992). Subtrochanteric fractures of the femur. In *Skeletal Trauma: Fractures, Dislocations, Ligametous Injuries,* B. D. Browner, J. B. Jupiter, A. M. Levine, and P. G. Trafton (Eds.), pp. 1485–1524. W. B. Saunders, Philadelphia.

Rutherford, W. H. (1985). The medical effects of seat-belt legislation in the United Kingdom: A critical review of the findings. *Archives of Emergency Medicine* 2:221–223.

Ryan, M. D. and J. J. Henderson (1992). The epidemiology of fractures and fracture-dislocations of the cervical spine. *Injury* 23:38–40.

Saadet, S., N. Rashidi-Ranjbar, M. Rasouli, and V. Rahimi-Movaghar (2011). Pattern of skull fracture in Iran: Report of the Iran National Trauma Project. *Ulus Travma Acil Cerrahi Derg* 17(2):149–151.

Sadek-Kooros, H. (1972). Primitive bone fracturing: a method of research. *Amer Antiquity* 37(3):369–382.

Safdar, N. and J. G. Meechan (1995). Relationship between fractures of the mandibular angle and the presence and state of eruption of the lower third molar. *Oral Surgery, Oral Medicine, Oral Pathology, Oral Radiology and Endodontics* 79:680–684.

Sakellaridis, T., A. Stamatelopoulos, E. Andrianopoulos, and P. Kormas (2004). Isolated first rib fracture in athletes. *British Journal of Sports Medicine* 38:e5–e7.

Saks, M. and D. Faigman (2005). Expert evidence after Daubert. *Annual Review of Law and Social Science* 1:105–130.

Salter, R. and W. Harris (1963). Injuries involving the epiphyseal plate. *J Bone Joint Surg [Am]* 45:587–622.

Salter, R. B. and W. R. Harris (1963). Injuries involving the epiphyseal plate. *Journal of Bone and Joint Surgery [Am]* 45:587–622.

Sanders, R. (1992). Patella fractures and extensor mechanism injuries. In *Skeletal Trauma: Fractures, Dislocations, Ligamentous Injuries*, B. D. Browner, J. B. Jupiter, A. M. Levine, and P. G. Trafton (Eds.), pp. 1685–1716. W. B. Saunders, Philadelphia.

Sanders, R., P. Fortin, T. DiPasquale, and A. Walling (1993). Operative treatment in 120 displaced intra-articular calcaneal fractures. Results using prognostic computed tomography scan classification. *Clinical Orthopaedics and Related Research* 290:87–95.

Sangeorzan, B. J., S. K. Benirschke, V. Moshe, K. A. Mayo, and S. T. Hansen (1989). Displaced intra-articular fractures of the tarsal navicular. *Journal of Bone and Joint Surgery [Am]* 71:1504–1510.

Sangeorzan, B. J. (1991). Midfoot fractures. Paper presented at the American Academy of Orthopaedic Surgeons Comprehensive Foot and Ankle Course, San Francisco.

Sasso, R. C. (2001). C2 dens fractures: Treatment options. *Journal of Spinal Disorders* 14(5):455–463.

Sauer, N. (1998). The timing of injuries and manner of death: Distinguishing among antemortem, perimortem, and postmortem trauma. In *Forensic Osteology: Advances in the Identification of Human Remains* (2nd ed.), K. Reichs (Ed.), pp. 321–332. Charles C Thomas, Springfield, IL.

Sawazaki, R., S. Lima Jr., L. Asprino, R. Moreira, and M. deMoraes (2010). Incidence and patterns of mandibular condyle fractures. *J Oral and Maxillofac Surg* 68(6):1252–1259.

Sawyer J. R., M. Beebe, A. T. Creek, M. Yantis, D. K. Kelly, and W. C. Warner (2012). Age-related patterns of spine injury in children involved in all-terrain vehicle accidents. *Journal of Pediatric Orthopaedics* 32:435–439.

Scalea, T., A. Goldstein, T. Phillips, S. J. A. Sclafani, T. Panetta, J. McAuley, and G. Shaftan (1986). An analysis of 161 falls from a height: the "jumper syndrome." *Journal of Trauma* 26:706–712.

Scharplatz, D. and M. Allgower (1976). Fracture dislocation of the elbow. *Injury* 7:143–159.

Schatzker, J. and M. Tile (1987). *The Rationale of Operative Fracture Care*. Springer-Verlag, New York.

Schatzker, J. (1987a). Fractures of the distal end of the humerus. In *The Rationale of Operative Fracture Care*, J. Schatzker and M. Tile (Eds.), pp. 71–87. Springer-Verlag, Berlin.

_____ (1987b). Fractures of the olecranon. In *The Rationale of Operative Fracture Care*, J. Schatzker and M. Tile (Eds.), pp. 89–95. Springer-Verlag, Berlin.

_____ (1987c). Subtrochanteric fractures of the femur. In *The Rationale of Operative Fracture Care*, J. Schatzker and M. Tile (Eds.), pp. 217–234. Springer-Verlag, Berlin.

_____ (1987d). Supracondylar fractures of the femur. In *The Rationale of Operative Fracture Care*, J. Schatzker and M. Tile (Eds.), pp. 255–273. Springer-Verlag, Berlin.

_____ (1987e). Fractures of the tibial plateau. In *The Rationale of Operative Fracture Care*, J. Schatzker and M. Tile (Eds.), pp. 279–295 Springer-Verlag, Berlin.

Schatzker, J. (1992). Tibial plateau fractures. In *Skeletal Trauma: Fractures, Dislocations, Ligamentous Injuries*, B. D. Browner, J. B. Jupiter, A. M. Levine, and P. G. Trafton (Eds.), pp. 1745–1769 W. B. Saunders, Philadelphia.

Schippers, J., P. Konings, W. Hassler, and B. Sommer (1995). Typical and atypical fractures of the odontoid process in young children. *Acta Neurochirurgica* 138:524–530.

Schmidek, H. H., D. A. Smith, and T. K. Kristiansen (1984). Sacral fractures. *Neurosurgery* 15:735–746.

Schmidt, C. and S. Symes (2008). *The Analysis of Burned Human Remains.* Elsevier Ltd.

Schmidt, C. W. (2008). Forensic dental anthropology: issues and guidelines. In *Technique and Application in Dental Anthropology*, J. D. Irish and G. C. Nelson (Eds.), pp. 266–292. Cambridge University Press, Cambridge, MA.

Schneider, D. and A. Nahum (1972). Impact studies of facial bones and skull. In *Proceedings of the 16th Stapp Car Crash Conference*, pp. 186–203, Detroit, MI.

Schneider, R. C. and E. A. Kahn (1956). Chronic neurological sequelae of acute trauma to the spine and spinal cord. *Journal of Bone and Joint Surgery* 38:985–997.

Schneider, R. C. (1985). Biomechanics of facial bone injury: Experimental aspects. In *The Biomechanics of Trauma*, A. M. Nahum and J. Melvin (Eds.), pp. 281–299. Appleton-Century-Crofts, Norwalk, CT.

Schweich, P. and G. Fleisher (1985). Rib fractures in children. *Pediatric Emergency Care* 1(4):187–189.

Schwend, R., C. Werth, and A. Johnston (2000). Femur shaft fractures in toddlers and young children: Rarely from child abuse. *J Pediatric Orthop* 20(4):475–481.

Schwobel, M. G. (1987). Avulsion fractures of tibial tubercle: A typical sports injury in adolescents. *Zeitschrift fur Kinderchirurgie* 42:181–183.

Seelig, M. and L. F. Marshall (1985). Biomechanics of head injury: Clinical aspects. In *Biomechanics of Trauma*, A. M. Nahum and J. Melvin (Eds.), pp. 225–243. Appleton-Century-Crofts, Norwalk, CT.

Seeman, W. R., G. Siebler, and H. G. Rupp (1986). A new classification of proximal humeral fractures. *European Journal of Radiology* 6:163–167.

Seinsheimer, F. (1978). Subtrochanteric fractures of the femur. *Journal of Bone and Joint Surgery [Am]* 60:300–306.

_____ (1980). Fractures of the distal femur. *Clinical Orthopaedics and Related Research* 153:169–179.

Seitz, W. H. and R. F. Papandrea (2002). Fractures and dislocations of the wrist. In *Rockwood and Green's Fracutes in Adults* (5th ed.), H. J. Bucholz (Ed.). Lippincott, Williams and Wilkins, Philadelphia.

Shackleford, S., L. Nguyen, T. Noguchi, L. Stathyavagiswaran, K. Inaba, and D. Demetriades (2011). Fatalaties of the 2008 Los Angeles train crash: Autopsy findings. *Am J Disaster Med* 6(2):127–131.

Shahim, F., P. Cameron, J. J. McNeil (2006). Maxillofacial trauma in major trauma patients. *Australian Dental Journal* 51(3):225–230.

Shapiro, R., A. S. Youngberg, and S. L. Rothman (1973). The differential diagnosis of traumatic lesions of the occipito-axial segment. *Radiologic Clinics of North America* 11:505–526.

Shaw, B., M. Kelleen, A. Shaw, W. Oppenheim, and M. Myracle (1997). Humeral shaft fractures in young children: Accident or abuse? *Journal of Pediatric Orthopaedics* 17(3):293–297.

Shaw, J. L. (1971). Bilateral posterior fracture dislocation of the shoulder and other trauma caused by convulsive seizures. *Journal of Bone and Joint Surgery [Am]* 53:1437–1440.

Shelton, W. R. and S. T. Canale (1979). Fractures of the tibia through the proximal tibial epiphyseal cartilage. *Journal of Bone and Joint Surgery [Am]* 61:167–173.

Shepherd, F. J. (1882). A hitherto undescribed fracture of the astragulus. *Journal de Anatomie et de la Physiologie* 18:79–81.

Sheridan, D. and K. Nash (2007). Acute injury patterns of intimate partner violence victims. *Trauma Violence* 8:281.

Sherk, H. H. and J. T. Nicholson (1970). Fractures of the atlas. *Journal of Bone and Joint Surgery [Am]* 52:1017–1024.

Sherr-Lurie, N., G. M. Bialik, A. Ganel, A. Schindler, and U. Givon (2011). Fractures of the humerus in the neonatal period. *Israel Medical Association Journal* 13:363–365.

Shkrum, M. J., R. N. Green, and E. S. Nowak (1989). Upper cervical trauma in motor vehicle collisions. *Journal of Forensic Sciences* 34:381–390.

Shrader, M. W. (2007). Proximal humerus and humeral shaft fractures in children. *Hand Clinics* 23:431.

———— (2008). Pediatric supracondylar fractures and pediatric physeal elbow fractures. *Orthopaedic Clinics of North America* 39:163–171.

Shults, R., S. Wiles, M. Vajani, and J. Helmkamp (2005). All-terrain vehicle-related nonfatal injuries among young riders: United States, 2001–2003. *Pediatrics* 116(5): e608–e612.

Siebenrock, K. A. and C. Gerber (1993). The reproducability of classification of fractures of the proximal end of the humerus. *Journal of Bone and Joint Surgery [Am]* 75:1751–1755.

Siegal, D. B. (1995). The boxer's fracture: Angulated metacarpal neck fractures of the little finger. *Journal of the Southern Orthopaedic Association* 4:32–37.

Sieradzki, J. and J. Sarwark (2008). Thoracolumbar fracture-dislocation in child abuse: Case report, closed-reduction technique and review of the literature. *Pediatric Neurosurgery* 44:253–257.

Sigurdardottir, K., S. Haldorsson, and J. Robertsson (2011). Epidemiology and treatment of distal radius fractures in Raykjavik Icelandic study from 1985. *Acta Orthopaedica* 82:494–498.

Silla, A. and J. Luoma (2012). Main characteristics of train-pedestrian fatalities on Finnish railroads. *Accident Analysis and Prevention* 45:61–66.

Silvennoinen, U., T. Ilzyka, C. Lindqvist, K. Oikarinen (1992). Different patterns of condylar fractures: An analysis of 382 patients in a 3-year period. *Journal of Oral and Maxillofacial Surgery* 50:1032–1037.

Simmonds, S. L., M. F. Whelan, and J. Basseches (2011). Nonsurgical pneumoperitoneum in a dog secondary to blunt force trauma to the chest. *J Vet Emerg Crit Care (San Antonio)* 21(5):552–557.

Simoni, P., R. Ostendorf, and A. J. Cox (2003). Effect of air bags and restraining devices on the pattern of facial fractures in motor vehicle crashes. *Archives of Facial Plastic Surgery* 5:113–115.

Simonsen, J. (1983). Injuries sustained from high-velocity impact with water after jumps from high bridges. *American Journal of Forensic Medicine and Pathology* 4:139–142.

Simonson, C., P. Barlow, N. Dehennin, M. Sphel, M. Toppet, D. Murillo, and S. Rozenberg (2007). Neonatal complications of vacuum-assisted delivery. *Obstetrics and Gynecology* 109(3):626–633.

Simpson, K. and B. Knight (1985). *Forensic Medicine* (9th ed.). Edward Arnold, Baltimore.

Siram, S. M., V. Sonalke, O. B. Bolorunduro, W. R. Greene, S. Z. Geerald, D. C. Chang, E. E. Cornwell, and T. A. Oyetunji (2011). Does the pattern of injury in elderly pedestrian trauma mirror that of the younger pedestrian? *Journal of Surgical Research* 167:14–18.

Sitter, P. (2000). Dress for success: USPA's 1999 fatality summary. *Parachutist* 41:30–37.

Skedros, J. G. (2012). Interpreting load history in limb-bone biomechanical foundations. In *Bone Histology: An Anthropological Perspective*, C. Crowder and S. Stout (Eds.), pp. 153–220. CRC Press, Boca Raton, FL.

Skellern, C., D. Wood, A. Murphy, and M. Crawford (2000). Non-accidental fractures in infants: Risk of further abuse. *J Pediatr Child Health* 36:590–592.

Skinner, M. and G. S. Anderson (1991). Individualization and enamel histology: A case report in forensic anthropology. *Journal of Forensic Sciences* 34:939–948.

Slauterbeck, J. R., M. S. Shapiro, S. Liu, and G. A. M. Finerman (1995). Traumatic fibular shaft fractures in athletes. *American Journal of Sports Medicine* 23:751–754.

Smeets, A., S. Robben, and M. Meradji (1990). Sonographically detected costochondral dislocation in an abused child: A new sonographic sign to the radiological spectrum of child abuse. *Pediatric Radiology* 20:566–567.

Smith, D. K. and P. M. Murray (1996). Avulsion fractures of the volar aspect of triquetral bone of the wrist: A subtle sign of carpal ligament injury. *American Journal of Roentgenology* 166:609–614.

Smith, E. and D. Farole (2009). *Profile of Intimate Partner Violence Cases in Large Urban Counties.* Bureau of Justice Statistics.

Smith, M. D., J. D. Burrington, A. D. Woolf (1975). Injuries in children sustained in free falls: an analysis of 66 cases. *Journal of Trauma* 15:987–991.

Sneppen, O., S. B. Christensen, O. Krogsoe, and J. Lorentzen (1977). Fracture of the body of the talus. *Acta Orthopaedica Scandinavica* 48:317–324.

Snyder, R. E., S. V. Hanagud, A. M. Jones, T. Grubbe, and P. McFeeley (1984). Forensic biomedical and engineering investigations of fatal trauma attributed to seat failure and rotational acceleration in a light aircraft crash. In *Human Identification: Case Studies in Forensic Anthropology*, T. A. Rathbun and J. E. Buikstra (Eds.), pp. 185–207. Charles C Thomas, Springfield, IL.

Sojat, A., T. Meisami, G. Sandor, and C. Clokie (2001). Epidemiology of mandibular fractures treated at the Toronto General Hospital: A review of 246 cases. *J Can Dent Assoc* 67(11):640–644.

Solan, M., R. Rees, and K. Daly (2002). Current management of torus fractures of the distal radius. *International Journal of the Care of the Injured* 33:503–506.

Sonoda, T. (1962). Studies on the strength for compression, tension, and torsion of the vertebral column. *Journal of the Kyoto Prefecture Medical University* 71:659–662.

Spencer, D. (1981). Upper cervical injuries in infants. *Journal of Forensic Science Society* 21:145.

Sperry, K. and R. Pfalzgraf (1990). Inadvertant clavicular fractures caused by the "chiropractic" manipulations of an infant: An unusual form of pseudoabuse. *Journal of Forensic Sciences* 35:1211–1216.

Spevak, M., P. Kleinman, P. Belanger, C. Primak, and J. Richmond (1994). Cardiopulmonary resuscitation and rib fractures in infants: A postmortem radiologic-pathologic study. *JAMA* 272(8):617–618.

Spiegel, P. G., J. W. Maat, D. R. Cooperman, and G. S. Laros (1984). Triplane fractures of the distal tibial epiphysis. *Clinical Orthopaedics and Related Research* 188: 74–89.

Spinas, E. and M. Altana (2002). A new classification for crown fractures of teeth. *Journal of Clinical Pediatric Dentistry* 26(3):225–231.

Spitz, W. (Ed.) (2005). *Spitz and Fisher's Medicolegal Investigation of Death: Guidelines for the Application of Pathology to Crime Investigation* (4th ed). Charles C Thomas, Springfield, IL.

Spitz, W. and R. Fisher (1980). *Medicolegal Investigation of Death: Guidelines for the Application of Pathology to Crime Investigation.* Charles C Thomas, Springfield, IL.

Sponseller, P. and C. Stanitski (2001). Fractures and dislocation. In *Rockwood and Wilkin's Fractures in Children,* B. Beaty and .J Kasser (Eds.), p. 981. Lippincott Williams and Wilkins, Philadelphia.

Stacey D. H., J. F. Doyle, and K. A. Gutowski (2008). Safety device use affects the incidence patterns of facial trauma in motor vehicle collisions: An analysis of the national trauma database from 2000 to 2004. *Plastic and Reconstructive Surgery Journal* 121:2057–2064.

Stanciu, C. and A. Dumont (1994). Changing patterns of scaphoid fractures in adolescents. *Canadian Journal of Surgery* 37:214–216.

Standring, S. (2008). *Gray's Anatomy: The Anatomical Basis of Clinical Practice* (40th ed.). Elsevier.

Stanitski, C. L. (1982). Low back pain in young athletes. *Physician and Sports Medicine* 10:77-83, 87–91.

Stanley, D., E. A. Trowbridge, and S. H. Norris (1988). The mechanisms of clavicular fracture: A clinical and biomechanical analysis. *Journal of Bone and Joint Surgery [Br]* 70:461–464.

Stauffer, E. D., H. Kaufer, and T. F. Kling (1984). Fractures and dislocations of the spine. In *Fractures in Adults,* C. A. Rockwood and D. P. Green (Eds.), pp. 987–1092. J. B. Lippincort, Philadelphia.

Stawicki, S., V. Gracias, S. Schrag, N. Martin, A. Dean, and B. Hoey (2008). The dead continue to teach the living: Examining the role of computed tomography and magnetic resonance imaging in the setting of postmortem examinations. *J Surg Educ* 65(3):200–205.

Stephens, N. G., A. S. Morgan, P. Corvo, and B. A. Bernstein (1995). Significance of scapular fracture in the blunt-trauma patient. *Annals of Emergency Medicine* 26:439–442.

Stewart, I. M. (1960). Jones fracture: Fracture of the base of the fifth metatarsal distal to the tuberosity. *Clinical Orthopaedics* 16:190–198.

Stewart, M. J. and L. W. Milford (1954). Fracture-dislocation of the hip. *Journal of Bone and Joint Surgery [Am]* 36:315–342.

Strack, G., G. McClane, and D. Hawley (2001). A review of 300 attempted strangulation cases. Part I: Criminal legal issues. *J Emerg Med* 21(3):303–309.

Strait, R., R. Siegel, and R. Shapiro (1995). Humeral fractures without obvious etiologies in children less than 3 years of age: When is it abuse? *Pediatrics* 96(4):667–671.

Stranc, M. and G. Robertson (1990). A classification of injuries of the nasal skeleton. *Ann Plast Surg* 2(6):468-474.

Strong, E., N. Pahlavan, and D. Saito (2006). Frontal sinus fractures: A 28-year retrospective review. *Otolaryngology-Head and Neck Surgery* 135(5):774–779.

Strouse, P. J., and C. L. Owings (1995). Fractures of the first rib in child abuse. *Pediatric Radiology* 197:763–765.

Sun, G. H., N. M. Shoman, R. N. Samy, and M. L. Pensak (2011). Analysis of carotid artery injury in patients with basilar skull fractures. *Otology and Neurotology* 32:882–886.

Sundra, M. and H. Carty (1994). Avulsion fractures of the pelvis in children: A report of 32 fractures and their outcome. *Skeletal Radiology* 23:85–90.

Swanson, T. V. and R. B. Gustilo (1993). Fractures of the humeral shaft. In *Fractures and Dislocations*, R. B. Gustilo, R. F. Kyle, and D. C. Templeman (Eds.), pp. 365–385. Mosby, St. Louis, MO.

SWGANTH.org (2011). Scientific Working Group for Anthropology. Date of download August, 2012.

Swischuk, L. E. (1992). Radiographic signs of skeletal trauma. In *Child Abuse: A Medical Reference* (2nd ed.), S. Ludwig and A.E. Kornberg (Eds.). Churchill Livingstone, New York.

Ta'ala, S. C., G. E. Berg, and K. Haden (2008). A Khmer Rouge execution method – evidence from Choeung Ek. In *Skeletal Trauma: Identification of Injuries Resulting from Human Rights Abuse and Armed Conflict*, E. H. Kimmerle and J. Baraybar (Eds.), pp. 196–199. CRC Press, Boca Raton, FL.

Tadj, A. and F. W. Kimble (2003). Fractured zygomas. *Australian and New Zealand Journal of Surgery* 73:49–54.

Taitz, J., K. Moran, and M. O'Meara (2004). Long bone fractures in children under 3 years of age: Is abuse being missed in emergency department presentations? *J Paediatr Child Health* 40:170–174.

Taleisnik, J. (1980). Post-traumatic carpal instability. *Clinical Orthopaedics and Related Research* 149:73–82.

Tavora, F., C. Crowder, C. C. Sun, and A. Burke (2008). Discrepencies between clinical and autopsy diagnoses. *Am J Clin Pathol* 129:102–109.

Taylor, K. (2001). *Forensic Art and Illustration.* CRC Press, Boca Raton, FL.

Taylor, M. T., B. Banerjee, and E. K. Alpar (1994). The epidemiology of fractured femurs and the effect of these factors on outcome. *Injury* 25:641–644.

Teasdall, R., F. H. Savoie, and J. L. Hughes (1993). Comminuted fractures of the proximal radius and ulna. *Clinical Orthopaedics and Related Research* 292:37–47.

Teh, J., M. Firth, A. Sharma, A. Wilson, R. Reznek, and O. Chan (2003). Jumpers and fallers: A comparison of the distribution of skeletal injury. *Clinical Radiology* 58(6):482–486.

Teisen, G. and T. Hjarbaek (1988). Classification of fresh fractures of the lunate. *Journal of Hand Surgery [Br]* 13:458–462.

Templeman, D. (1992a). Fractures of the acetabulum. In *Fractures and Dislocations*, R. B. Gustilo, R. F. Kyle, and D. C. Templeman (Eds.), pp. 757–781. Mosby, St. Louis, MO.

_____ (1992b). Fractures of the distal femur. In *Fractures and Dislocations*, R. B. Gustilo, R.F. Kyle, and D.C. Templeman (Eds.), pp. 981–995. Mosby, St. Louis, MO.

_____ (1992c). Fractures of the patella. In *Fractures and Dislocations*, R. B. Gustilo, R. F. Kyle, and D. C. Templeman (Eds.), pp. 897–900. Mosby, St. Louis, MO.

Tencer, A. F., R. Kaufman, K. Ryan, D. C. Grossman, M. B. Henley, F. Mann, C. Mock, F. Rivara, S. Wang, J. Augenstein, D. Hoyt, and B. Eastma (2002). Femur fractures in relatively low speed frontal crashes: The possible role of muscle forces. *Accident Analysis and Prevention* 34:1–11.

Tenenbein, M., M. H. Reed, and G. B. Black (1990). The toddler's fracture revisited. *American Journal of Emergency Medicine* 8:208–211.

Teresinski, G. and R. Madro (2002). Evidential value of injuries useful for reconstruction of the pedestrian-vehicle location at the moment of collision. *Forensic Science International* 128:127–135.

Thaller, S. and S. Mabourakh (1991). Pediatric mandibular fractures. *Ann Plast Surg* 26(6):511–513.

Thangavelu, A., R. Yoganandha, and A. Vaidhyanathan (2010). The association of third molars with mandibular angle fractures: A meta-analysis. *International J of Oral and Maxillofacial Surgery* 39(2):136–139.

Theivendrean, K., C. W. McBryde, and S. N. Massoud (2008). Scapula fractures: A review. *Trauma* 10:25–33.

Thierauf, A., S. Lutz-Bonengel, T. Sanger, S. Vogt, W. Rupp, and M. Grosseperdekamp (2012). Suicide by multiple blunt head traumatisation using a stone. *Forensic Science International* 214(1):e47–e50.

Thomas, A. P. and R. Birch (1983). An unusual hamate fracture. *Hand* 15:281–286.

Thomas, E. M., K. W. Tuson, and P. S. Browne(1974). Fractures of the radius and ulna in children. *Injury* 7:120–124.

Thomas, F. B. (1957). Reduction of Smith's fracture. *Journal of Bone and Joint Surgery [Br]* 39:463–470.

Thomas, S., N. Rosenfield, J. Leventhal, and R. Markowitz (1991). Long-bone fractures in young children: Distinguishing accidental injuries from child abuse. *Pediatrics* 88(3):471–476.

Thomas, T. T. (1905). Fractures of the head of the radius. *University of Pennsylvania Medical Bulletin* 18:184–197, 221–234.

Thomine, J. M. (1975). Les fractures ouvertes de squeulette digital dans les plaises de la main et des doigts. *Actual Chir Paris, Masson et Cit* pp. 776–780.

Thoren, H., T. Iizuki, D. Hallikainen, and Lindqvist (1992). Different patterns of mandibular fractures in children: An analysis of 220 fractures in 157 patients. *Journal of Cranio-Maxillo-Facial Surgery* 20:292–296.

Thornton, A. and C. Gyll (1999). *Children's Fractures*. Saunders, London.

Throckmorton, T. and J. E. Kuhn (2007). Fractures of the medial end of the clavicle. *Journal of Shoulder and Elbow Surgery* 16(1):47–54.

Tile, M. and G. F. Pennal (1980). Pelvic disruption: principles of management. *Clinical Orthopaedics and Related Research* 151:56–64.

Tile, M. (1987a). Fracture of the proximal humerus. In *The Rationale of Operative Fracture Care*, J. Schatzker and M. Tile (Eds.), pp. 31–59. Springer-Verlag, Berlin.

_____ (1987b). Fractures of the pelvis. In *The Rationale of Operative Fracture Care*, J. Schatzker and M. Tile (Eds.), pp. 133–172. Springer-Verlag, Berlin.

_____ (1987c). Fractures of the distal tibial metaphysis involving the ankle joint: The pilon fracture. In *The Rationale of Operative Fracture Care*, J. Schatzker and M. Tile (Eds.), pp. 343–369. Springer-Verlag, Berlin.

_____ (1987d). Fractures of the talus. In *The Rationale of Operative Fracture Care*, J. Schatzker and M. Tile (Eds.), pp. 409–432. Springer-Verlag, Berlin.

_____ (1987e). Fractures of the ankle. In *The Rationale of Operative Fracture Care*, J. Schatzker and M. Tile (Eds.), pp. 375–405. Springer-Verlag, Berlin.

Tile, M. (1988). Pelvic ring fractures: should they be fixed? *Journal of Bone and Joint Surgery [Br]* 70B:1–12.

Tintinalli, J. and M. Hoelzer (1985). Clinical findings and legal resolution in sexual assault. *Annals of Emergency Medicine* 14(5):447–453.

Tohyama H., K. Kutsumi, and K. Yasuda (2002). Avulsion fracture at the femoral attachment of the anterior cruciate ligament after intercondylar eminence fracture of the tibia. *American Journal of Sports Medicine* 30:279–282.

Tomczak, P. D. and J. E. Buikstra (1999). Analysis of blunt trauma injuries: Vertical deceleration versus horizontal deceleration injuries. *Journal of Forensic Sciences* 44(2):253–262.

Torg, J. S., H. Pavlov, L. H. Cooley, M. H. Cooley, M. H. Bryant, S. P. Arnoczky, J. Bergfeld, and L. Y. Hunter (1982). Stress fractures of the tarsal navicular: A retrospective review of twenty-one cases. *Journal of Bone and Joint Surgery [Am]* 64:700–712.

Tortosa, J., J. Martinez-Lage, and M. Pozo (2004). Bitemporal head crush injuries: Clinical and radiological features of a distinctive type of head injury. *Journal of Neurosurgery* 100(4):645–651.

Tossy, N., C. Mead, and H. M. Sigmond (1963). Acromioclavicular separations: Useful and practical classification for treatment. *Clinical Orthopaedics* 28:111–110.

Trafton, P. G., T. J. Bray, and L. A. Simpson (1992). Fractures and soft tissue injuries of the ankle. In *Skeletal Trauma: Fractures, Dislocation, Ligamentous Injuries*, B. D. Browner, J. B. Jupiter, A. M. Levine, and P. G. Trafton (Eds.), pp. 1871–1957. W. B. Saunders, Philadelphia.

Trafton, P. G. (1992). Tibial shaft fractures. In *Skeletal Trauma: Fractures, Dislocations, Ligamentous Injuries*, B. D. Browner, J. B. Jupiter, A. M. Levine, and P. G. Trafton (Eds.), pp. 1771–1869. W. B. Saunders, Philadelphia.

Transfeldt, E. E. and M. Aebi (1992). Fractures and dislocations of the cervical spine. In *Fractures and Dislocations,* R. B. Gustilo, R. F. Kyle, and D. C. Templeman (Eds.), pp. 647–676. Mosby, St. Louis, MO.

Tredwell, S. J., K. Van Petegham, and M. Clough (1984). Pattern of forearm fractures in children. *Journal of Pediatric Orthopedics* 4:604–608.

Trivellato, P. F. B., M. F. M. Arnez, C .E. Sverzut, and A. E. Trivellato (2011). A retrospective study of zygomatico-orbital complex and/or zygomatic arch fractures over a 71-month period. *Dental Traumatology* 27:135–142.

Truman, J. (2011). *National Crime Victimization Survey: Criminal Victimization, 2010.* Bureau of Justice Statistics.

Tuli, S., C. H. Tator, M. G. Fehlings, and M. Mackay (1997). Occipital condyle fractures. *Neurosurgery* 41:368–376.

Turk, E. E. and M. Tsokos (2005). Vehicle-assisted suicide resulting in complete decapitation. *American Journal of Forensic Medicine and Pathology* 26(3):292–293.

Turner, C. H. (2006). Bone strength: Current concepts. *Annals of the New York Academy of Science* 1068:429–446.

Turner, C. II and J. Turner (1999). *Man Corn: Cannibalism and Violence in the Prehistoric American Southwest.* University of Utah Press, Salt Lake City, UT.

Ubelaker, D. (1992). *Bones: A Forensic Detective's Casebook.* HarperCollins, NY.

Ubelaker, D. H. (1992). Hyoid fracture and strangulation. *Journal of Forensic Sciences* 37(5):1216–1222.

Ubelaker, D. H. and B. J. Adams (1995). Differentiation of perimortem and postmortem trauma using taphonomic indicators. *Journal of Forensic Sciences* 40:509–512.

Uva, J. L. (1995). Review: Autoerotic asphyxia in the United States. *Journal of Forensic Sciences* 40:574–581.

Varley, G. W., R. Spencer-Jones, P. Thomas, D. Andrews, A. D. Green, and D. B. Stevens (1993). Injury patterns in motorcycle road racers: Experience on the Isle of Man 1989–1991. *Injury* 24(7):443–446.

Vasilas, A., R. V. Grieco, and N. F. Bartone (1960). Roentgen aspects of injuries to the pisiform bone and pisotriquetral joint. *Journal of Bone and Joint Surgery [Am]* 42:1317–1328.

Vellet, A. D., P. H. Marks, P. J. Fowler, and T. G. Muntro (1991). Occult posttraumatic osteochondral lesions of the knee: Prevalence, classification and short-term sequelae evaluated with MR imaging. *Radiology* 178:271–276.

Verriest, J. P. (1984). Thorax and upper absomen: Kneumatics, tolerance levels and injury criteria. In *The Biomechanics of Injury Trauma,* B. C. Aldman and A. Chapon (Eds.), pp. 251–275. Elsevier Science, Amsterdam.

Verschueren, P., H. Delye, B. Depreitere, C. Van Lierde, B. Haex, D. Berckmans, I. Verpost, J. Goffin, J. Vander Sloten, and G. Van der Perre (2007). A new test set-up for skull fracture characterization. *Journal of Biomechanics* 40:3389–3396.

Vij, K. (2008). *Textbook of Forensic Medicine and Toxicology* (4th ed.). Elsevier, New Delhi.

Vikramaditya, P. (2001). Two cases of isolated first rib fractures. *Emerg Med J* 18:498–499.

Vikramaditya, P. P. (2001). Two cases of isolated first rib fracture. *Emergency Medicine Journal* 18:498–499.

Villa, P. and E. Mahieu (1991). Breakage patterns of human long bones. *J Human Evolution* 21:27–48.

Violence Policy Center (2011). *When men murder women: an analysis of 2009 homicide data – females murdered by males in single victim/single offender incidents.* http://www.vpc.org/studies/wmmw2011.pdf, date of download April, 2012.

Vives, M. J., S. Kishan, J. Asghar, B. Peng, M. F. Reiter, S. Milo, and D. Livingston (2008). Spinal injuries in pedestrians struck by motor vehicles. *Journal of Spinal Disorders and Techniques* 21:281–287.

Vogel, H. and V. G. Brogdon (2003). Beating. In *A Radiologic Atlas of Abuse, Torture, Terrorism, and Inflicted Trauma*, H. Vogel, B. G. Brogdon, and J. D. McDowell (Eds.), pp. 109–118. CRC Press, Boca Raton, FL.

Vogler, H., N. Westlin, D. Mlodzienski, and F. Moller (1995). Fifth metatarsal fractures: Biomechanics, classification, and treatment. *Clinics in Podiatric Medicine and Surgery* 12:725–747.

Vogt, M. T., J. H. Cauley, M. M. Tomaino, K. Stone, J. R. Williams, and J. H. Herndon (2002). Distal radius fractures in older women: A 10-year follow-up study of descriptive characteristics and risk factors the study of osteoporotic fractures. *Journal of the American Geriatric Society* 50(1):97–103.

Volk, A., P. Merkle, and M. Stevanovic (1995). Unusual capitate fracture: A case report. *J Hand Surg [Am]* 20(4):581–2.

Vuori, J. and H. Aro (1993). Lisfranc joint injuries: Trauma mechanisms and associated injuries. *Journal of Trauma* 35(1):40–45.

Waddell, J. P. (1979). Subtrochanteric fractures of the femur: A review of 130 patients. *Journal of Trauma* 19:582–591.

Walker, J. L., T. L. Greene, and P. A. Lunseth (1988). Fractures of the body of the trapezium. *Journal of Orthopeadic Trauma* 2:22–28.

Walker, P. L. (1997). Wife beating, boxing, and broken noses: Skeletal evidence for the cultural patterning of violence. In *Troubled Times: Violence and Warfare in the Past*, F. D. Martin (Ed.), pp. 145–179. Gordon and Breach, Amsterdam.

Waller, J. A. (1985). *Injury Control: A Guide to Causes and Prevention of Trauma.* Lexington Books, Lexington, MA.

Wallis, L. and I. Greaves (2002). Injuries associated with airbag deployment. *Emerg Med J* 19(6):490–493.

Walsh, H. P. J., C. A. N. McLaren, and R. G. Owen (1987). Galeazzi fractures in children. *Journal of Bone and Joint Surgery [Br]* 69:730–733.

Walsh, J. (2004). Fractures of the hand and carpal navicular bone in athletes. *Southern Medical Journal* 97(8):762–765.

Walz, F. (1984). Lower abdomen and pelvis, anatomy and types of injury. In *The Biomechanics of Impact Trauma*, B. Aldman and A. Chapon (Eds.), pp. 279–286. Elsevier Science, Amsterdam.

Wang, X., J. D. Mabrey, and C. Agarwal (1998). An interspecies comparison of bone fracture properties. *Biomedical Materials and Engineering* 8:1–9.

Ward, F. O. (1838). *Human Anatomy.* Renshaw, London.

Wassmund, M. (1934). Uber luxationsfrakturen de Kieferdelenks. *Deutsche Kieferch* 1:27–54.

Watanabe, T. (1972). *Atlas of Legal Medicine.* J. B. Lippincort, Philadelphia.

Watson-Jones, R. (Ed.) (1941). *Fractures and Other Bone and Joint Injuries* (2nd ed.). Williams and Wilkins, Baltimore.

Waugh, W. (1958). Ossification and vascularization of the tarsal navicular and their relation to Kohler's disease. *Journal of Bone and Joint Surgery [Br]* 40:765–777.

Weber, M., R. Risdon, A. Offiah, M. Malone, and N. Sebire (2009). Rib fractures identified at post-mortem examination in sudden unexpected deaths in infancy (SUDI). *Forensic Science International* 189(1–3):75–81.

Weber, E. R. and E. Y. Chao (1978). An experimental approach to mechanism of scaphoid waist fractures. *Journal of Hand Surgery [Am]* 3:142–148.

Wedel, V., G. Found, and G. Nusse (2013). A 37-year-old cold case identification using novel and collaborative methods. *Journal of Forensic Identification* 63(1):5–21.

Wehbe, M. and L. Schneider (1984). Mallet fractures. *J Bone and Joint Surgery [Am]* 66(5):658–659.

Weiner, S. and H. Wagner (1998). The material bone: Structure-mechanical function relations. *Annual Rev Materials Sciences* 28:271–298.

Wheatley, B. P. (2008). Perimortem or postmortem bone fractures? An experimental study of fracture patterns in deer femora. *Journal of Forensic Sciences* 53(1):69–72.

Wheeless III, C. (2012). *Wheeless' Textbook of Orthopaedics.* Duke University, Raleigh-Durham, NC.

White, A. A. and M. M. Panjabi (1978). The basic kinetics of the human spine – a review of past and current knowledge, *Spine* 3:12–20.

White, A. P., R. Hashimoto, D. C. Novell, and A. R. Vaccaro (2010). Morbidity and mortality related to odontoid fracture surgery in the elderly population. *Spine* 35:S146–S157.

White, T. (1992). *Prehistoric Cannibalism at Mancos 5MTUMR-2346.* Princeton University Press, Princeton, NJ.

Whittington, R. (1981). Motorcycle fatalities: Analysis of Birmingham coroner's records. *Injury* 12:267–273.

Wieberg, D. A. and D. J. Wescott (2008). Estimating the timing of long bone fractures: Correlation between the postmortem interval, bone moisture content, and blunt force trauma fracture characteristics. *Journal of Forensic Sciences* 53(5):1028–1034.

Wilber, J. J. and G. H. Thompson (1994). The multiply injured child. In *Skeletal Trauma in Children*, N. E. Green and M. F. Swiontkowski (Eds.), pp. 65–98. W. B. Saunders, Philadelphia.

Wilkins, B. (1997). Head injury: abuse or accident? *Arch Dis Child* 76:393–397.

Williams, D. J. (1981). The mechanisms producing fracture-separation of the proximal humeral epiphysis. *Journal of Bone and Joint Surgery [Br]* 63:102–107.

Wilson, F. C. (1984). Fractures and dislocations of the ankle. In *Fractures in Adults*, C. A. Rockwood and D. P. Green (Eds.), pp. 1665–1701. J. B. Lippincott, Philadelphia.

Wilson, P. (1933). Fractures and dislocation in the region of the elbow. *Surgery, Gynecology and Obstetrics* 56:335–359.

Winquist, R. and S. T. Hansen (1980). Comminuted fractures of the femoral shaft treated by intramedullary nailing. *Orthopedic Clinics of North America* 11:633–648.

Winquist, R., S. T. Hansen, Jr., and D. K. Clawson (1984). Closed intramedullary nailing of femoral fractues: A report of five hundred and twenty cases. *Journal of Bone and Joint Surgery [Am]* 66:529–539.

Wolfe, S. E. and L. D. Katz (1995). Intra-articular impaction fractures of the phalanges. *Journal of Hand Surgery [Am]* 20:327–333.

Wood-Jones, F. (1913). The ideal lesion produced by judicial hanging. *Lancet* 1(4662): 53.

World Health Organization (1978). *Application of the International Classification of Diseases to Dentistry and Stomatology (ICD-DA)*, pp. 88–89. World Health Organization, Geneva.

Worlock, P., M. Stower, and P. Barbor (1986). Patterns of fractures in accidental and non-accidental injury in children: A comparative study. *British Medical Journal* 293:100–293.

Worn, M. (2007). Rib fractures in infancy: Establishing the mechanisms of cause from the injuries: A literature review. *Med Sci Law* 47:200–21.

Wright, G., A. Bell, G. McGlashan, and R. R. Welbury (2007). Dentoalveolar trauma in Glasgow: An audit of mechanism and injury. *Dental Traumatology* 23:226–231.

Wu, V., H. Huff, and M. Bhandari (2010). Pattern of physical injury associated with intimate partner violence in women presenting to the emergency department: A systematic review and meta-analysis. *Trauma, Violence, & Abuse* 11(2):71–82.

Wurtz, L. D., F. A. Lyons, and C. A. Rockwood, Jr. (1992). Fracture of the middle third of the clavicle and dislocation of the acromioclavicular joint: A report of four cases. *Journal of Bone and Joint Surgery [Am]* 74:133–137.

Wyatt, J., T. Squires, G. Norfolk, and J. Payne-James (2011). *Oxford Handbook of Forensic Medicine.* Oxford University Press, Oxford.

Wyrsch, R. B., K. P. Spindler, and P. R. Stricker (1995). Scapular fracture in a professional boxer. *Journal of Shoulder and Elbow Surgery* 4:395–398.

Yee, E. S., A. N. Thomas, and P. C. Goodman (1981). Isolated first rib fracture: Clinical significance after blunt chest trauma. *Annals of Thoracic Surgery* 32:278–283.

Yoganandan, N. and F. Pintar (2004). Biomechanics of temporo-parietal skull fractures. *Clin Biomech* 19(3):225–239.

Yoganandan, N., F. Pintar, A. Sances, P. J. Walsh, C. Ewing, D. Thomas, and R. Snyder (1995). Biomechanics of Skull Fracture. *Journal of Neurotrauma* 12(4):659–668.

Yokoo, S. (1952). The compression test upon the diaphysis and the compact substance of the long bones of human extremities. *Journal of the Kyoto Prefecture Medical University* 51:291.

Young, J. W. R. and A. R. Burgess (1987). *Radiologic Management of Pelvic Ring Fractures.* Urban and Schwarzberg, Baltimore and Munich.

Young, M. H. (1973). Long-term consequences of stable fractures of the thoracic and lumbar vertebral bodies. *Journal of Bone and Joint Surgery [Br]* 55:295–330.

Zandi, M., M. Saleh, S. R. S. Houseini (2011). Are facial injuries caused by stumbling different from other kinds of fall accidents? *Journal of Craniofacial Surgery* 22(6):2388–2392.

Zeigler, D. W. and N. Agarwal (1994). The morbidity and mortality of rib fractures. *Journal of Trauma* 37:975–979.

Zephro, L. (2012). *Determining the Timing and Mechanism of Bone Fracture in Bovine Bone, Department of Anthropology*. Department of Anthropology, University of California, Santa Cruz, CA.

Zettas, J. P., P. Zettas, and B. Thanasophon (1979). Injury patterns in motorcycle accidents. *Journal of Trauma* 19(11):833–836.

Zhu, B. L., S. Oritani, K. Ishida, L. Quan, S. Sakoda, M. Q. Fujita, and H. Maeda (2000). Child and elderly victims in forensic autopsy during a recent 5 year period in the southern half of Osaka city and surrounding areas. *Forensic Science International* 113:215–218.

Zimmerman, R. A. and L. T. Lilaniuk (1981). Computed tomography in pediatric head trauma. *Neuroradiology* 8:257–271.

Zingg, M., K. Laedrach, J. Chen, K. Chowshury, T. Vuillemin, F. Sutter, and J. Raveh (1992). Classification and treatment of zygomatic fractures: A review of 1,025 cases. *Journal of Oral and Maxillofacial Surgery* 50:778–790.

Zuckerman, J. D., K. J. Koval, and F. Cuomo (1993). Fractures of the scapula. *Instructional Course Lectures* 42:271–281.

Zwipp, H. and H. Tscherme, H. Thermann, and H. Weber (1993). Osteosynthesis of displaced intraarticular fractures of the calcaneus: Results in 123 cases. *Clinical Orthopaedics and Related Research* 290:76–86.

SUBJECT INDEX